Transforming Nursing Education Through Problem-Based Learning

Elizabeth Rideout, Ph.D, RN

Associate Professor, School of Nursing

Faculty of Health Sciences

McMaster University

Hamilton, Ontario, Canada

JONES AND BARTLETT PUBLISHERS

Sudbury, Massachusetts

BOSTON   TORONTO   LONDON   SINGAPORE

World Headquarters
Jones and Bartlett Publishers
40 Tall Pine Drive
Sudbury, MA 01776
978-443-5000
www.jbpub.com
info@jbpub.com

Jones and Bartlett Publishers Canada
2406 Nikanna Road
Mississauga, ON L5C 2W6
CANADA

Jones and Bartlett Publishers International
Barb House, Barb Mews
London W6 7PA
UK

Library of Congress Cataloging-in-Publication Data

Rideout, Elizabeth.
  Transforming nursing education through problem-based learning / Elizabeth Rideout.
    p. cm.
  Includes bibliographical references and index.
  ISBN 0-7637-1427-5 (alk. paper)
   1. Nursing—Study and teaching. 2. Problem-based learning. I. Title.

RT73 .R49 2001
610.73'071'1–dc21

                               00-064517

Production Credits
Acquisitions Editor: Penny Glynn
Associate Editor: Christine Tridente
Production Editor: AnnMarie Lemoine
V. P., Manufacturing and Inventory Control: Therese Bräuer
Cover Design: AnnMarie Lemoine
Design and Composition: Carlisle Communications, Ltd.
Printing and Binding: Malloy Lithographing
Cover Photograph © Photodisc

Printed in the United States of America
03 02 01   10 9 8 7 6 5 4 3 2

CONTENTS

Preface vii

Acknowledgments xi

Contributors xiii

CHAPTER 1

Nursing Education for the Twenty-First Century 1

Catherine Tompkins

CHAPTER 2

The Problem-Based Learning Model of Nursing 21
Education

Elizabeth Rideout and Barbara Carpio

CHAPTER 3

Facilitating Self-Directed Learning 51

Dauna Crooks, Ola Lunyk-Child, Chris Patterson,
and Jeannette LeGris

CHAPTER 4

Facilitating Small Group Learning 75

Gerry Benson, Charlotte Noesgaard,
and Michele Drummond-Young

CHAPTER 5

Facilitating Information Management Skills   **103**
and Dispositions

Liz Bayley, Neera Bhatnagar, and Patricia Ellis

CHAPTER 6

Fostering Reflection and Reflective Practice   **119**

Barbara Brown, Nancy Matthew-Maich, and Joan Royle

CHAPTER 7

Developing Problems for Use in Problem-Based   **165**
Learning

Michele Drummond-Young and E. Ann Mohide

CHAPTER 8

The Faculty Role in Problem-Based Learning   **193**

Angela C. Wolff and Elizabeth Rideout

CHAPTER 9

Evaluating Student Learning   **215**

Elizabeth Rideout

CHAPTER 10

Developing Clinical Opportunities and Resources   **239**
for Problem-Based Learning

Joan A. Royle, Wendy Sword, Margaret Black,
Barbara Brown, and Tracy Carr

CHAPTER 11

Developing Learning and Library Resources   **259**

Janice Bignell, Hallie Groves, and Liz Bayley

CHAPTER 12

Standardized Patients as an Educational Resource   **281**

Andrea Baumann and Elizabeth Rideout

CHAPTER 13

Problem-Based Learning in Master's Degree   **293**
Education

Constance M. Baker

CHAPTER 14

Using Problem-Based Learning in Distance Education   **311**

Otto H. Sanchez-Sweatman

CHAPTER 15

Introducing Problem-Based Learning: A Process of   **325**
Adoption or Adaptation?

Barbara Carpio

Index   **339**

PREFACE

Nursing—along with the environments in which nurses work—has been changing rapidly. These changes in nursing practice necessitate changes in nursing eduction. Among the various strategies proposed, one approach that has attained considerable prominence is problem-based learning (PBL). Since its development in the late sixties at the medical school at McMaster University in Canada, PBL has spread to many institutions worldwide and has been adopted in a variety of professional education settings. To date the bulk of writing about problem-based learning, its implementation, and its curricular implications has dealt with its use in medical education. Similarly, conferences on PBL were once the domain solely of medical educators. This is no longer the case. It has steadily become recognized as one of the most important recent trends in nursing education and one of the most promising ways of equipping nurses with the attributes they need.

With the growing interest in PBL among nurse educators worldwide comes the need for a book that will be a comprehensive guide and resource for anyone considering its implementation in nursing education. This book is a project of faculty members at the School of Nursing at McMaster University, where problem-based learning has been used in all nursing courses since the mid-seventies. The Institute for Nurse Educators, held annually at McMaster, attracts participants from around the world who wish to learn about and experience the PBL method. McMaster nursing faculty members have conducted workshops on PBL in Canada, the United States, Great Britain, Chile, Thailand, Sweden and Japan. In virtually every instance there have been requests for written materials that describe not only the process of PBL but also the strategies and resources needed to implement it successfully. The Nursing Education Research Unit (NERU) at McMaster was established in 1995 to explore a range of questions related to nursing education, and to focus in particular on the process and outcomes of problem-based, self-directed, small-group learning. Altogether these experiences led the faculty, and particularly those involved in NERU, to make a commitment to this project.

The first chapter discusses how the roles and education of nurses have changed over the past several decades, and indicates why the problem-based model is particularly relevant to today's needs. Chapter 2 contains an overview of the model itself. In the subsequent four chapters various core features and outcomes of the problem-based approach are described. Together, these chapters indicate how the model provides the educational experiences that lead to the outcomes required by nurses now and in the foreseeable future. Chapter 3 focuses on self-directed learning and its importance within PBL. It describes the challenges new learners face in self-directed learning, and the strategies their teachers can use to facilitate the independent and interdependent learning of students. The fourth chapter, on small group learning, deals with the structure, function and process of small problem-based learning groups, and how these tend to be different from those of small groups in other educational approaches. In the fifth chapter the need for the development by students of information management skills is discussed. Being computer literate has begun to be described as a necessary outcome for all nursing graduates; however, it is particularly relevant to PBL, where students must acquire current information to bring to their small group tutorials. This skill, in turn, helps students to become competent and committed lifelong learners. The final chapter in this section discusses the importance of critical reflection and the relevance of PBL in developing critically reflective practitioners. One other desired outcome of nursing education that has been much discussed in the literature is critical thinking. Since the centrality of critical thinking within the PBL model is evident throughout this book, and since there is abundant literature on critical thinking and methods to facilitate it within educational programs generally, we chose not to include a separate chapter on that topic in this book.

Chapters 7–12 focus on the resources required to implement the PBL model effectively. The first resource to be considered is the actual problems to be presented to students. These are essential to learning outcomes and must be derived from the desired curriculum of study. In Chapter 7 the process of problem development is described, from identification of the content to be included in the problems to the details of their development. In the next chapter, the role of the teacher in the PBL model is presented, along with the faculty development programs that have been found useful. In Chapter 9 we turn to the question of evaluation of students in a PBL setting. Although the principles here are not dissimilar to those that can guide any student evaluation, there are a number of evaluation methods that have evolved for use specifically with the PBL model. These methods are presented and examples provided.

Chapter 10 deals with clinical nursing courses. Clinical courses have always had an inevitable "problem-based" focus, since in each clinical experience students are learning to assess patients and families and help them address present and potential problems. This chapter deals with the particular ways that the PBL model helps students meet the expectations for learning specific to clinical settings. Chapter 11 provides an overview of various resources required for effective use of the PBL model in nursing and describes four of them in some detail: a library, an anatomy laboratory, a clinical skills laboratory, and a computer laboratory. In Chapter 12, another important resource, the standardized patient, is presented. The development of standardized patients programs, and the training and use of standardized patients today, are described in a way that will allow readers to plan and implement such a program.

In Chapter 13 the focus shifts to the emerging use of the PBL model in graduate level education. A summary of the literature is presented, describing the current use of PBL in master's programs in nursing. Chapter 14 explores the use of case- and problem-based learning in distance education in nursing. A brief overview of the various distance modalities is followed by a review of research on the effectiveness and level of acceptance by students and faculty of problem- and case-based learning through distance education formats. The final chapter of the book deals with the process of institutional change required for implementation of the PBL model into a nursing program. Implications for administrators, faculty and students are described.

A particular strength of this book is its integration of relevant theory, research and practical information. This book will be an invaluable resource for nursing faculty contemplating the use of the PBL model. As well, this book is intended to be useful to nursing students in PBL settings, who are required to adapt to a learning milieu that is usually quite different from anything they have previously encountered. Students of education generally will also find here a wide-ranging discussion of an important development in professional education.

ACKNOWLEDGMENTS

T he first acknowledgment must go to the nursing students at McMaster University from whom the contributors to this book have learned about what they believe continues to be an exciting, challenging and effective approach to nursing education. Without our ongoing experiences and our reflection on those experiences, PBL might well be described only in academic terms rather than as the dynamic learning process through which personal and professional growth for students and faculty is ongoing.

The superb editorial skills of Barbara Patterson, wise and wonderful secretary in the School of Nursing at McMaster, along with her attention to detail, commitment to the project and belief that it could be done, were essential to the fruition of our plans. Many thanks are also extended to the other staff members, in particular Betty McCarthy and Sharon Baptist.

This book is very much a collaborative effort, in the spirit of the model of education we are describing. The idea for a book on PBL arose from an international conference on nursing education that was hosted by McMaster University School of Nursing in June, 1995. At that time it became apparent that a book on the PBL model in nursing education was needed. The faculty members who contributed to this book worked together to move the project from idea to implementation and I thank each of them for their ongoing commitment and participation. I met Connie Baker from Indiana University at a PBL conference in Montreal and she brought her enthusiasm and experience with the model to the book, joining the many McMaster contributors.

To my husband, David Palmer, a very large thank you for accepting an absentee wife in the final months of preparing the manuscript and for providing invaluable assistance in a number of ways.

The excellent assistance of Christine Tridente of Jones and Bartlett and Janet Kiefer of Carlisle Communications is also acknowledged. The prompt responses to myriad questions and the general level of support throughout the publication process have been much appreciated.

Elizabeth Rideout

CONTRIBUTORS

Constance M. Baker, B.S.N., M.A., Ed.M., Ed.D.
Professor, Nursing Administration
Indiana University
Indianapolis, IN

Andrea Baumann, B.Sc.N., M.Sc.N., Ph.D.
Professor, Associate Dean,
Health Sciences (Nursing)
McMaster University School of Nursing
Hamilton, ON

Liz Bayley, B.A., M.L.S.
Assistant Clinical Professor
Head of Systems/Curriculum Integration
Coordinator, Health Sciences Library
McMaster University
Hamilton, ON

Gerry Benson, B.N., M.Sc.
Assistant Professor
McMaster University School of Nursing
Hamilton, ON

Neera Bhatnagar, B.Sc., M.L.T.S.
Reference Librarian, Public Services
Health Sciences Library
McMaster University
Hamilton, ON

Janice E. Bignell
Coordinator, Learning Resources
Education Services
McMaster University
Hamilton, ON

Margaret Black, B.Sc.N., M.S.N., Ph.D.
Associate Professor
McMaster University School of Nursing
Hamilton, ON

Barbara Brown, B.Sc.N., B.A., M.Sc.N.
Associate Professor
McMaster University School of Nursing
Hamilton, ON

Barbara Carpio, B.Sc.N., M.Sc.N., M.Sc. (T)
Associate Professor
McMaster University School of Nursing
Hamilton, ON

Tracey Carr, B.Sc.N, M.B.A. (C)
Administrator/Placement Coordinator,
B.Sc.N. Program
McMaster University School of Nursing
Hamilton, ON

Dauna Crooks, B.Sc.N., M.Sc.N., DNS
Associate Professor
McMaster University School of Nursing
Hamilton, ON

Michele Drummond-Young, B.Sc.N., M.H.Sc.
Assistant Professor
McMaster University School of Nursing
Hamilton, ON

Patricia Ellis, B.Sc., M.Sc.
Associate Professor
McMaster University School of Nursing
Hamilton, ON

Hallie Groves, Dip.RT, B.Sc., M.Sc., PhD.
Associate Professor
McMaster University School of
Rehabilitation Science
Hamilton, ON

Jeannette LeGris, B.N., M.H.Sc.
Assistant Professor
McMaster University School of Nursing
Hamilton, ON

Ola Lunyk-Child, B.Sc.N., M.Sc.N., Ph.D. (C)
Assistant Professor
McMaster University School of Nursing
Hamilton, ON

Nancy Matthew-Maich, B.Sc.N., M.Sc.(T)
Professor, Department of Nursing
Mohawk College of Applied Arts and
Technology
Hamilton, ON

E. Ann Mohide, B.Sc.N., M.H.Sc., M.Sc.
Associate Professor, School of Nursing
& Associate Member,
Clinical Epidemiology & Biostatistics
McMaster University
Hamilton, ON

Charlotte Noesgaard, B.N., M.Sc.N.
Assistant Professor
McMaster University School of Nursing
Hamilton, ON

Chris Patterson, B.Sc., B.Sc.N., M.Sc.N.
Assistant Professor
McMaster University School of Nursing
Hamilton, ON

Elizabeth Rideout, B.N., M.H.Sc., M.Sc., Ph.D.
Associate Professor
McMaster University School of Nursing
Hamilton, ON

Joan A. Royle, B.Sc.N., M.Sc.N.
Associate Professor
McMaster University School of Nursing
Hamilton, ON

Otto Sanchez-Sweatman, M.D., M.Sc., Ph.D.
Assistant Professor
McMaster University School of Nursing
Hamilton, ON

Wendy Sword, B.Sc.N., M.Sc.(T.), Ph.D.
Assistant Professor
McMaster University School of Nursing
Hamilton, ON

Catherine Tompkins, B.Sc.N., M.Ed., Ph.D.
Associate Professor and Chair,
B.Sc.N. Program
McMaster University School of Nursing
Hamilton, ON

Angela Wolff, B.Sc.N., M.S.N.
Continuing Education Coordinator
Registered Nurses Association of
British Columbia
Vancouver, BC

Nursing Education for the Twenty-First Century 1

Catherine Tompkins

As university nursing education moves into the first decade of this new century, nurse educators must critically examine their roles in preparing future nurses for a health care environment impacted by a panoply of technological, demographic, intellectual, moral, and economic complexities. In doing so, we have the opportunity, and indeed the moral imperative, to graduate nurses who will be able to ask and seek to answer the questions that these challenges pose for their patients, their communities, their profession, as well as their own personal lives.

To educate means "to give intellectual, moral, and social instruction to a pupil; to train or instruct for a particular purpose" (Oxford English Dictionary, 1996). Nursing education for the twenty-first century must embrace a model of education "which integrates moral reasoning and ethical values with technical [and I would add, intellectual] expertise" (National League for Nursing [NLN], 1989, p. 3). Only such a model will adequately prepare graduates to face the challenges head on, put their knowledge into action to enable their patients and communities to move to health and healing, and enable the profession to grow and mature.

NURSING IN THE TWENTY-FIRST CENTURY

Many of the challenges that nursing will confront as the profession moves into the twenty-first century are as yet unknown. However, there are some changes that have significant implications for nursing which have been predicted with a degree of certainty, including:

- Changing demographics of the population in the Western world highlighted by a growing proportion of elderly persons, and increasing numbers of people living with chronic illnesses and disabilities;
- More knowledgeable health care consumers who insist on full participation in health care decisions;
- Increasing use and complexity of information, communications, and health care technology;
- Emphasis on prevention of illness and maintenance of health;

1

- The impact of the "shrinking" globe and resultant globalization;
- Increasing demographic and cultural diversity;
- Growing awareness of the relationship between health and wellness and the environment;
- Major transitions in the ways in which health care is funded and delivered.

Change has always surrounded us but never in history has the rapidity and complexity of change been so profound. Few of us who graduated a generation ago recognize the classrooms and health care settings that are so different from those that supported our learning and early days of practice. As the health care delivery system engages in the process of re-invention, so too must nursing re-invent itself—not only to respond to the changes that inevitably will result in roles and working environments, but to ensure that nursing plays a significant role in determining the changes that will ensue.

O'Neil (1998) highlights six trends that he concludes will characterize health care delivery in the United States in the twenty-first century:

1. More integrated health care systems to, in part, respond to consumer (purchaser) demands for accountability for cost and quality and to reduce excess capacity;
2. New, more intensively managed systems that will be focused on system values of cost reduction, consumer satisfaction, and demonstrable quality outcomes;
3. Demand for more evidence-based data about performance that will be weighed against objective standards of cost, satisfaction, and quality;
4. Movement of service provision outside of high-cost hospital systems to sites where low cost, high quality, and satisfaction can be achieved;
5. More emphasis on and effective management of the use of information and communications technology. O'Neil predicts that "technology is likely to be the single most important resource in the eventual reengineering of the core processes of health care, transforming both the clinical and nonclinical dimensions of care" (1998, p. 6). Technology will also be a means through which the patient and consumer gain knowledge of the health care system;
6. A shift in the emphasis from the biomedical to the psychosocial-behavioral aspects of health and health care, increasing opportunities for approaches to improve health and treat diseases that fall outside the biomedical realm.

This changing landscape of health care will necessitate a change in the roles, responsibilities, educational requirements, and employment patterns of nurses. As the acuity of hospital settings soars and increasing numbers of patients receive care outside of traditional health care delivery settings, as growing numbers of nurses are being diverted away from direct patient care and into roles in training and supervision of staff, and as nurses face external demands to determine and provide cost-effective, quality nursing care, nursing graduates will require new sets of competencies for practice.

Lindeman (2000) cites the views of four sources regarding the future of nursing practice in the twenty-first century. McBride's (1999) new paradigm of nursing practice includes:

- Nursing at the patient's side wherever the patient is located;
- Outcomes oriented practice;
- Emphasis on triaging needs, being mindful of costs;
- Emphasis on mortality, limiting morbidity, and maximizing functioning and quality of life;
- Nursing which not only includes direct care but also promoting self-care, directing care given by others, designing population-based health care programs, and managing patient services;
- Provision of primary care;
- Managing lifestyle change.

The PEW Health Professions Commission (O'Neil and PEW, 1998) presents 21 competencies that in many ways overlap with those cited by McBride (1999) but that also include embracing a personal ethic of social responsibility and service, exhibiting ethical behavior in all professional activities, and continuing to learn and help others learn.

A United States Department of Labor report identified the following eight universal job skills as required by the nurse of the future: helping/instructing others, leadership/persuasiveness, problem solving/creativity, initiative, work as part of a team, frequent public contact, manual dexterity, and physical stamina (Eagles, 1999).

Finally, Lindeman (2000) summarizes a project conducted by the Nebraska Nurses Association and the Nebraska Board of Nursing to identify initial and continued competencies for the nursing workforce. While the competencies required by the nurse of the future are consistent with those identified by McBride (1999), the Nebraska project cited increased assessment skills and patient teaching skills as among the most important and identified flexibility and creativity as essential personal attributes (Burbach and Exstrom, 1999).

Valainis (2000) has identified nine competencies for the baccalaureate prepared nurse, succinctly capturing the essential qualities embedded in those cited above. For Valainis, the competent twenty-first century nurse:

- Independently practices nursing and evaluates her/his own performance;
- Identifies gaps in knowledge and plans appropriate professional development activities to keep current with changes in practice and to solve practice problems;
- Assesses patient needs from the patient's point of view and empowers patients/families to actively participate in the care to the extent they are able;

- Manages care across facility boundaries by providing patients/families with continuity of services and consistency of message;
- Synthesizes the knowledge and skills of nursing with those of public health science to promote the health of the community (specific populations or aggregates);
- Ensures cost-effective, quality care;
- Differentiates nursing functions from those of other professional and nonprofessional health disciplines, articulates nursing functions clearly to others, and practices collaboratively;
- Exerts leadership in ensuring nursing's unique contribution to policy development in the areas of preventative and remedial aspects of illness, cooperating with other professions in planning for positive health from all levels from community to international;
- Supports peers in improving nursing skills already in existence and developing new nursing skills.

Clearly these competencies and those developed by other nurse visionaries in practice, education, and professional organizations have common themes that will challenge nurse educators as they seek to develop educational programs that prepare graduates for twenty-first century nursing. Nursing education programs need to develop self-directed lifelong learners who have the capacity to know themselves; who have an ethic of service; and who have the flexibility and creativity to work with informed and empowered patients, families, groups, and communities to meet their needs in a variety of health care settings. Educators must be able to help students look beyond the traditional boundaries of health care to consider the broad determinants of health, and to understand and be able to influence public and health care policy. They must facilitate the development of skills in teaching, leadership, supervision, and political action; and the capacity to identify best practices, to assess consumer/patient satisfaction, and to use and contribute to research to improve the quality of outcomes. In an increasingly diverse environment, their graduates must be culturally competent and open to moving beyond the biomedical model to embrace healing tools and practices used long before the advent of modern medicine, as well as embracing the technological advances of the future.

The nurse of this century will continue to encounter career paths trod in the twentieth century including those of direct care clinicians in all health care settings, consultants, administrators, educators, case managers, primary health care providers, advanced practice nurses, clinical nurse specialists, and independent practitioners. However, untraveled, and not yet envisioned, paths lie before us as change hurls us ever forward. Our graduates must be prepared to take nursing into new and uncharted territory. They must be prepared to ask and answer new questions for the profession and for quality health care.

Thus, nursing education is faced with a formidable challenge. The PEW Health Professions Commission in the United States concluded that "at the present time most of the nation's educational programs remain oriented to prepare individuals for yesterday's health care system and not for the demands of the new health care system" (Lindeman, 2000, p. 9). What will it take to move nursing knowledge from a twentieth century perspective to that of the twenty-first century?

NURSING KNOWLEDGE FOR THE TWENTIETH CENTURY

The history of university nursing education is less than a century old and as we approach our second century it is important to consider what Alligood (1997) refers to as eras of nursing knowledge. These eras reflect the emphases that have influenced, and been influenced by, the history of the profession and the development of nursing education (Meleis, 1991).

While Nightingale recognized nursing as a discipline with responsibilities and knowledge distinct from medicine, it was not until the early decades of the twentieth century that there emerged an explicit awareness of the need for specialized knowledge to guide the profession of nursing. At the turn of the twentieth century, nursing education was under the control of hospitals. Hospital administrators (most often physicians) and the apprenticeship model for nursing training emphasized practice based on rules, procedures, and tradition (Ashley, 1976). Nursing leaders, however, maintained a commitment to Nightingale's ideals and, increasingly, reliance on medical knowledge and skills was deemed to be insufficient for the emerging profession. The *curriculum era* of the 1920s and 1930s resulted in an expansion of nursing curricula beyond medical knowledge to include what were known as the nursing arts (social sciences and specific nursing procedures) (Alligood, 1997). The development of college and university nursing programs in the United States and Canada also occurred during this period, heralding the shift in focus from primarily a training model to an educational model for the discipline of nursing.

This movement of nursing into schools of higher learning led to the *research era* of nursing knowledge (Alligood, 1997). Emerging in the 1940s and 1950s, this era reflected the belief that only through nursing research would a suitable body of knowledge be generated as the basis for nursing practice. Scholarship and dissemination of knowledge were emphasized and, in an effort to increase the "scientific" status of the profession, reference to the "art" of nursing was virtually lost. Indeed, what were previously referred to as nursing arts laboratories, where students learned and practiced procedures, became known as skills laboratories. While this change in name for the rooms in which students learned and practiced how to offer nursing care may seem insignificant at first glance, it reflects an important shift in thinking about what nurses do from a more holistic act emphasizing, by definition, creativity, imagination, and aesthetics, to acts characterized by technical expertise.

Reflecting this newly adopted culture of university-based nursing education, the research era heralded increasing opportunities for graduate education in nursing. Overlapping with the research era (Meleis, 1991), the *graduate education era* dawned, supported by the identified need for nurse scientists to generate nursing research. Whereas many nurse educators previously sought higher education in "softer" disciplines traditionally associated with the arts (education, anthropology, sociology, and philosophy), as doctoral education in nursing flourished by the end of the 1970s in the United States and the 1980s in Canada, educators increasingly identified with the science of nursing. Undergraduate education began to focus on introducing student nurses to research as a basis for their practice and for their future professional education.

It was also during the 1970s that nurse theorists began publishing their work in response to the critique that nursing research was lacking a conceptual foundation. The *theory era* was ushered in by the Nursing Educator Theory Conference in 1978 and flourished through the 1980s and 1990s (Alligood, 1997). The early phase of this era emphasized theory development. Nurse theorists developed models, frameworks, and theories in an attempt to define the essence of nursing and nursing practice. Theory utilization has been the emphasis of the later phase of this era as a recognition developed that education, research, and theory were not ends in themselves, but tools for nursing practice. Selected nursing theories were adopted as frameworks for curricula by many nursing education programs while others assumed a more pluralistic approach, introducing their students to a variety of theories. Theory-based practice continued to be foundational for many nursing education programs.

Looking ahead, Alligood (1997) proposed that what will be needed for the new age of nursing is the utilization and testing of theory/knowledge within a critical thinking framework. Theory and research together will lead to a science that will inform practice to meet the future needs of nursing clients.

Linked with this prediction (but not included in Alligood's 1997 work), the current era of nursing knowledge is that of *evidence-based practice.* Grounded within the larger framework of knowledge acquisition for provision of quality health care, this era reflects the effort to identify and apply the best available evidence to a specific clinical situation. Schools of nursing in the waning years of the last decade emphasized the skills required for evidence-based nursing practice which have included literature search strategies and critical appraisal of the identified literature.

While this framework for the development of nursing knowledge is helpful in understanding our past and our present, authors (both within nursing and in other fields) have identified significant changes in understanding that I believe suggest yet other eras of knowledge that will be significant for nursing as the profession enters the twenty-first century. Unlike the sequential development of areas of focus for nursing knowledge as presented by Alligood (1997), these new developments are occurring simultaneously, thus challenging educators to assume a complex multidimensional perspective.

THE EMERGING ERA OF KNOWLEDGE FOR TWENTY-FIRST CENTURY NURSING PRACTICE

Carper's (1978) discussion of ways of knowing and her equal valuing of aesthetic, ethical, personal, and empirical ways of knowing in nursing marked the beginning of a series of discussions in the nursing literature that held significant implications for the discipline. Increasingly some nurse theorists and educators called for a return to what they perceived as the philosophical base of nursing knowledge—caring (Watson, 1999; Leininger and Watson, 1990). The positing of a return to the heart of nursing led to the *era of moral/ethical knowing.*

As early as 1979, Curtin suggested that the purpose of nursing is not scientific but moral—"the welfare of other human beings" (p. 2). The core of Bevis and Watson's caring curriculum is the assumption that "caring is informed moral action that adamantly resists reducing persons (students or patients) to the moral status of object (Gadow, 1985, 1988; Watson, 1985)" (1989, p. 42). Freire captures the essential quality of personal and moral knowing in education in the following:

> ... to transform the experience of education into a matter of simple tech-
> nique is to impoverish what is fundamentally human in this experience:
> namely, its capacity to form the human person. If we have any serious re-
> gard for what it means to be human, the teaching of contents cannot be
> separated from the moral formation of the learners. To educate is essen-
> tially to form. (1998, p. 39)

Stephen Brookfield based his book *Developing Critical Thinkers: Challenging Adults to Explore Alternative Ways of Thinking and Acting* on the premise that "Being a critical thinker is part of what it means to be a developing person, and fostering critical thinking is crucial to creating and maintaining a healthy democracy" (1987, p. 1). Involving much more than skills of logical analysis, critical thinking implies being aware of the assumptions foundational to our actions and responses, paying attention to the context within which our actions and ideas originate, questioning single answers to problems and claims to universal truths, and being open to alternative ways of looking at and acting in the world. The moral imperative of adults is not only to fully develop themselves as individuals, but also to contribute to the growth of a more democratic society.

This freeing from extant ways of thinking has been linked with emanci-patory learning. Freire's earlier work, *Pedagogy of the Oppressed* (1970), described the emancipatory outcomes of liberatory education, and it is arguably the most well-known work in the area of education. However, much of what has been written in recent nursing literature in this area cites Habermas' work in critical social theory. Habermas (1971, 1979) defines three areas of human interest that are essential to a functioning society:

1. Technical interests arise from the instrumental work that must be done by societies. These interests are guided by empirical-analytical knowledge that provides explanatory and predictive power and allows technical control of the world.
2. Practical interests are concerned with language, communication, and intersubjectivity and are guided by historical-hermeneutic knowledge that provides understanding and shared interpretation of meaning. Such knowledge allows us to understand social-cultural phenomena and to gain reciprocal understanding between individuals and groups.
3. Emancipatory (critical) interests are concerned with social equity, freedom, and justice. These are guided by knowledge discovered through a process of becoming aware of competing power structures and social inequity (conscientization).

In a world where the disparity in distribution of power is becoming ever greater, in cities with growing numbers of disenfranchised citizens, and in health care environments where difficult decisions must be made in an era of decreasing resources, the nurse must recognize the critical interests of her clients and of her own profession. In order to provide ethical care that is grounded in a social justice frame, nurses must use not only empirical and hermeneutic knowledge but also critical knowledge to challenge the status quo, to advocate for, and more importantly, support the individuals, families, and communities with whom they work to become empowered for their own health.

Nurses will be compelled to consider broad issues that influence the well-being of individuals and populations such as the health of the environment; poverty; social inequity based on gender, ethnicity, race, sexual orientation, physical and mental ability, age, and other attributes that define "difference"; and even issues of war and peace. Political competence, action, and activism will be skills required by nurses for the twenty-first century. Going beyond knowledge of and skill in policy analysis and development that is a component of most current educational programs, political activism and an ethic of service will be a requirement of ethical/moral nursing practice for the future health care environment.

Such ethical practice requires that practitioners engage in personal knowing. Only through awareness of the self can nurses examine their values and beliefs and come to new understandings. Work in both critical thinking and reflective practice evidences this changing emphasis from theory/knowledge-based practice to self-awareness-based praxis and, in doing so, defines the era of personal knowing.

Personal knowing involves knowing the self in order to become a therapeutic instrument of healing within an interpersonal relationship. Chinn and Kramer (1999) present a model in which personal knowing arises from two critical questions, Do I know what I do? Do I know what I know? Brookfield's (1987) work in critical thinking and reflection adds two elements to these questions, Why do I do what I do? How do I know what I know? Through an inner reflective process, we come to understand our "selves" and identify and question our assumptions and our "taken for granted" responses to situations and circumstances—we become *self*-conscious. "Reflection is an occasion for the student's intervention in examining and changing life. . . . "learning begins with taking the self as the first—but not the last—objective of knowledge" (Aronowitz, 1998, pp. 9 and 12).

Part of the process of personal knowing is developing curiosity, which Freire (1998) refers to as the "cornerstone of learning and growth" (p. 79). "Curiosity is what makes me question, know, act, ask again, recognize" (p. 81). This imperative of curiosity and questioning inherent in reflective learning and practice requires that we engage critically and thoughtfully in whatever we are doing. Schön (1983) refers to the process of "reflection-in-action" which he views as "central to the 'art' by which practitioners sometimes deal well with situations of uncertainty, instability, uniqueness, and value conflict" (p. 50)—situations that nurses confront in their everyday practice.

As nurses or nurse educators, faced with challenges and the myriad tasks that are demanded of us in a time of receding resources and support, we are at risk of going into "auto-pilot" (Palmer, Burns, and Bulman, 1994). We may practice and teach by rote, by tradition, by standardized care plans, by scripted lectures—unquestioning and unconscious. However, the risk in this type of practice is not only losing the individual patient or student in the process but also losing our "selves." While we may complete the required tasks, our "self" is no longer a part of the nursing or teaching relationship. Through self-knowing we engage in nurturing and respecting the power of the self. Through self-knowing, we develop the capacity for self-direction.

Personal knowing is not a process that takes place in isolation for we only know and create our "selves" in relation to others. It is an "unfolding process that is grounded in the context of everyday experience, in relationship with others" (Chinn and Kramer, 1999, p. 171). Thus, there is no separate "self"— no objective being that can be separate from those with whom we are in a relationship, whether it is a relationship within the context of research, the context of education, or that of nursing practice.

It was in the early 1980s that the qualitative/quantitative debate in nursing research reached its peak and the challenge to "objectivity" began. Post-modern philosophies and their rejection of duality began to appear in the nursing literature shifting the focus of knowing from the objective to the relational, from the mechanistic to the holistic. The *era of relational and holistic knowing* presents a significant challenge for nurse educators, as it is no longer sufficient for our students and graduates to attain factual knowledge about the "other."

Relational knowing for nursing has impacted on our view of the essential nature of the relationship between the patient and the nurse. Traditionally seen as a helper-helpee relationship characterized by an objective stance assumed by the nurse, in order to be professional and unbiased, the essence of the nurse-patient relationship is changing. Terms like *authenticity, transpersonal, caring,* and *transcendent* pepper the current nursing literature and belie the notion (indeed, the possibility) of separateness. The patient cannot be known independent of the nurse, the student cannot be known independent of the teacher.

Hall and Allan (1994) discuss the concept of self-in-relation, which they perceive to be the core of holistic nursing practice. Grounded within the philosophy of traditional Chinese medicine, the four dynamics that nurture self-in-relation are:

1. Caring by giving which requires presence, involvement, and mutual sharing—a giving to one another that affirms the value and purpose of each life.
2. Empowerment of both individuals within a relationship where value is given to reciprocity and that which each brings to the relationship.
3. An understanding of the value of human life, which develops as each person in the relationship engages in the quest of finding meaning in life and thus further develops the self.
4. A sense of community, which is deemed to be the most important yet most elusive aspect of holistic healing practice. Within a caring community, self-in-relation can develop (Hall and Allan, 1994, Chinn and Kramer, 1999).

Closely linked with the concept of relational knowing is that of holistic knowing. Traditionally, knowledge has been broken down into discrete parts. We research by examining parts of the whole—limiting, to as much a degree as possible, confounding variables that will influence the study results. We teach by components. The curriculum is a set of building blocks; each block, while not necessarily discrete, is a part of the whole. Once the particulars of each block are attained and understood, the whole can be understood. Such reductionism and mechanistic thinking has been challenged in the latter decades of the twentieth century. However, Cartesian dualism of the mind and the body remained virtually unchallenged throughout twentieth century health care practice and research.

As we enter the twenty-first century, the nursing profession is moving beyond our modern roots within the Western biomedical model to incorporate thousands of years of traditional healing knowledge from our Aboriginal, Asian, Latin, African, and northern European ancestors. Some theorists see this movement as a "return to our roots" (Fontaine, 2000, p. ix). Indeed, Nightingale was acutely aware of the "interconnections between and among all dimensions of the personal, the public, and the political . . ." (Watson, 1999, p. 263) and nursing's imperative to view the patient as a whole being. However, ethnocentrism and a commitment to viewing health from a purely biomedical perspective has resulted in twentieth century nursing straying from Nightingale's insightful vision.

Our increasingly diverse community of health care consumers demands that we move beyond a "cure" focus for health to also consider healing within an integrative framework that includes the mind-body-spirit-environment as an indivisible whole. Watson's (1979, 1985, 1999) work in the science of human caring and Roger's (1970) concept of the unitary person introduced holistic understanding of the client to nursing in the latter decades of the twentieth century but their visions have remained marginal within nursing practice. As the new century dawns, it is time to re-visit the holistic frameworks that recognize the inseparability of the body-mind-spirit, the individual and the environment, health and illness, and the nurse and the client.

Within this frame of relational knowing, the reality of increasing diversity within our health care practice presents a very different problem. The western world is experiencing a period of profound social change—widening cultural diversity, the "graying" of the population, increasing numbers of people living with disabling conditions, families that are constituted in ways that do not resemble the traditional Western nuclear family, growing numbers of people living in poverty, communities that reflect health care and social values and issues outside of the status quo. Within a relational knowing context, the individual persons, families, and communities reflected within this new reality no longer are seen as the "other," the foreign, the unusual, the deviant, but are known in relation to ourselves. A shift in focus occurs, transforming the lens from one searching for difference, to one seeking that which we have in common, that which unifies us as a larger community seeking health and healing.

Capra (1996) suggests that a community that is aware of the interdependence of its members will be enriched by diversity. That diversity will enrich both the relationships within the community, the community as a whole and the individual members within it. "In such a community information and ideas flow freely through the entire network, and the diversity of interpretations and learning styles—even the diversity of mistakes—will enrich the entire community" (p. 304).

But these principles have only been reflected minimally within the traditional nursing classrooms and within the nursing profession. While there is an increase in the numbers of students from diverse ethnic, racial, social, and cultural backgrounds seeking entry into the profession of nursing, the literature (and professional experience) tells us that the diversity within the nursing profession remains inadequate to meet the needs of our changing population. It also reflects that "minority students" struggle more to succeed within our value-laden curricula. Outlaw (1997) calls for a "diversity agenda" for nursing for the twenty-first century in which she refers to developing cultural competence for practice and research. Ferguson's (1997) book *Educating the 21st Century Nurse: Challenges and Opportunities* ventures that what may define nursing in the future will be its ability, as a profession, to respond to health care needs within diverse environments. In order to do so, nurses need to develop an attitude of openness and not just a tolerance, but an affinity, for change, uncertainty, and difference.

We can no longer rely on the traditional truths that sustained us through the twentieth century. At one time it was sufficient for nurses to have a certain knowledge base, for example, to know that the average body temperature was 37°C—to know that facts were "true." However, in the latter part of the twentieth century, the volume of new knowledge exploded and continues to explode at a stunning rate. There are few facts that remain unchallenged. The established truths that supported nursing education and practice in the curriculum era have been thrown into suspicion. Many of these truths are being challenged over and over again by new scientific discoveries, new strains of diseases, new treatment methodologies (many alien to the traditional Western model), new ideologies for health care, changing roles of health care providers and their clients, and new understandings of all aspects of health, illness, the environment, and working life.

We have entered the *era of multiple truths.* Uncertainty and constant change characterize the external environment within which the nursing profession and its educational programs are developing. As early as the 1960s, the impact of seeming whirlwinds of change was acknowledged. "The only people who will live successful in tomorrow's world are those who can accept and enjoy temporary systems" (Farson, 1969 as cited in Ferguson, 1997, p. xxiii). Making a personal paradigm shift to embracing uncertainty and change will be essential to survival in a world of shifting truths.

Valentine (1998) suggests that Deepak Chopra's thesis *The Seven Spiritual Laws of Success* provide an exemplar for this transformation in perspective— "And what is the known? The known is our past. The known is nothing other than the prison of past conditioning. There is no evolution in that. . . . Uncertainty, on the other hand, is the fertile ground of pure creativity and freedom. . . . Relinquish your attachment to the known, step into the unknown, and you will step into the field of all possibilities" (Chopra, 1994 cited in Valentine, pp. 338–339).

Finally, we are being challenged by the *era of technological knowing.* As increasingly complex technology is introduced into the health care environment, nurses must acquire and master the skills required for competent management of that technology while maintaining a holistic focus on the patient and family. Perhaps more importantly, technological development is presenting health care with intellectual, social, ethical, and moral issues that were unimaginable in the last century.

The human genome project has allowed us, in President Bill Clinton's words, to "learn the language in which God created life" (Talaga and Papp, 2000). Computer technology allows instantaneous communication around the world, websites provide health care practitioners and consumers with information and education from a wide variety of perspectives, advances in robotics allow surgeons to perform surgical procedures deemed "miracles" a few decades ago, and genetic engineering promises to eliminate many disabling conditions and illnesses. As a result of these technological advances, it is predicted that the average age for survival in the Western world will increase dramatically.

New technologies will also result in health care becoming portable—allowing diagnoses to be made and health care to be provided distant from traditional health care institutions. Patient interaction with the health care system will be very different than the face-to-face contact that currently characterizes our therapeutic interactions (Given, Given, and DeVoss, 1997). Technologically competent health care consumers are even now presenting to their practitioners with knowledge gleaned from the Internet and a desire to be more involved in managing their health care. Nurses and physicians are required to help their patients analyze and interpret the health/illness information they have acquired. As the public increasingly becomes aware of the range of resources available to them, they are requesting a choice in terms of their health care provider. New health care specialists are evolving—health educators, health technology specialists, holistic physicians, palliative care specialists—in response to the demands of the informed consumer.

However, health care cannot totally become a market-driven system based on consumer demand. Combined with ongoing efforts in cost-containment by governments, such technological possibilities will challenge health care professionals to make difficult choices. Requirements for cost-effectiveness, mechanisms of gate-keeping, and controlled referral systems will limit the access to technology. Patients and families who are not able to access technology or to function effectively within a high-tech environment will be disadvantaged and marginalized (Given, Given, and DeVoss, 1997). Thus, as well as developing technical competence with the new machines that will support patients in monitoring and regaining health and wellness, nurses will be challenged with developing new knowledge in the areas of informatics and education of patients in the effective access and use of health care information. They will also be faced with the moral obligation to address the ethical questions that use of technology will inevitably evoke and to confront the inequitable access to its "miracles".

TEACHING METHODOLOGIES FOR THIS NEW ERA

This shift to personal and moral knowing and the rejection of the objective world within a context of a "high tech" health care (and educational) environment has significant implications for how nursing education is implemented. The hegemony of Tylerian behaviorist learning theory has been evident in the curricula and methods of teaching in most North American schools of nursing. For more than 50 years, lists of behavioral objectives, learning outcomes that could only be determined through objectively observable and measurable behaviors, and teacher-student relationships characterized by a hierarchical one-way transmission of knowledge have been the hallmarks of the behaviorist nursing curriculum.

In the late 1980s Bevis and Watson (1989) introduced a new paradigm for nursing education that challenged institutionalized behaviorism. While accepting the value of the behaviorist approach for aspects of nursing that require memorization and skill acquisition, these forward thinking nurse educators began to question the adequacy of the tenets of the behaviorist paradigm for professional nursing education. As we recognize that learning is more than acquisition of knowledge, we acknowledge that teaching is more than the transferring of knowledge from the teacher to the student. Teaching in the new era of nursing education requires a more egalitarian relationship, genuineness, a willingness to know ourselves and to be open to change and growth, and skill in fostering inquiry and dialogue.

"To know how to teach is to create possibilities for the construction and production of knowledge rather than to be engaged simply in a game of transferring knowledge. . . . In other words, I ought to be aware of being a critical and inquiring subject in regard to the task entrusted to me, the task of teaching and not that of transferring knowledge" (Freire, 1998, p. 49).

Heidegger (1968) asserts that teaching is more difficult than learning, not because teachers must possess and transmit large bodies of knowledge and facts but because the task of the teacher is not to teach, but to "let learn." Indeed, if the teacher-student relationship is genuine, according to Heidegger, "there is never a place in it for the authority of the know-it-all . . . " (1968, p. 15).

Conceptualizing education in this way requires a change in fundamental relationships between teachers and students. Clayton and Murray (1989) entitle their chapter on teaching "Faculty-student relationships: Catalytic connection." While this title embodies an inherently appealing alliteration, an examination of the definition of catalysis reflects that it is something that brings about a change without changing itself. However, teaching within the new paradigm of relational knowing and intersubjectivity requires recognition that both the teacher and the taught are changed through the process of learning. "Education takes place when there are two learners who occupy somewhat different spaces in an ongoing dialogue. But both participants bring knowledge to the relationship, and one of the objectives of the pedagogic process is to explore what each knows and what they can teach each other" (Aronowitz, 1998, p. 8).

Students enter the learning situation with their unique life experiences and an essential moment in the learning process is when they critically evaluate what they know and what they value. Skill in facilitating this process is key for successful teaching within this new paradigm. Brookfield and Preskill (1999) present discussion as a powerful educational tool to help students (and their teachers) develop an awareness of and appreciation for the multiplicity of views and perspectives that reflect the complexity of human experience. Through the opportunity for students to have their voices heard and their views valued, to speak and to listen, to give and to receive, these authors declare that the goal of discussion mirrors that of democracy—"to nurture and promote human growth" (p. 3). Through the collaborative and cooperative process which occurs in discussion, students are exposed to new points of view, are challenged to expand their horizons, come to mutual understanding, and "a collective wisdom emerges that would have been impossible for any of the participants on their own" (p. 4).

In the nurse-patient relationship, the goal is to understand the lived experience and world of the patients and through the collective wisdom of the nurse and the patient, to work together towards health and wellness. Only through developing the skills of listening, developing self-awareness, and valuing of another's perspective will students acquire the capacity for effective therapeutic relationships with their patients. Teachers within this educational paradigm, through their interactions with their students, model the authentic, humanistic connections that are the foundation of the nurse-patient relationship.

"The reciprocal learning between teachers and students is what gives educational practice its gnostic character. . . . It is artistic and moral . . ." (Freire, 1998, p. 67). This esoteric, mystical nature of the process of education is consistent with work in the area of teaching within a philosophy of caring (Bevis and Watson, 1989; Leininger and Watson, 1990; Watson, 1999). "There ought be no list of what to teach because education for the new age is not about content, *it is about soul, it is about process*" (author's italics) (Moccia, 1989, p. xi).

This caring imperative for nursing education is made more complex by the demands for access to education within the context of the technological advances which allow teaching in the "absence of physical presence" (Diekelmann, 2000). Correspondence classes, tele- and videoconferencing, faculty travel to off-site campus classrooms, and video and television-based learning have been and continue to be used to provide distance education. Interactive Web-based learning is the newest addition to the repertoire of media in which education is taking place. This technology-based methodology will allow education to be provided anywhere in the world, where and when it is wanted, thereby increasing access to continuing, graduate, and basic education for nursing. Some initial research has shown no differences in student learning outcomes upon completion of Web-based and traditional learning (Yucha and Princen, 2000; DeAmicis, 1997; White, 1992), and the argument has been offered that the skills gained in Web-based instruction may be more important than the content covered in the course because of the potential influence the Web has on our everyday lives (Fleming and Levie, 1993). However, the consequence of the absence of physical presence has yet to be examined.

Just as technology-based care challenges health care providers, new pedagogical methodologies require a re-visioning of the teacher and student roles. Diekelmann (2000) reflects on the struggles and rewards of being a distance teacher as they lose their "familiar landmarks and touchstones" (p. 51). So too do students lose their familiar roles, assumptions, and learning strategies as they venture into an alien learning environment.

The educational possibilities offered through distance education are as yet unknown and untested. "Distance education may be the place to push the edges of what constitutes schooling, learning and teaching and to create new pedagogies for the changing instructional landscape as nursing education enters the new millennium" (Diekelmann, 2000, p. 52).

CONCLUSION

Bevis and Watson (1989) recognized the importance of designing learning environments that "enable nursing graduates to be more responsive to societal needs, more successful in humanizing the highly technological milieus of health care, more caring and compassionate, more insightful about ethical and moral issues, more creative, more capable of critical thinking, and better able to bring scholarly approaches to client problems and issues and to advocate ethical positions on behalf of patients" (p. 1).

In the following chapters problem-based learning will be described as a model to meet the challenges that face nurse educators in their task of assisting student nurses to develop the scientific, aesthetic, moral/ethical, personal, and technical knowledge and expertise to meet the challenges that face nurse educators in their task of assisting student nurses to develop the scientific, aesthetic, moral/ethical, personal and technical knowledge and expertise to meet the needs of the health care consumer of the future. As will be detailed in these chapters, problem-based, small group, self-directed, and reflective learning provides the environment in which students and teachers learn together, in which extant knowledge is challenged through dialogue, in which students develop self-awareness through reflection, and in which there are "hands-on" opportunities for nursing praxis.

As Chinn and Kramer acknowledge in their fifth, heavily revised, edition of *Theory and Knowledge*, "Praxis—thoughtful reflection and action that occur in synchrony—comes from the whole of knowing and knowledge in nursing practice" (1999, p. 1). Rooted in critical social theory, praxis means "acting with awareness, a simultaneous doing while reflecting on the doing, always shifting what is done, based on insights from reflection" (Chinn and Kramer, 1999, pp. 207–208). While the more commonly used term—practice—represents maintaining the status quo (doing what has always been done, following the procedure manual, using the standardized care plan), praxis implies a very different approach to nursing. Nursing becomes a prospective process involving not only what we know, but who we are. Only if we are successful in engaging students in knowing in each of the areas of knowledge will we prepare them for thoughtful, critical praxis. Only if they engage in praxis will they help envision and shape the future of their patient's lives, their communities, their own lives as nurses, and the future of the profession.

The challenge is ours, as nurse educators, to engage in teaching praxis— to become critically aware of the values that underlie our curriculum, our teaching strategies, our evaluation measures, our dialogue with our students—

to engage in synchronous reflection and action to create and shape nursing education. If we are successful, we will have prepared our graduates to venture onto the untraveled paths into the limitless unknown of twenty-first century health care.

REFERENCES

Alligood, M. R. (1997). The nature of knowledge needed for nursing practice. In M. R. Alligood and A. Marriner-Tomey (Eds.), *Nursing Theory: Utilization & Application*. St. Louis: Mosby.

Alligood, M. R. and Marriner-Tomey, A. (Eds.) (1997). *Nursing Theory: Utilization & Application*. St. Louis: Mosby.

Aronowitz, A. (1998). Introduction. In P. Freire, *Pedagogy of Freedom: Ethics, Democracy, and Civil Courage*. New York: Rowman & Littlefield.

Ashley, J. (1976). *Hospitals, Paternalism, and the Role of the Nurse*. New York: Teachers College Press.

Bevis, E. O. and Watson, J. (1989). *Toward a Caring Curriculum: A New Pedagogy for Nursing*. New York: National League for Nursing.

Brookfield, S. (1987). *Developing Critical Thinkers: Challenging Adults to Explore Alternative Ways of Thinking and Acting*. San Francisco: Jossey-Bass.

Brookfield, S. and Preskill, S. (1999). *Discussion as a Way of Teaching: Tools and Techniques for Democratic Classrooms*. San Francisco: Jossey-Bass.

Burbach, V. and Exstrom, S. (1999). Continued competency in Nebraska: Process and progress. *Issues: A Newsletter of the National Council, 20*(2), 5–11.

Capra, F. (1996). *The Web of Life*. New York: Anchor Books.

Carper, B. (1978). Fundamental patterns of knowing in nursing. *Advances in Nursing Science, 1*(1), 13–23.

Chinn, P. L. and Kramer, M. K. (1999). *Theory and Nursing: Integrated Knowledge Development* (5th ed.). St. Louis: Mosby.

Chopra, D. (1994). *The Seven Spiritual Laws of Success: A Practical Guide to the Fulfillment of Your Dreams*. San Rafael, CA: Amber-Allen Publishing, The New World Library.

Clayton, G. M. and Murray, J. P. (1989). Faculty-student relationships: Catalytic connection. In N.L.N., *Curriculum Revolution: Reconceptualizing Nursing Education*. New York: National League for Nursing.

Curtin, L. (1979). The nurse as advocate: A philosophical foundation for nursing. *Advances in Nursing Science, 1*(3), 1–10.

DeAmicis, P. A. (1997). Interactive videodisc instruction is an alternative method for learning and performing a critical nursing skill. *Computers in Nursing, 15*(3), 155–158.

Diekelmann, N. (2000). Technology-based distance education and the absence of physical presence. *Journal of Nursing Education, 39*(2), 51–52.

Eagles, Z. E. (1999). Career transitions: Your future in nursing. *Nurse Week, 12,* 14–15.

Farson, R. (1969). How can anything that feels so bad be so good? *Saturday Review of Literature* (Sept. 6), 20–21.

Ferguson, V. D. (1997). *Educating the 21st Century Nurse: Challenges and Opportunities.* New York: National League for Nursing.

Fleming, M. and Levie, W. H. (1993). *Instructional Message Design: Principles from the Behavioral and Cognitive Sciences* (2nd ed.). Engelwood Cliffs, NJ: Educational Technology Publications.

Fontaine, K. L. (2000). *Healing Practices: Alternative Therapies for Nursing.* New Jersey: Prentice Hall.

Freire, P. (1970). *Pedagogy of the Oppressed* (M. Bergman Ramos, trans.). New York: Seabury Press.

Freire, P. (1998). *Pedagogy of Freedom: Ethics, Democracy, and Civil Courage* (P. Clarke, trans.). New York: Rowman & Littlefield.

Gadow, S. (1985). Nurse and patient: The caring relationship. In Bishop & Scudder (Eds.), *Caring, Curing, Coping.* Tuscaloosa: University of Alabama Press.

Gadow, S. (1988). Covenant without cure: Letting go and holding on in chronic illness. In J. Watson and M. A. Ray (Eds.), *The Ethics of Care and the Ethics of Cure: Synthesis in Chronicity.* New York: National League for Nursing.

Given, B. A., Given, C. W., and DeVoss, D. N. (1997). The education of nurses for the future—Caring for those with chronic health problems. In V. D. Ferguson, *Educating the 21st Century Nurse.* New York: National League for Nursing.

Habermas, J. (1971). *Knowledge and Human Interests* (J. Shapiro, trans.). Boston: Beacon Press.

Habermas, J. (1979). *Communication and the Evolution of Society* (T. McCarthy, trans.). Boston: Beacon Press.

Hall, B. A. and Allan, J. D. (1994). Self in relation: A prolegomenon for holistic nursing. *Nursing Outlook, 42,* 110.

Heidegger, M. (1968). *What Is Called Thinking?* (F. Weick and J. Gray, trans.). New York: Harper & Row.

Leininger, M. and Watson, J. (Eds.) (1990). *The Caring Imperative in Education.* New York: National League for Nursing.

Lindeman, C. A. (2000). The future of nursing education. *Journal of Nursing Education, 39*(1), 5–12.

McBride, A. B. (1999). Breakthroughs in nursing education: Looking back, looking forward. *Nursing Outlook, 47*(3), 114–119.

Meleis, A. I. (1991). *Theoretical Nursing: Development and Progress* (2nd ed.) Philadelphia: J. B. Lippincott.

Miller, B. K., Haber, J., and Byrne, M. W. (1990). The experience of caring in the teaching-learning process of nursing education: Student and teacher perspectives. In M. Leininger and J. Watson (Eds.). *The Caring Imperative in Education.* New York: National League for Nursing.

Moccia, P. (1989). Preface. In E. O. Bevis and J. Watson. *Toward a Caring Curriculum: A New Pedagogy for Nursing.* New York: National League for Nursing.

National League for Nursing (1989). *Curriculum Revolution: Reconceptualizing Nursing Education.* New York: National League for Nursing.

Noddings, N. (1984). *Caring: A Feminine Approach to Ethics and Moral Development.* Berkeley: University of California Press.

O'Neil, E. N. (1998). The changing health care environment. In E. O'Neil and J. Coffman (Eds). *Strategies for the Future of Nursing.* San Francisco: Jossey-Bass.

O'Neil, E. N. and the PEW Health Professions Commission (1998). *Recreating Health Professional Practice for a New Century.* San Francisco: Pew Health Professions Commission.

Outlaw, F. (1997). A call for scholarly inquiry on human diversity. In V. D. Ferguson, *Educating the 21st Century Nurse.* New York: National League for Nursing.

Palmer, A., Burns, S., and Bulman, C. (1994). *Reflective Practice in Nursing: The Growth of the Professional Practitioner.* Oxford: Blackwell Science.

Rogers, M. E. (1970). *A Theoretical Basis of Nursing.* Philadelphia: F. A. Davis.

Schön, D. A. (1983). *The Reflective Practitioner: How Professionals Think in Action.* New York: Basic Books.

Talaga, T. and Papp, L. (2000, June 27). "Geneticists Open New Chapter in Book of Life." *The Toronto Star,* p. A1.

Valainis, B. (2000). Professional nursing practice in an HMO: The future is now. *Journal of Nursing Education, 39*(1), 13–20.

Valentine, N. M. (1998). Nursing's New World—A Guide for Taking Professional and Personal Responsibility to Make Health Care Better in the Next Century. In V. D. Ferguson, *Educating the 21st Century Nurse.* New York: National League for Nursing.

Watson, J. (1979). *Nursing and the Philosophy and Science of Caring.* Boston: Little Brown.

Watson, J. (1985). Nursing: *Human Science and Human Care.* Norwalk, CT: Appleton-Century-Crofts.

Watson, J. (1988). *Nursing: Human Science and Human Care: A Theory of Nursing.* New York: National League for Nursing.

Watson, J. (1999) *Postmodern Nursing and Beyond.* New York: Churchill Livingstone.

White, E. M. (1992). *Assessing Higher Order Thinking and Communication Skills in College Graduates Through Writing.* Commissioned paper. Washington, DC: National Centre for Education Statistics. ERIC Document Publication No. 340767.

Yucha, C. and Princen, T. (2000). Insights Learned from Teaching Pathophysiology on the World Wide Web. *Journal of Nursing Education, 39*(2), 68–71.

The Problem-Based Learning Model of Nursing Education

Elizabeth Rideout and Barbara Carpio

A compelling case for change in nursing education has been made in the previous chapter, a change that has been written about and debated widely since the mid-1980s. There is a consensus that new models of education are required for nurses to develop the knowledge, skills, and abilities to be critical thinkers, independent decision makers, lifelong learners, effective team members, and competent users of new information technologies. Above all, they must be reflective practitioners, able to identify their own strengths and take action to overcome limitations. A review of the literature indicates that nurse educators have responded in varying degrees to the challenge to prepare practitioners who have the desired qualities. Some educational programs have incorporated a more reflective component into their otherwise traditional programs, on the grounds that learning to critique one's actions will assist learners to develop greater critical thinking and enhance awareness of self and the environment (Atkins and Murphy, 1993; Baker, 1996; Jones, 1995; Saylor, 1990). Other programs have tried to encourage more in-depth, "meaningful" learning in traditional curricula by the use of strategies such as concept mapping (Irvine, 1995).

However, in the few reports of major shifts in the philosophy, structure, and process of nurse-education curricula, problem-based learning (PBL) has emerged as the most promising approach to pursue. Most programs that have adopted PBL are in Australia, where it is now used by the majority of schools of nursing (Creedy, Horsfall, and Hand, 1992; Doring, Bramwell-Vial, and Bingham, 1994; Heliker, 1994; Little and Ryan, 1988; McMillan and Dwyer, 1989; Ryan and Little, 1991; Townsend, 1990a, 1990b). Indeed, the only previous book devoted to PBL in nursing describes the curriculum from Griffith University in Queensland (Alavi, 1995). There are also published reports of PBL use in—among others—Canada (Brandon and Majumdar, 1997; Rideout, 1999), England (Frost, 1996; Grandis, Long, and Mountford, 1999), Hong Kong (Tiwari, 1999; Tang, Lai, Arthur, and Leung, 1999), South Africa (Uys and Gwele, 1999), the United States (Amos and White, 1998; Miller and Lee, 1999; White, Amos, and Kouzekanani, 1999), and Wales (Andrews and Jones, 1996).

This chapter presents an overview of the PBL Model and the outcomes of the method, while subsequent chapters describe in more detail the strategies required to produce the outcomes and the resources required for implementation. We begin with a brief review of PBL in the context of educational theory. Following this we will present an easy-to-follow guide to the practical use of problem-based learning. PBL in essence consists of a number of steps through which students progress in order to achieve learning objectives. Although in practice different educational programs may use a somewhat different series or number of steps, there are discernible commonalities in the process. Our intent is that any teacher/learner group could begin to use the model after reviewing the process as described in this chapter. A sample problem is also included. The final section of the chapter contains a review of the literature on the outcomes and effectiveness of the problem-based model.

THE PBL MODEL DEFINED

Problem-based learning (PBL) was developed originally as an alternative approach to the education of physicians (Barrows and Tamblyn, 1980; Barrows, 1996) and first implemented at McMaster University School of Medicine in Canada in 1969 (Neufeld and Barrows, 1974; Schmidt, Lipkin, deVries, and Greep, 1989). Since then PBL has spread world-wide in medical education and its use has been reported in several other disciplines in higher education besides nursing, such as architecture (Kingsland, 1996), business (Stinson & Milter, 1996), engineering (Woods, 1996), mathematics (Seltzer, Hibert, Maceli, Robinson, and Schwartz, 1996), occupational and physiotherapy (Saarinen and Salvatori, 1994), and science (Allen, Duch, & Groh, 1996) as well as in elementary and secondary education (Jaramillo, 1999; Kang, 1999).

Although some authors suggest that the definition of PBL remains elusive, essential and common characteristics of PBL emerge from any description of the model. The first and essential characteristic of PBL is described by Boud (1985): "The principal idea behind problem-based learning is that *the starting point for learning should be a problem,* a query or a puzzle that the learner wishes to solve" (p. 13). In this respect Ross (1991) contrasts PBL with traditional approaches: "This approach turns the normal approach found in university and college programs on its head. In the normal approach, it is assumed that learners have to have the knowledge required to approach a problem before they can start to work on the problem; here, the knowledge arises from the work on the problem" (p.36). Doing things this way around, according to Walton and Matthews (1989), avoids the tendency of traditional methods to place undue emphasis on material for memorization, and instead develops learning for "capability" rather than simply for the sake of acquiring knowledge.

A second essential characteristic is the *student-centered nature* of the approach, with its emphasis on self-directed learning (SDL). Students are presented with problems that contain a number of concepts and issues, and they have considerable control over—and responsibility for—their choice of which issues to pursue, their identification of individual learning needs, and their selection of resources to use. Synthesizing and presenting their research to others, and participating in self-evaluation are additional expected SDL behaviors of students in the PBL model. The emphasis in this student-centered, as contrasted with teacher-centered approach is on "learning to learn," so they can meet the lifelong need to adapt to contemporary knowledge, challenges, and problems they will encounter in the future (Glasgow, 1997).

Third, although problem-based learning has been adapted for use in large groups (Allen et al., 1996), it was originally conceived to take place in small groups and this remains the method of choice in most programs. Learners normally meet together in groups of 5–10, most often with a faculty member present, to work through the presented problems. The small-group face-to face nature of the process encourages learners to develop the skills and abilities to work together in groups.

In summary, the essential characteristics of PBL are:

- A curriculum organized around problems that are relevant to desired learning outcomes, rather than organized by topics or disciplines
- Conditions that facilitate small-group work, self-directed learning, independent study, functional knowledge, critical thinking, lifelong learning, and self-evolution.

Central to any definition of PBL is the term *problem,* which forms the starting point of the learning endeavor. The use of this term raises difficulty for some people otherwise attracted to PBL, since it may imply that nursing consists exclusively of dealing with problems, thus overemphasizing illness rather than health, and focusing on patients' difficulties rather than strengths. As well, it may be seen as implying an overly simple emphasis on *solutions* to problems rather than an exploration of them. However, within the PBL approach the term *problem* usually encompasses any situation relevant to learning to be a nurse: a situation or circumstance in a particular setting where specific kinds of knowledge and understanding have to be applied to provide explanation and elicit appropriate action (Barrows and Tamblyn, 1980; Dolmans and Schmidt, 1996; Walton and Matthews, 1989). Although alternate terms have been suggested, such as situation-focused learning, context-based learning, and inquiry-based learning, the general consensus is that the term *problem* best describes the starting point for the learning process.

A second issue that often arises in discussions of the PBL Model is whether it is applicable to clinical courses within professional education, or only to the theoretical components. Although the majority of writing about PBL has focused on its use in classroom settings, the model is equally applicable to clinical teaching since, in reality, clinical nursing courses (and those in medicine, physiotherapy and even engineering) have traditionally been problem-based. Learners work in clinical settings, with real people, dealing with real-life issues. Subsequent chapters, and Chapter 10 in particular, will therefore make reference to its use in both settings although the emphasis will be on classroom examples since they represent the most significant departure from traditional educational practice.

A third commonly debated issue is the extent to which a curriculum must be problem-based, and the evidence suggests that this can vary considerably (Barrows, 1986; Ross, 1991). As originally conceived, PBL was a philosophy of education that required that the entire curriculum be developed around problems, and such curricula continue to be defined as *completely integrated* (Barrows, 1988; Creedy et al., 1992). Examples of completely integrated curricula have been described in nursing (Alavi, 1995), medicine (Neufeld and Barrows, 1974), and physical and occupational therapy (Saarinen and Salvatori, 1994; Solomon, 1994). At the other extreme are programs where only a small minority of courses use PBL within a curriculum that is otherwise more traditional and information-oriented (Khoiny, 1996; Miller and Lee, 1999; Stern, 1995). This is often the situation when one or two faculty members learn about PBL and choose to use it in their own courses. In some instances, this prompts a curriculum review and a decision to increase the number of PBL courses. In other cases, PBL continues to be the choice of only a minority of instructors.

Between these two extremes are *hybrid curricula,* where several PBL courses are offered along with courses presented in a more traditional way (Armstrong, 1991). This is the situation in the School of Nursing at McMaster University, where PBL has been the dominant approach since the mid-1970s. The present curriculum includes three types of courses: *nursing* courses, both clinical and theoretical, which comprise 60 percent of the curriculum and use PBL throughout; *health sciences* courses (including biological sciences, population health, and research), which use a combination of approaches but are not predominantly problem-based; and *elective* courses, chosen by the individual student from the entire range of university offerings to complement their study of nursing. Learners can make the transition between PBL and traditional methods with planned support.

Thus, a considerable range exists in the extent to which PBL may be implemented within a curriculum and the decision to adopt the model appears to depend on many factors, including administrative and faculty commitment and the availability of resources.

THEORETICAL FOUNDATION OF PROBLEM-BASED LEARNING

The theoretical underpinnings of PBL were not well articulated in the early literature (Barrows and Tamblyn, 1980; Spaulding and Cochran, 1991). In fact the model appears to have arisen from the personal experiences and beliefs of a few medical educators (Barrows, 1996) and can perhaps be said to have had nontheoretical beginnings. However, as the method has evolved, and as commentary on it has multiplied, increasing attention has been paid to its connections with educational theories and theorists, and a substantial theoretical as well as practical base for the approach may now be claimed.

John Dewey and Jerome Bruner

Problem-based learning appears to reflect the views of the famous proponent of "progressive education," John Dewey, who declared: "There is no point in the philosophy of progressive education which is sounder than its emphasis upon the importance of the participation of the learner in the formation of the purposes which direct his activities in the learning process" (Dewey, 1938, p. 67). In PBL tutorials learners are able to identify learning issues and use learning resources that meet their individual objectives. Schmidt (1993) argues that PBL's emphases on problem analysis prior to information gathering and on self-directed learning activities were influenced by Bruner's notion of intrinsic motivation as a force that drives people to learn more about their world (Bruner, 1977). Albanese and Mitchell (1993) have also noted the connections between PBL and Bruner's theory of discovery (or inquiry) learning, in which he suggested that learning is enhanced when learners actively participate in the process and when learning is organized around a problem.

Cognitive Psychology and PBL

The congruence between PBL and learning theory grounded in cognitive psychology has also been described by Schmidt et al., (1989) and expanded upon by Schmidt alone (1993). He puts forward five principles that support PBL as a method for acquiring new information: activation of prior knowledge; elaboration of knowledge; encoding specificity, or the restructuring of knowledge to fit the problem presented; epistemic curiosity; and the contextual dependency of learning.

Activation of prior knowledge presupposes the use of earlier knowledge in understanding new information. Since learning, by its nature, has a restructuring character, prior knowledge and the way it is structured in the long-term memory will influence new learning. Schmidt suggests PBL uses this principle, as learners are asked to review what they already know about a problem before proceeding.

The claim that *elaboration of knowledge* is a principle that supports PBL is based on the work of L. M. Reder (discussed in Schmidt et al., 1989), who contends that elaborations provide redundancy in the memory structure and redundancy is both a safeguard against forgetting and an aid to rapid retrieval. Elaboration of knowledge is stimulated in PBL as learners formulate and criticize hypotheses about a given problem, discuss the relevant evidence with other learners, and present summaries of information they have researched.

Encoding specificity refers to the resemblance between the situation in which something is learned and the situation in which it is applied. As Schmidt et al. (1989) state: "successful retrieval of information in the future is promoted when the retrieval cues that are to reactivate the information are encoded together with that information" (1989, p. 106). In PBL, learners learn about patient issues in relation to problems that they will encounter in clinical practice.

Schmidt proposes that *epistemic curiosity* or intrinsic interest is congruent with problem-based learning, since group discussion promotes the clarification of one's own point of view when confronted with other perspectives.

Schmidt's last principle is that of the *contextual dependency of learning.* He sees PBL as an application of the principle that the ability to activate knowledge in the long-term memory and to make it available for use depends on *contextual cues.* Information learned in a particular context will be more likely to be retrieved when the same context is present in the future. In PBL information is learned in relation to commonly encountered problems, and thus information retrieval should be triggered when similar problems are confronted in the practice setting.

Constructivism and the Work of Lev Vygotsky

A further theoretical perspective on PBL is offered by constructivist episte-mology, a recently developed area of learning theory rooted in the work of Lev Vygotsky and his followers (Vygotsky, 1978, 1987). The central tenet of constructivism is that knowledge is "constructed" by the learner's cognitive activity in continuous interaction with participation in the social community of which the learner is a member. Learning takes place through active partic-ipation in social interactions with more knowledgeable individuals while engaged in relevant and meaningful activity. Learners receive assistance through interactions characterized by such activities as directing, modeling, questioning, and providing cognitive structuring and feedback, until they are able to perform without assistance or guidance. Learning must be "trans-formed" to the individual level so that self-regulation occurs, allowing movement to a higher level of both competency and independence.

Constructivism provides a theoretical rationale for PBL in two ways. First, PBL also places learning within a social context. Learners meet together with a tutor to work on meaningful problems related to their chosen area of practice. They work collaboratively as they discuss issues and assist each other in making connections between new ideas and prior knowledge, creating new meanings as they complete their tasks. Second, the roles of tutors and students in PBL are congruent with the constructivist paradigm in which more capable or knowledgeable persons assist but do not dominate the activ-ities and experiences of the learner. In PBL each student is responsible for his or her learning and the tutor and other learners are responsible for assisting each student to achieve optimal learning. The tutor has the addi-tional responsibility of providing clear task and goal structures and facilitating the learning process through consultation, assisting with collaborative interactions, and providing feedback to participants.

THE PBL MODEL IN ACTION

The PBL Model has been implemented in various ways over the 30 years since it was first developed, including using PBL in large groups of 20 or more learners rather than the usual 5 or 10 (Allen et al., 1996; Rangachari, 1996; Woods, 1996), using peers as facilitators in place of faculty (Solomon and Crowe, 1999), and dealing with a new problem each session rather than using a single problem as the focus of learning for several sessions (Charlin, Mann, and Hansen, 1998). Nonetheless, the original process described by Barrows and Tamblyn (1980) remains the most commonly used, in which learners meet weekly or biweekly in groups of five to ten with a faculty tutor present. Learners work through problems in a systematic way to accomplish learning objectives they have identified, and each problem occupies learners for a minimum of two sessions. Evaluation of learning outcomes is a central feature of the process, and includes assessment of both individual accomplishment and the group's ability to work effectively. It is important to emphasize that there is a considerable amount of terminology associated with learning about and implementing the PBL Model. It is useful to develop a Glossary of Terms so that faculty members and students use the same terms, decreasing the likelihood of confusion (Table 2.1).

Table 2.1 *PBL Glossary of Terms*

Data gap	Information about the client, context, and/or the health care situation that has not yet been revealed at a given point. Data gaps may be "filled" by referring to the chart data: the health history and findings from the physical exam included in the paper problem package.
Essential content	Content that must be covered in the curriculum at a specific time, that is, specific Level II content to be covered in the Level II PBL nursing course.
Hypothesis	May begin as an educated guess or hunch as a means of initial questioning. It often is used to begin the exploratory stage of clinical reasoning. A hypothesis should be based on existing knowledge and/or data from the scenario. As clinical reasoning continues, the hypothesis should be developed formally. Often hypotheses are used to drive the data gathering, identify knowledge gaps, and formulate learning issues.
Independent learning	The individual student takes on the responsibility for learning activities. These activities are determined by the student's learning issues, learning preference, and learning style.

continued

Table 2.1 *PBL Glossary of Terms   continued*

Interdependent learning	The small group takes over the responsibility of the teaching-learning tasks. This may involve any of the steps of PBL, that is, developing group learning objectives in order to bridge research knowledge gaps.
Issues	These may be factors or points of view that relate to the situation, that is, the stage of human growth and development of the identified clients, ethical dilemmas, and adaptation to illness.
Knowledge gap	Information needed in order to continue with exploratory phases of clinical reasoning and problem solving, for example, natural course of an illness; effectiveness; role of the nurse. It also is necessary to bridge the knowledge gap to develop reasoning and knowledge about a given area.
Learning issues	A knowledge gap identified for further study. Learning issues are refined in the process of examining knowledge gaps.
Learning resources	Any person, place (e.g., organization), or thing (e.g., book, article, video) that contributes to the students' knowledge about the learning issues.
Paper problem package	A comprehensive learning package used to facilitate PBL which, in this case, is related to clinical concepts and skills. The paper problem package includes a series of scenarios, student and tutor guides, chart data, health history, lists of concepts, the learning concept grid, resource list, and a feedback form.
Scenario	The context within which the health care problem and the client exist. There is usually more than one scenario in each paper problem package. In general, the scenarios are presented in chronological order.
Self-directed learning	This is a student-centered process by which learning needs are established through mutual assessment and participative decision making. First, the students decide what they want *and* need to learn. However, the tutor must provide guidance to ensure the appropriate course and curriculum objectives and essential content are met within these learning needs. The learning activities may include inquiry, independent study, and experiential techniques. The amount of tutor guidance varies with the student's ability to identify appropriate learning needs and prioritize the learning issues.

The actual process of the PBL Model is variously described as consisting of seven steps, as used in health sciences programs at Maastricht University in the Netherlands (Schmidt, 1983), six steps in the Harvard Medical School model (Davis and Harden, 1999), and the five steps originally defined by Barrows and Tamblyn (1980). However, there is consensus that in response to a presented problem learners should take actions roughly as outlined in Table 2.2 and described below.

Table 2.2 *Steps of the PBL Process*

1. The problem is presented to the group, terms are reviewed, and hypotheses generated.

2. Learning issues and information sources are identified.

3. Information gathering and independent study occur.

4. The knowledge acquired is discussed and debated critically.

5. Knowledge is applied to the problem in a practical way.

6. Reflection on the content and process of learning occurs.

Table 2.3 *A Sample PBL Scenario*

Scenario I

Eric, an 18-month-old boy, was brought to the emergency department at 4:30 P.M. by his mother. He had been vomiting and had diarrhea for the past 48 hours. He also had a fever and was flushed and listless. He has just been admitted to the Pediatric Unit. You are the nurse admitting him to the unit. He is clinging to his mother and cries as you approach him.

First, *the problem is presented* before any preparation or study has occurred. Typically, several problems will have been developed for a particular course, and students will be able to choose which problem to tackle at a particular time. Each problem consists of anything from one to four patient scenarios; in the case of multiple scenarios, these represent a sequence of developments concerning the same patient situation. In addition to the scenarios, each problem includes relevant chart data along with a tutor guide listing intended learning issues. If a standardized (simulated) patient is available for interview by the students at some point in the process, information about this is also included in the *problem package*. Initially, however, the students are given only the scenario. The scenario presented usually consists of a brief written description of a patient situation such as might be encountered by a practicing professional (Table 2.3). There are of course alternative ways of presenting the scenario, such as a video clip from a patient interview.

The group begins by identifying terms and concepts that are unfamiliar to some or all members. Terms that are unfamiliar to some students may be known to others, and so the process of information sharing begins at this stage. Alternatively, the students may have resources with them to consult for quick definitions. (If the faculty tutor is an expert in areas of knowledge required, the group may ask for information. However, if the tutor provides information, it should be only in the form of isolated items of knowledge, since the tutor's role is not to be the transmitter of information but instead the facilitator of student-directed learning.) If no one in the group has knowledge about unfamiliar terms or concepts, these are noted as learning issues to be pursued.

Next, learners work together to generate a number of possible hypotheses to explain the patient's situation. Students use previous knowledge, as well as their own ideas, opinions, and common sense, to produce possible explanations. Knowledge gaps and areas requiring exploration become apparent at this stage. Through this discussion learners *identify learning issues*, that is, what the individuals and the group need to understand better in order to proceed with the problem. A useful resource to assist students (especially beginning students) in generating hypotheses and learning issues is the "Let's Hypothesize" board game (Ingram, Ray, Landeen, and Keane, 1998). Students use dice to make their way around a board with spaces that correspond to six categories of hypotheses: physical, psychological, social, developmental, spiritual/cultural, and political/economic. As they land on a space, they must generate a hypothesis or learning issue related to the category. The game continues until the first player reaches the finish line. The game is a useful approach of assisting students to conceptualize issues within a scenario in a broad and holistic way. An example of the issues identified for the Eric problem is presented in Table 2.4.

At this point the information to be gathered normally relates to the patient's *generic* situation (for example, asthma, methods of birth control, legal issues regarding child abuse), rather than specific information about the *actual* patient in the scenario. Learners are encouraged to obtain first the kind of knowledge they would need to have in order eventually to work effectively with the specific patient situation. They may also begin to identify *data gaps* which relate specifically to the patient in the scenario.

It is essential that the learning issues be made clear and specific enough at this point to allow the students to gather useful and relevant information. Possible learning resources to be used are also often discussed at this stage. Depending on the nature of the problem, students may decide to consult content experts, library resources, computerized information, or community

Table 2.4   *Learning Issues and Data Gaps Identified During Step 2 of the PBL Process*

• Growth and development of 18-month-old

• Possible dehydration—signs/symptoms/assessment

• Altered electrolyte balance

• Family issues—Mom is alone. Single Mom? Other children? Work? Social support? Financial stresses? Coping? Knowledge of health care needs of child?

• Day care—safety issues, benefits to children

• Causes of vomiting and diarrhea in 18-month-old

• Treatment for dehrydration

• Hospitalization-anxiety for Mom and Eric—nursing actions to reduce anxiety

• Role of the pediatric nurse

members. Since PBL groups usually meet either weekly or biweekly, students need "unscheduled time" available between meetings for required *information-gathering and independent study.*

When the group meets again, having completed the research, the *knowledge acquired is discussed and debated critically.* During this process the group may identify further gaps in knowledge (i.e., additional learning issues to be pursued), or the learners may find themselves ready to apply their knowledge to the presenting patient. At this point in the PBL process learners usually need further details about the patient and his or her situation. This detail is generally referred to as chart data and contains, at a minimum, demographic data, past and current health history, and further information about the current presenting situation. (A portion of the chart data available for Eric is presented in Table 2.5.) Learners may obtain this information in one of a number of ways. They may want to interview a standardized patient, who will provide the information through a history and physical examination conducted by the learners. Alternatively, the data may be available as a resource package in the library, and reviewing and summarizing that data may be an objective for the next meeting. In some groups, learners chose to role-play, with the chart data made available to one student acting as a patient while other learners take on the role of interviewer.

At this point the learners may be able to explain fully the phenomena identified in the problem scenario, or more likely they will identify additional learning issues that require another period of individual study. It is not enough, however, simply to accumulate relevant information, for the process now requires students to *apply what they have learned to the problem in a practical way.* This may mean, for example, developing a plan for teaching the patient and family, or designing a long-term plan of care.

The final step of the process consists of *reflecting on the content and process of learning* that has occurred and thus integrating it into the student's existing knowledge and skills. It is suggested that this stage is critical to ensure the retrieval of what has been learned when a similar situation or problem is encountered in the future (Davis and Harden, 1999). At this point learners also discuss the process they used in their group, identifying what worked well and what they would like to change before going on to the next problem. The quality and quantity of learning, and the functioning of both individual members and the group as a whole, are scrutinized at this time through formative evaluation by individuals, peers, and faculty. This process also emphasizes that primary responsibility for the learning attained by the group and its members rests with the learners, under the guidance of a faculty tutor.

In the specific context of nursing, a curriculum using the above procedure needs to be based on a series of priority health problems that incorporate content identified as important or essential to the practice of nursing, and in accordance with the competencies specified by provincial, state, and national governing bodies. The use of the PBL process described above encourages students to regard nursing practice as evidence-based and

Table 2.5 *A Sample of the Patient Data for Eric Burns*

Pediatric Admission Data Base—Nursing	
A. Admission data	Admitted from ER
	Carried by mother
B. Brief history from parent/child's point of view	Began being fussy at night 5 days ago
	No appetite the next day
	Noisy breathing, began vomiting 2 days ago
	No energy, diarrhea for 2 days
	Fever today, T = 40°C(R), given Tylenol
	Phoned doctor today, advised to go to ER
C. Health history	Well child, no previous hospitalizations
	Had been in contact with child at day care who had diarrhea
	Immunizations up to date
D. Profile of child	Feeds himself table food, good appetite
	Vision, hearing, mobility—normal
	Not toilet trained, wears diapers
	Sleeps 10 hours/night, bedtime 8 P.M.
	Has bedtime story, sleeps alone
E. Adjustment to hospital	Anxious, upset, crying
	Mother cooperative
	Only child, single mom
	Grandparents will probably visit
F. Nursing assessment	T = 39.2°C P = 130 R = 28
	BP 90/50 Wt. 25 lbs
	Lethargic
	Good air entry, no crackles noted
	Skin flushed, no bruises, no rashes
	Mucous membrane—dry
G. General assessment	Febrile, lethargic child, needs rehydration
	Mother concerned and anxious

requiring the application of both critical thinking and continuous learning. PBL is designed to produce graduates who take responsibility for their own learning and who become accustomed to scrutinizing their effectiveness both as learners and eventually as health care professionals. The self-directed learner of today is the reflective practitioner of the future.

As this overview of the PBL Model indicates, there are many changes required in the roles of students and faculty members, and in the curriculum as a whole. All of these areas will be discussed in detail in later chapters. Let us turn now to the issue of its effectiveness.

DOES IT WORK? INVESTIGATIONS OF THE PBL MODEL

Having described a typical PBL session and acknowledged the many issues to be considered in implementing the model, we will now consider the main question raised by educators interested in PBL: *Does it work?* The adoption of PBL by more and more programs within an increasing number of disciplines has resulted in a profusion of studies designed to answer that question. A body of research has explored student and faculty experiences, perceptions, and satisfaction with the model, while research that addresses the positive and negative outcomes of this learning approach can be divided into studies that explored three main themes: the accumulation of knowledge, decision making and clinical practice ability, and self-directed and lifelong learning. It is noteworthy that there is a dearth of published research that looks at other purported outcomes of the PBL Model of particular interest to nurse educators, such as critical thinking, reflective practice, and teamwork. There is much to be done to truly determine the effectiveness of the model.

Student Satisfaction with the PBL Model

Studies of student perceptions of their learning environments have often accompanied the introduction of PBL into a program of study, and they have generally compared the experiences of learners (most often medical learners) in student-centered and/or problem-based curricula with those experiencing a more conventional curriculum approach. Some have used quantitative measures (Clarke, Feletti, and Engel, 1984; Moore-West, Harrington, Mennin, Kaufman, and Skipper, 1989; Bernstein, Tipping, Bercovitz, and Skinner, 1995; Kaufman and Mann, 1997) while others have employed qualitative methods of data collection (Davis, 1994; Ishida, 1995; Khoiny, 1995; Stern, 1995). Altogether this has been an area of interest to researchers seeking to understand the strengths and limitations of problem-based learning.

Quantitative Studies

Clarke et al. (1984) used the 58-item Medical School Learning Environment Survey in a cross-sectional study of student perceptions of a newly introduced problem-based curriculum across the years of the program. The scale, assessed as both reliable and valid, is comprised of the following seven subscales: flexibility, student-student interaction, emotional climate, support-iveness, meaningful life experience, organization, and breadth of interest. Overall mean scores of the learners in the problem-based curriculum were higher than those of learners in traditional programs in other universities and, although PBL scores did become less favorable over the years in the program, they indicated a persistently favorable educational environment. In a similar study, Moore-West and her colleagues at the University of New Mexico (1989) evaluated their problem-based, student-centered approach to medical education by comparing learners in the PBL curriculum with those enrolled in the existing traditional approach being offered within the same university. Learners were compared on perceived level of stress and attitudes toward the learning environment. The latter were assessed using a modified version of the instrument used by Clarke et al. (1984). Their findings were that learners in the problem-based group perceived the emotional climate of the program and the interpersonal relationships among learners to be better in their program than did the learners in the traditional group, although perceptions of both student groups were progressively less positive over time in the program.

Further evidence of positive responses from learners to the PBL approach comes from Bernstein et al., in their 1995 study of attitudes and experiences of medical learners before and after a five-week session where they used the PBL approach for the first time in their medical education. Responses to a questionnaire designed for the study revealed a statistically significant shift to a more positive perception of PBL at completion of the course. Learners described the advantages of PBL as better retention and reinforcement of learning; more enjoyable, stimulating, and interesting; enhancement of interpersonal skills; and learners learn how to learn rather than memorize. Learners expressed concerns about acquiring required knowledge, both before and after the PBL experience, indicating this is an ongoing issue in the PBL approach despite the overall positive perception associated with it.

Kaufman and Mann (1997) focused their attention on student attitudes to one component of medical education—basic sciences—among learners in a PBL compared to a conventional lecture-based program. Learners were surveyed about the importance of basic science knowledge for clinical practice and the level of satisfaction with the learning method to which they were exposed using a questionnaire developed by the investigators. The authors found a statistically significant difference in favor of the PBL group.

Two recent studies (Rideout, 1998; Rideout et al., 2000) used the Course Experience Questionnaire to explore perceptions of learners pursuing baccalaureate degrees in nursing. The 38-item CEQ consists of 6 subscales, each with satisfactory reliability and identified through factor analysis, namely independence, tutors, expectations, assessment, workload, and outcomes, as well as one item that assessed overall satisfaction with the program. In the first study conducted with all students enrolled in the 4-year BScN program at McMaster University, the learners indicated overall high levels of satisfaction in all areas and there were significant differences among learners in levels of the program in two areas. Learners in beginning levels of the program were significantly more likely than their counterparts in senior levels to agree with statements that student assessment is based on memorization and testing of content. Senior level students were more likely to agree with statements about the intended outcomes of the program, including developing problem-solving and analytic skills and the ability to work in teams, manage their workload, and communicate effectively.

In the second study, Rideout et al. (2000) compared the perceptions of graduating students in two nursing programs, one using the PBL Model (McMaster University) and the other. employing a more conventional approach to nursing education (University of Ottawa). The students undertaking the PBL program were more satisfied with their educational experience than their counterparts in the conventional program, indicating higher satisfaction with tutors, level of independence, assessment, and program outcomes, but no difference in relation to workload or clarity of expectations.

Qualitative Studies

Although perceptions can be explored using quantitative measures, the use of more open-ended approaches is also important in any investigation of thoughts and feelings (Cohen and Manion, 1989). Six recent studies were identified that used qualitative approaches to explore the experiences of learners in programs that incorporated student-centered problem-based pedagogy.

Ishida (1995) studied the responses to problem-based learning of Japanese, Filipino, and mixed-ancestry learners enrolled at the University of Hawaii School of Nursing ($N=17$), due in part to her hunch that non-Caucasian learners might report different responses to PBL than their Caucasian counterparts. Inquiry-focused learning was the philosophy underlying the BScN curriculum where PBL was used in some courses within the program, while other strategies such as lecture/discussion and computer-assisted learning were employed in other courses. To determine the level of satisfaction with the PBL component of the program, learners were asked to choose between PBL and lecture/discussion for subsequent courses in their program and to give reasons for their choice. A majority of informants (71 percent) selected PBL, and cited as reasons the level of involvement, opportunity for "student direction," flexibility, independence, and the relationships developed between learners and faculty. The learners also identified some limitations with the method, among them the time required to figure out the different expectations among faculty in the courses, the lack of security that the information they were sharing was accurate, and the conflicts that sometimes arose in the learning groups. Ishida also expressed surprise that learners from a variety of ethnic backgrounds found PBL "congenial and supportive of their learning" (p. 110).

Khoiny (1995) investigated the perceptions of PBL among nurse practitioner learners ($N=15$) who participated in four PBL sessions that took place within a curriculum that was otherwise traditional, with lectures and clinical practice used as the methods of teaching. Data were collected using two methods: a PBL attitude questionnaire consisting of open-ended questions developed by the investigator; and focus group interviews conducted with all participating learners. In response to the question, "If you had a choice between lecture and PBL, which one would you choose, and why?" most learners expressed a preference for the PBL approach, stating they felt more involved in discussion and that it was more active, more fun, and more practical. They also commented that, although they liked the interactive nature of the PBL sessions and their relevance to clinical practice, they obtained more information in a shorter period of time when the lecture method was used. Other weaknesses mentioned by respondents were similar to those reported by Ishida and included: the sense that some learners did not prepare enough, concerns about having learned all the important content, and the lack of immediate answers to questions raised in the group. Khoiny concludes that the PBL Method was perceived in a positive way but that concerns remained on the part of learners about the depth and breadth of learning obtained.

A third qualitative study examined the interactions of a group consisting of six medical learners and two facilitators in the first year of an integrated PBL program (Davis, 1994). Data were collected using participant observation, informal interviewing, document analysis, and videotaping. Learners described the program as enjoyable, holistic, active, social, and everything they hoped it would be, while the facilitators commented that the joy of learning was obvious in the learners. No concerns with the approach were reported, leading Davis to conclude that the PBL approach is viewed positively by both learners and faculty.

Stern (1995) found that occupational therapy learners enrolled in a PBL course within a traditional program attributed many positive benefits to the PBL approach, including enhancing their professional behavior, helping them integrate the various elements of their academic program, enhancing their clinical reasoning skills, and providing personal benefit or gain. Learners were overwhelmingly positive about the experience and no negative comments about PBL were reported.

Rather than explore the overall perceptions of learners, Solomon and Finch (1998) chose to investigate the stressors experienced by learners entering a fully integrated PBL program leading to a degree in physiotherapy at McMaster University. Learners kept a journal throughout the first unit of study, where they recorded what they had learned, what had contributed to learning, and what had impeded learning. Sixty-five percent of learners identified uncertainty about the breadth and depth of knowledge and time pressures as stressors. Other stressors identified, in order of frequency, were: lack of confidence in the PBL approach, misunderstanding of PBL and the faculty role, unrealistic expectations of self, demands of group learning, heavy workload, stress related to search for resources, tutorial evaluation, and group panic. Although all learners in the program had undergone a rigorous admissions process, including a personal interview and, therefore, were well-informed about the educational approach used, the data from this study indicates that PBL poses stress for new learners, and this needs to be recognized and dealt with to help smooth the transition from more conventional methods of learning.

Finally, Rideout (1998) used open-ended questions and in-depth interviews with learners enrolled in a 4-year Bachelor of Science in Nursing program to explore their perceptions of learning in the program where PBL is used in all nursing courses, which comprise 60 percent of the total curriculum. Although learners expressed high levels of satisfaction with the program and commented in particular about the freedom and personal choice the approach allowed, they also identified challenges associated with: (1) the methods of assessment used (they asked for more formal testing and fewer essays/papers); (2) the perceived lack of clarity and a sense of inconsistency of expectations among faculty; and (3) concerns about the breadth and depth of their learning, particularly as they prepared for their nurse registration examinations.

Faculty Perceptions of PBL

Faculty perceptions and attitudes toward PBL, like those expressed by students, are generally positive. Faculty who were interviewed by Maxwell and Wilkerson (1990) before and after they participated as tutors for the first time in the newly introduced PBL curriculum at Harvard University reported that the experience was much more positive than they expected and the opportunity to interact on a more personal level with learners was the chief source of satisfaction. Other benefits included a sense of personal growth and accomplishment derived from the experience. In a similar study of student and faculty perceptions of PBL conducted at the time PBL was introduced at the University of Toronto, Bernstein et al. (1995) found virtually all the attitudes expressed by students were shared by faculty, who commented they found the interaction between themselves and the learners more collegial, fun, easy, engaging, and relaxed than in the traditional program. They also commented on the benefits they derived from learning a new approach to teaching.

Vernon (1995) corroborated the positive attitudes of faculty in his survey of tutors from 22 American and Canadian medical schools that use PBL in all or part of their programs. Respondents rated PBL more positively than traditional methods overall, and differences were noted in five of eight areas explored, namely student interest and enthusiasm, faculty interest, personal satisfaction, student reasoning, and preparation for clinical practice. Learning efficiency was judged to be equal in both methods and the traditional method was judged superior for learning factual knowledge in the basic sciences. When asked what tutors liked best and least about PBL, student contact, student motivation, group atmosphere, and self-directed learning were all identified as positive aspects of PBL. Time requirements of faculty, poor student motivation, student evaluation problems, lack of structure and faculty control, and problems with integration of basic science knowledge were all noted as the most disliked features of PBL.

Summary of Student and Faculty Perceptions of PBL

In summary, all these studies together indicate that the PBL approach is viewed positively by students and faculty. These findings emerge from data collected using a variety of methods, including fixed-choice and open-ended questionnaires, and personal and group interviews. Both learners and faculty described PBL as enjoyable, interactive, relevant, practical, and holistic. Limitations with the method were also noted by learners, including a lack of confirmation that they were learning the essential content, a belief that group process issues were sometimes problematic, and the sense that different tutors sometimes had different expectations of learners. The few negative comments from faculty related to the lack of efficiency of the method (in terms of tutor time and student learning), difficulties with student evolution, and loss of tutor control. Generally, the areas of concern or issues for improvement were few, leaving the impression that PBL is viewed in a uniformly positive way by participants, whether students or faculty.

Outcomes of the PBL Model

Three meta-analyses published in 1993 provide comprehensive reviews of the literature in this area. A brief overview of the purpose and process of these three reviews will be presented in the following section, followed by their findings, supplemented by the most recent literature about the outcomes of the PBL model. All the findings will be summarized according to the questions posed commonly by those interested in but still sceptical about PBL, namely:

- How does the *accumulation of knowledge* of PBL learners compare to that of learners in conventional curricula?
- Do learners in PBL programs develop the same, higher or lower levels of *clinical decision making and clinical practice skills* compared to their counterparts in conventional curricula?
- Do PBL learners demonstrate increased *self-directed learning* behaviors and involvement in *lifelong learning* as compared to learners from conventional curricula?

Descriptions of the Meta-Analyses

Albanese and Mitchell (1993) identified all studies in the medical education literature from 1972 to 1992 that had problem-based learning in the title, and included for analysis all those for which information was provided about scope of the intervention, type of study design, number of PBL participants, and specific outcome measures and results. A meta-analysis strategy was used where effect sizes as well as p-values were reported. It is noteworthy that details about the type of PBL (integrated, hybrid, limited to one course) or the quality of PBL (e.g., level of functioning of the small groups or even size of group) were not addressed by the reviewers.

The second review was conducted by Vernon and Blake (1993), concurrently with that of Albanese and Mitchell, and for the same stated purpose: "This period of heightened interest (in PBL) is a good time to summarize what we can demonstrate about the possible outcomes of PBL in general" (p. 550). Analysis was conducted on "all identifiable research on health-related educational programs that contained a significant PBL emphasis" (p. 550), while studies that were "purely descriptive and afforded no comparison of any sort" (p. 551) were excluded. A meta-analysis strategy using 22 research reports on 14 programs employed common techniques such as calculating effect sizes for original research results, supplemented with "vote counts" (and associated sign tests). Like Albanese and Mitchell, they do not describe the "PBL intervention" in detail.

The third review, conducted by Berkson (1993), included literature on the theoretical foundations of PBL as well as empirical and experimental data, in order to "examine whether the faith in PBL embodied by (these) prestigious endorsements can find support in the current literature" (p. S79). She summarized the data (101 references are included) according to specified questions and reached conclusions based on the findings of the various studies reviewed. Her findings are therefore descriptive and were not subjected to statistical analysis.

Thus a quite similar literature was reviewed for similar purposes in three reviews conducted and published within months of each other. Now, what of their results?

Accumulation of Knowledge

Albanese and Mitchell (1993) examined studies that compared the academic performance of learners in PBL and traditional curricula on specific standardized tests (e.g., the National Board of Medical Examiners Parts 1 and 11, an examination taken by all medical learners in the United States) and reached the following conclusion: "Thus, while the expectation that PBL learners will not do as well as conventional learners on basic science tests appears to be generally true, it is not always true" (p. 57). Vernon and Blake (1993) also used data from studies of student performance on similar standardized tests and concluded that "these ES (effect size) data suggest a significant trend favouring traditional teaching methods" (p. 556). Berkson (1993) compared academic achievement of traditional and PBL medical learners by examining studies that had used a wide array of measures of knowledge acquisition (true/false questions, multiple choice questions, rating scores, and qualifying or licensing exams) and concluded that "no one has been able to demonstrate an important advantage of one curriculum over the other" (p. S80). Berkson's conclusions should be viewed with caution since the studies she examined used such a variety of measures of academic achievement, included no statistical analysis, and instead reported results of the various studies as "PBL slightly better," "PBL slightly worse," or "equivalent outcome."

In a post-1992 study with nursing learners, Newman (1995) compared the knowledge of learners enrolled in PBL with those in a non-PBL approach in one course within a conventional BScN curriculum. Scores on the final examination, which consisted of multiple choice and short answer questions, were slightly but nonsignificantly higher for the non-PBL approach on the multiple choice questions, while PBL learners scored slightly higher on the short answer questions, but again the differences were nonsignificant. Thus, one curriculum approach was not favored over the other. These results should be viewed conservatively since they are based on one course only within a total 4-year nursing program.

Solomon and colleagues compared the performance of physiotherapy learners from an integrated PBL program with those from a program that has introduced PBL into some senior courses within an otherwise traditional curriculum (Solomon, Binkley, and Stratford, 1996). Learners performed equally well on a multiple choice examination that included basic science and clinical science questions, with the PBL learners attaining slightly higher scores that were not statistically significant. Distlehorst and Robbs (1998) presented their comparison of the performance of medical students enrolled in one of two curricular tracks at the Southern Illinois University Medical School, one a conventional approach and the other completely integrated PBL. Using the United States Medical Licensing Examination as the measure of knowledge, they found no significant difference between the groups. In a recent study, Kaufman and Mann (1999) also compared the performance of medical students from a PBL with those from a conventional curriculum. They looked at students' results on a number of tests of knowledge achievement at three time intervals and concluded that the performance at all three times was equivalent in the two groups.

Rideout et al. (2000), in their study comparing nursing students from a PBL curriculum with those from a conventional curriculum, found the PBL students scored significantly higher on their self-assessments of nursing knowledge, particularly in the areas of individual, family, and community assessment; communication; teaching/learning; and the health care system. No significant differences were found on an objective measure of knowledge, the National Nursing Registration Examination, although there was a slight trend in favor of the conventional students.

Altogether the evidence from these reviews concerning academic achievement is slightly in favor of non-PBL programs when the outcome is measured using traditional fixed choice examinations, although the more recent research does not suggest there is any significant difference.

Decision Making and Clinical Practice Ability

To answer this question, Albanese and Mitchell (1993) included in their analysis seven studies that compared the clinical ratings by faculty supervisors of graduates of PBL compared to conventional curricula. In all the studies, "ratings by faculty were either more positive for learners in the PBL curriculum or nonsignificantly different from the ratings of the conventional group" (p. 65). They went on to state: "High clinical ratings would not be expected if PBL residents had deficits in their diagnostic acumen" (p. 67). Vernon and Blake (1993) also used studies that compared clinical perform-ance on one or more measures, most often observations of behavior with real or simulated patients, and they reached a conclusion similar to that of Albanese and Mitchell, namely, that PBL learners exhibited better clinical performance than did learners from conventional programs.

More recent evidence supports the findings reported in the three meta-analyses. Perceptions of medical education were compared among learners and graduates from three Dutch medical schools, one of which was a PBL school and the others conventional (Busari, Scherpbier, and Boshuizen, 1997). Participants completed self-assessments on their overall satisfaction with their learning, as well as their interpersonal, communication, and clinical patient management skills. Respondents from the PBL program felt more satisfied with their training and better prepared in interpersonal and commu-nication skills, but reported no difference from those from traditional schools in their ability to manage clinical situations. Although the authors acknowl-edged the limitations of a study that relied on self-assessments, differences did emerge that could be considered indicative of the different curricula of the three universities.

In their study comparing the clinical functioning of students from PBL and conventional tracks within the same medical school, Distlehorst and Robbs (1998) looked at measures of performance in the clinical clerkship and found the PBL students scored systematically higher, although the effect sizes were not large. They concluded the most important outcome of their study was demonstrating that students completing the fully integrated PBL curriculum were not in any way disadvantaged, and that they performed well in their clinical rotations.

Blake and Parkison (1999) examined the appraisals by clinical faculty members of the clerkships of medical students completing a newly estab-lished PBL curriculum. The assessments were generally favorable, and the particular strengths of the PBL students compared to the previous cohorts of students included clinical reasoning and problem-solving skills, history-taking ability, and knowledge of pathophysiology. Although this study is limited by the retrospective nature of data collection and the subjective nature of the information, the findings are similar to those of other studies of the effects of PBL on clinical knowledge and skills.

In the Rideout et al. study (2000) there were no statistically significant differences in the perceived abilities of nursing students in conventional and PBL curricula in four areas of clinical functioning: clinical decision making; collaboration; communication; and self-directed activity, although there was a trend toward greater preparedness in the latter two areas.

Self-Directed and Lifelong Learning Behaviors

Studies that compared the time used in self-study and the use of library resources were reviewed to determine similarities and differences in self-study behaviors between PBL and other learners. Albanese and Mitchell (1993) reviewed three relevant studies and concluded that PBL learners reported higher library utilization rates and were more likely to study in the library than at home and to use a wider variety of written materials. No clear pattern emerged in relation to time spent in study. Albanese and Mitchell conclude that "PBL learners are substantially more likely to use the library and library resources to study" (p. 62).

Berkson (1993) reviewed the same three studies as Albanese and Mitchell and, like them, concluded that PBL learners used a wider variety of resources and checked out more books from the library than did conventional learners. She questioned the meaning of this difference and concluded that evidence is still lacking to support the premise that "the practice of self-directed learning in the context of a PBL curriculum enhances self-directed learning skills, thus maximising the probability of the quality of learning continuing once the student has graduated and throughout a physician's career" (p. S84). Furthermore, Berkson states: "The post-graduate practice of self-directed learning strategies may prove more dependent on the proximity of available resources, peer expectations, role models, the physicians' profile, and time constraints than on 'putative' skills previously acquired or refined in a PBL or traditional curriculum" (p. S84).

Vernon and Blake (1993) reviewed four studies that provided data on the use of various learning resources by learners in PBL and conventional programs and concluded that "PBL learners (1) placed more emphasis on journals and on-line literature searches as resources and (2) made greater use of the library" (p. 557). They did not comment on the possible relationships between these findings and the likelihood of engaging in lifelong learning behaviors.

A recent study by Deretchin, Hamilton, Hawkins, and Contant (1999) compared medical students from a hybrid PBL program (termed a mixed-format) with those from a conventional program and found the former group used a greater quantity and quality of resources, and rated the contribution of such resources to their learning as higher. The authors concluded that the mixed-format curriculum in "support of lifelong learning is guardedly encouraging" (p. 177).

All three review articles reported a dearth of research exploring similarities or differences between PBL and conventional curricula in promoting lifelong learning, while conceding that it is a difficult construct for which to develop measures. All three refer to the study by Shin, Haynes, and Johnston (1993) where McMaster and University of Toronto graduates were compared 5–10 years post-graduation on their use of current treatments for hypertension. McMaster graduates were more likely to use newer treatments than those from the University of Toronto. There was consensus that the study was not well designed, in that no pretest was included and McMaster graduates may have received a better grounding in the management of hypertension since it is an area of expertise in research at McMaster.

CONCLUSION

There is a growing amount of literature on the benefits and limitations of PBL compared to conventional curricula. To date the studies have almost unanimously used medical students from diverse programs. Some conclusions can be drawn from the available literature. First, there has been a slight trend in the studies reported to somewhat better performance on standard examinations by students from conventional curricula compared to those from PBL programs, although this trend is not evident in the most recent studies. Second, learners from PBL curricula tend to be rated somewhat better in regards to their clinical performance, with the difference especially evident in their interpersonal communication. Finally, the evidence clearly supports increased library use and use of a wider variety of library resources by PBL learners. However, the relationships among library/resource use and the outcomes of knowledge, clinical practice, and lifelong learning have not been reported.

Wolf (1993) summarizes the research reported in the three meta-analyses reviewed above, with the following critique: "(1) there is a paucity of good-quality studies and evidence available regarding the hypothesis that PBL produces learning and/or learners different than or superior to those derived from traditional approaches; (2) results often are incomplete and poorly reported in the existing primary research reports; and (3) there is a tremendous need for well-designed creative primary research-evaluation studies that examine important, clinically relevant behaviors and outcomes" (p. 544).

There continues to be a need for research that examines the process and outcomes of PBL, indicating that the call for research made by Wolf in 1993 is still relevant in 2000. Furthermore, there must be research that explores the particular areas of interest to nurses who are incorporating the PBL Model. Because of its purported effectiveness in preparing the inquiring, reflective, knowledgeable, and collaborative nurse required for the world of nursing practice today and in the future, research must be initiated that investigates these outcomes. However, as the empirical evidence accrues that will support or question the PBL Model, we must acknowledge that students and faculty view the PBL Model positively, describe an array of benefits that derive from its use and, without exception, indicate they would not revert to the more conventional teacher-centered and subject-driven approaches still current in the majority of nursing programs. In the following chapters, the several foci of student learning in the PBL Model are described in detail, the resources to support learning are presented, and some of the newer applications of the model are outlined.

REFERENCES

Alavi, C. (1995). *Problem-Based Learning in a Health Sciences Curriculum.* London: Routledge.

Albanese, M. A. and Mitchell, S. (1993). Problem-based learning: A review of literature on its outcomes and implementation issues. *Academic Medicine, 68,* 52–81.

Allen, D. E., Duch, B. J., and Groh, S. E. (1996). The power of problem-based learning in teaching introductory science courses. In L. Wilkerson and W. M. Gijselaers (Eds.), *Bringing Problem Based Learning to Higher Education: Theory and Practice.* San Francisco: Jossey-Bass.

Amos, E. and White, M. J. (1998). Problem-based learning. *Nurse Educator, 23*(2), 11–14.

Andrews, M. and Jones, P. R. (1996). Problem-based learning in an undergraduate nursing program: A case study. *Journal of Advanced Nursing, 23,* 357–365.

Armstrong, E. G. (1991). A hybrid model of problem-based learning. In D. Boud and G. Feletti (Eds.), *The Challenge of Problem-Based Learning.* New York: St. Martin's.

Atkins, S. and Murphy, K. (1993). Reflection: A review of the literature. *Journal of Advanced Nursing, 18,* 1188–1192.

Baker, C. R. (1996). Reflective learning: A teaching strategy for critical thinking. *Journal of Nursing Education, 35*(1), 19–22.

Barrows, H. S. (1986). A taxonomy of problem-based learning methods. *Medical Education, 20,* 481–486.

Barrows, H. S. (1988). *The Tutorial Process.* Springfield, IL: Southern Illinois University Press.

Barrows, H. S. (1996). Problem-based learning in medicine and beyond: A brief overview. In L. Wilkerson and W. M. Gijselaers (Eds.), *Bringing Problem Based Learning to Higher Education: Theory and Practice.* San Francisco: Jossey-Bass.

Barrows, H. S. and Tamblyn, R. M. (1980). *Problem-Based Learning: An Approach to Medical Education.* New York: Springer.

Berkson, L. (1993). Problem-based learning: Have the expectations been met? *Academic Medicine, 68*(10), S79–S88.

Bernstein, P., Tipping, J., Bercovitz, K., and Skinner, H. A. (1995). Shifting students and faculty to a PBL curriculum: Attitudes changed and lessons learned. *Academic Medicine, 70*(3), 245–247.

Blake, R. L. and Parkison, L. (1999). Faculty evaluation of the clinical performances of students in a problem-based learning curriculum. *Teaching and Learning in Medicine, 10*(2), 69–73.

Boud, D. (1985). Problem-Based Learning in Education for the Professions. Sydney, Australia: HERDSA.

Brandon, J. E. and Majumdar, B. (1997). An introduction and evaluation of problem-based learning in health professions education. *Family and Community Health, 20*(1), 1–15.

Bruner, J. S. (1977). *The Process of Education.* Cambridge, MA: Harvard University Press.

Busari, J. O., Scherpbier, J. J. A., and Boshuizen, H. P. A. (1997). Comparative study of medical education as perceived by students at three Dutch universities. *Advances in Health Sciences Education, 1*, 141–151.

Charlin, B., Mann, K., and Hansen, P. (1998). The many faces of problem-based learning: A framework for understanding and comparison. *Medical Teacher, 20*, 323–330.

Clarke, R. M., Feletti, G. I., and Engel, C. E. (1984). Student perceptions of the learning environment in a new medical school. *Medical Education, 18*, 321–325.

Cohen, L. and Manion, L. (1989). *Research Methods in Education.* New York: Routledge.

Creedy, D., Horsfall, J., and Hand, B. (1992). Problem-based learning in nursing education: An Australian view. *Journal of Advanced Nursing, 17*, 727–733.

Davis, S. S. (1994). *Problem-Based Learning in Medical Education: A Qualitative Study of Curriculum Design and Students Experience in an Experimental Program.* Unpublished doctoral dissertation, Ohio State University.

Davis, M. H. and Harden, R. M. (1999). AMEE medical education guide No.15: Problem-based learning: A practical guide. *Medical Teacher, 21*(2), 130–140.

Deretchin, L. F., Hamilton, R. J., Hawkins, J., and Contant, C. F. (1999). Learning behaviors in a mixed traditional and problem-based learning curriculum. *Education for Health, 12*(2), 169–179.

Dewey, J. (1938). *Logic, the Theory of Inquiry.* New York: Holt.

Distlehorst, L. H. and Robbs, R. S. (1998). A comparison of problem-based learning and standard curriculum students: Three years of retrospective data. *Teaching and Learning in Medicine, 10*(3), 131–137.

Dolmans, D. and Schmidt, H. (1996). The advantages of problem-based curricula. *Post-graduate Medical Journal,* 535–538.

Doring, A., Bramwell-Vial, A., and Bingham, B. (1994). Staff comfort/discomfort with problem-based learning: A preliminary study. *Nurse Education Today,* 263–266.

Frost, M. (1996). An analysis of the scope and value of problem-based learning in the education of health professionals. *Journal of Advanced Nursing, 24*, 1047–1053.

Glasgow, N. (1997). *New Curriculum for New Times: A Guide to Student Centred, Problem-Based Learning.* Thousand Oaks, CA: Corwin Press.

Grandis, S., Long, G., and Mountford, B. (1999). Back to core values: An integrated whole course approach through enquiry based learning (EBL). In J. Conway, D. Melville, and A. Williams (Eds.), *Research and Development in Problem-based Learning, Volume 5.* Callaghan, Australia: PROBLARC.

Heliker, D. (1994). Meeting the challenge of the curriculum revolution: Problem-based learning in nursing education. *Journal of Nursing Education, 33,* 45–47.

Ingram, C., Ray, K., Landeen, J., and Keane, D. R. (1998). Evaluation of an educational game for health sciences students. *Journal of Nursing Education, 37*(6), 240–246.

Irvine, L. M. C. (1995). Can concept mapping be used to promote meaningful learning in nurse education? *Journal of Advanced Nursing, 21,* 1175–1179.

Ishida, D. N. (1995). *Learning preferences among ethnically diverse nursing students exposed to a variety of collaborative learning approaches including problem-based learning.* Unpublished doctoral dissertation, University of Hawaii.

Jaramillo, R. (1999). We got our kicks on route 66: A PBL case study. In J. Conway, D. Melville, and A. Williams (Eds.), *Research and Development in Problem-Based Learning.* Callahan, Australia: PROBLARC.

Jones, P. R. (1995). Hindsight bias in reflective practice: An empirical investigation. *Journal of Advanced Nursing, 21,* 783–799.

Kang, I. (1999). Sociomoral development: A case study of an elementary school. In J. Conway, and A. Williams (Eds), *Themes and Variations in PBL.* Callahan, Australia: PROBLARC.

Kaufman, D. M. and Mann, K. V. (1997). Basic science in problem-based learning and conventional curricula: Students' attitudes. *Medical Education, 31,* 177–180.

Kaufman, D. M. and Mann, K. V. (1999). Achievement of students in a conventional and problem-based (PBL) curriculum. *Advances in Health Sciences Education, 4,* 245–260.

Khoiny, F. E. (1995). *The Effectiveness of Problem-Based Learning in Nurse Practitioner Education.* Unpublished doctoral dissertation, University of Southern California.

Kingsland, A. J. (1996). Time expenditure, workload, and student satisfaction in problem-based learning. In L. Wilkerson and W. M. Gijselaers (Eds.), *Bringing Problem-Based Learning to Higher Education: Theory and Practice.* San Francisco: Jossey-Bass.

Little, P. and Ryan, G. (1988). Educational change through problem-based learning. *Australian Journal of Advanced Nursing, 5*(4), 31–35.

Maxwell, J. A. and Wilkerson, L. (1990). A study of non-volunteer faculty in a problem-based curriculum. *Academic Medicine, 65*(9), S13–S14.

McMillan, M. A. and Dwyer, J. (1989). Changing times, changing paradigm: The MacArthur experience. *Nurse Education Today, 9,* 93–99.

Miller, J. and Lee, V. (1999). A pilot program of problem-based learning with undergraduate students to foster critical thinking and transition to professional nursing practice. In J. Conway, D. Melville, and A. Williams (Eds.), *Research and Development in Problem-based Learning, Volume 5.* Callaghan, Australia: PROBLARC.

Mohide, E. A. and Drummond-Young, M. (1996). *Developing Paper Problems for Small Group Learning in Baccalaureate Nursing Programmes: A Survey.* In Global Connection in Learning, First International Conference of the Nursing Education Research Unit, McMaster University, Hamilton, ON, June.

Moore-West, M., Harrington, D. L., Mennin, S. P., Kaufman, A., and Skipper, B. J. (1989). Distress and attitudes toward the learning environment: Effects of a curriculum innovation. *Teaching and Learning in Medicine, 1*(3), 151–157.

Neufeld, V. and Barrows, H. (1974). The "McMaster" philosophy: An approach to medical education. *Journal of Medical Education, 49*(11), 1040–1050.

Newman, M. G. (1995). *A Comparison of Nursing Students in Problem-Based and the Lecture Method.* Unpublished master's thesis, University of Alberta, Edmonton, AB.

Rangachari, P. K. (1996). Twenty-up: Problem-based learning with a large group. In L. Wilkerson and W. M. Gijselaers (Eds.), *Bringing Problem-Based Learning to Higher Education: Theory and Practice.* San Francisco: Jossey-Bass.

Rideout, E. (1998). *The Experience of Learning and Teaching in a Non-Conventional Nursing Curriculum.* Unpublished doctoral dissertation, University of Toronto.

Rideout, E. (1999). Doing it: The roles, influences and behaviors of tutors. In J. Conway and A. Williams (Eds.), *Themes and Variations in PBL.* Callaghan, Australia: PROBLARC.

Rideout, E., England-Oxford, V., Brown, B., Fothergill-Bourbonnais, F., Ingram, C., Benson, G., Ross, M., and Coates, A. (2000). A comparison of problem-based and conventional curricula in nursing education. Submitted to *Advances in Health Sciences.*

Ross, B. (1991). Toward a framework for problem-based curricula. In D. Boud and G. Feletti (Eds.), *The Challenge of Problem-Based Learning.* New York: St. Martin's.

Ryan, G. and Little, P. (1991). Innovations in a nursing curriculum. In D. Boud and G. Feletti (Eds.), *The Challenge of Problem-Based Learning.* New York: St. Martin's.

Saarinen, H. and Salvatori, P. (1994). Education of occupational and physiotherapists for the year 2000: What, no anatomy course? *Physiotherapy Canada, 46,* 81–86.

Saylor, C. R. (1990). Reflection and professional education: Art, science, and competency. *Nurse Educator, 15*(2), 8–11.

Schmidt, H. G. (1983). Problem-based learning: Rationale and description. *Medical Education, 17,* 11–16.

Schmidt, H. G. (1993). Foundations of problem-based learning: Some explanatory notes. *Medical Education, 27,* 422–432.

Schmidt, H. G., Lipkin, M., deVries, M. W., and Greep, J. M. (Eds.) (1989). *New Directions for Medical Education: Problem-Based Learning and Community-Oriented Medical Education.* New York: Springer-Verlag.

Seltzer, S., Hilbert, S., Maceli, J., Robinson, E., and Schwartz, D. (1996). An active approach to calculus. In L. Wilkerson and W. M. Gijselaers (Eds.), *Bringing Problem-Based Learning to Higher Education: Theory and Practice.* San Francisco: Jossey-Bass.

Shin, J., Haynes, R., and Johnson, M. E. (1993). Effect of problem-based, self-directed undergraduate education on lifelong learning. *Canadian Medical Association Journal, 148,* 79–88.

Solomon, P. (1994). Problem-based learning: A direction for physical therapy education? *Physiotherapy Theory and Practice, 74,* 528–533.

Solomon, P. E., Binkley, J., and Stratford, P. W. (1996). A descriptive study of learning processes and outcomes in two problem-based curriculum designs. *Journal of Physical Therapy, 10*(2), 72–76.

Solomon, P. and Crowe, J. (1999). Evaluation of a model of student peer tutoring. In J. Conway and A. Williams (Eds.), *Themes and Variations in PBL.* Callaghan, Australia: PROBLARC.

Solomon, P. and Finch, E. (1998). A qualitative study identifying stressors associated with adapting to problem-based learning. *Teaching and Learning in Medicine, 10*(2), 58–64.

Spaulding, W. B. and Cochran, J. (1991). *Revitalizing Medical Education: Mc-Master Medical School, the Early Years, 1965–1974.* Hamilton, ON: BC Decker.

Stern, P. (1995). *Case-Based Learning in Occupational Therapy: A Case Study of Student Perceptions.* Unpublished doctoral dissertation, University of Virginia.

Stinson, J. E. and Milter, R. G. (1996). Problem-based learning in business education. In L. Wilkerson and W. H. Gijselaers (Eds.), *Bringing Problem-Based Learning to Higher Education: Theory and Practice.* San Francisco: Jossey-Bass.

Tang, C., Lai, P., Arthur, D., and Leung, S. F. (1999). How do students prepare for traditional and portfolio assessment in a problem-based learning curriculum? In J. Conway and A. Williams (Eds.), *Themes and Variations in PBL.* Callaghan, Australia: PROBLARC.

Tiwari, A. (1999). The effect of problem-based learning on students' approach to learning: A study of student nurse educators in Hong Kong. In J. Conway and A. Williams (Eds.), *Themes and Variations in PBL.* Callaghan, Australia: PROBLARC.

Townsend, J. (1990a). Problem-based learning. *Nursing Times, 86*(14), 61–62.

Townsend, J. (1990b). Teaching/learning strategies. *Nursing Times, 86*(23), 66–68.

Uys, L. R. and Gwele, N. S. (1999). A descriptive analysis of the process of problem-based teaching/learning. In J. Conway and A. Williams (Eds.), *Themes and Variations in PBL* Callaghan, Australia: PROBLARC.

Vernon, D. T. A. (1995). Attitudes and opinions of faculty tutors about problem-based learning. *Academic Medicine, 70*(3), 216–223.

Vernon, D. T. A. and Blake, R. L. (1993). Does problem-based learning work? A meta-analysis of evaluative research. *Academic Medicine, 68,* 550–563.

Vygotsky, L. S. (1978). *Mind in Society: The Development of Higher Psychological Processes.* (M. Cole, V. John-Steiner, S. Scribner, and E. Souberman, Eds.). Cambridge, MA: Harvard University Press.

Vygotsky, L. S. (1987). *The Collected Works of LS Vygotsky.* (R. W. Rieber and A. S. Carton, Eds.). New York: Plenum.

Walton, H. J. and Matthews, M. B. (1989). Essentials of problem-based learning. *Medical Education, 23,* 542–558.

White, M. J., Amos, E., and Kouzekanani, K. (1999). Problem-based learning: An outcomes study. *Nurse Educator, 24*(2), 33–36.

Wolf, F. M. (1993). Problem-based learning and meta-analysis: Can we see the forest for the trees? *Academic Medicine, 68*(7), 542–544.

Woods, D. (1996). Problem-based learning for large classes in chemical engineering. In L. Wilkerson and W. M. Gijselaers (Eds.), *Bringing Problem-Based Learning to Higher Education: Theory and Practice.* San Francisco: Jossey-Bass.

Facilitating Self-Directed Learning

Dauna Crooks, Ola Lunyk-Child, Chris Patterson, and Jeannette LeGris

A s we enter the new millennium, continued change in both our personal and professional lives is inevitable. In particular, health care providers and educators will be faced with increasing complexities within their respective systems. One approach to learning will not meet the needs of health professionals being educated to deliver evidence-based care, nor will one educational method meet the needs of students with varied backgrounds and learning styles. Nevertheless, problem-based learning (PBL), with its emphasis on self-directed learning (SDL), is an appropriate method for developing the attitudes and skills to cope with ever-changing environments. Through self-directed learning, students identify their own goals and needs, plan strategies to meet those needs and evaluate their progress. This chapter will examine self-directed learning by: (1) exploring the competencies needed to become a self-directed learner; (2) identifying a process for developing the required competencies; and (3) outlining several key educational strategies that promote these competencies. The issues and challenges that emerge in working with students as they become self-directed learners will also be addressed.

FOUNDATIONS OF SELF-DIRECTED LEARNING

Self-directed learning is grounded in humanistic, deterministic, constructivist, and transformative philosophies which build upon and compliment each other. Humanism views men and women as self-interpreting beings whose goal is to find meaning in their lives through perceptions and experiences. This philosophy acknowledges the abilities of learners to identify, within a learning context, those aspects of their lives that are meaningful and valuable to them. In SDL, individuals have freedom, within the boundaries of the curriculum goals and outcomes, to determine educational choices, and are ultimately responsible and accountable for the learning that occurs. Determinism emphasizes learners' responsibilities to the educational process and their ability to use skills of critical evaluation.

Constructivists view knowledge as something that learners must construct for themselves in order to understand, predict, and control their environment (Blais, 1988; Candy, 1991; Creedy, Horsfall, and Hand, 1992). Constructivists propose that individuals acquire meaningful knowledge when they investigate independently. When a state of "not knowing" occurs, and previous frameworks cannot explain observations about a phenomenon, individuals are challenged to create new cognitive constructions; working from a base of what they already know. In other words, they merge newly acquired knowledge with old learning, which is a core tenet of problem-based self-directed learning.

Learning accompanied by thoughtful reflection creates change, since both the structure and process of learning are changed by each and every learning experience. As learners develop their knowledge and skill base, they are encouraged to explore and use frameworks for learning. This exploration of approaches to learning, combined with an ongoing examination of beliefs, values, and experiences, leads to change which is internalized and attains personal and intrinsic meaning. This process is defined by Mezirow (1985, 1991) as transformative. For transformation to occur, students need to be free to act and experience control over their learning destiny. This freedom is at the core of the PBL Model.

DEFINITION OF SELF-DIRECTED LEARNING

Despite the obvious appeal of the self-directed approach for educators and students, there still remains considerable ambiguity around the definition and implementation of this type of learning. However, the definition of Knowles (1975) remains useful since it is both broad and descriptive:

> Self-directed learning is a process in which individuals take the initiative, with or without the help of others, in diagnosing their learning needs, formulating learning goals, identifying human and material resources for learning, choosing and implementing appropriate learning strategies, and evaluating learning outcomes. (p. 18)

Andragogy or adult learning theory is central to SDL, since the basic assumption is that adults want to learn and have the attributes and motivation to take responsibility for their own learning (Knowles, 1986). SDL can occur within one's personal world and/or within the formal educational system, as is the case when problem-based SDL is used in nursing education. Whichever the instance, students are active in and responsible for their learning within the educational process.

There is some controversy about whether in fact SDL means students determine not only *how* they will learn but also *what* they will learn. Norman (2000) suggests that SDL is an oxymoron when applied to health professional education, since he takes the position that SDL must, by definition, call for students to choose the content. Judging by our experience in nursing education, this is not necessarily so. A self-directed approach can be applied because students, although they are given considerable choice, exercise that choice within boundaries dictated by curriculum guidelines. The problems for study are developed based on content selected through a process that is described in Chapter 8. Still there is considerable opportunity for choice: students can decide the order in which they consider the specific problems available within a course of study; they determine the particular learning issues they wish to explore; they select the learning resources they use; they often choose the topic and sometimes the method of evaluation; and they participate in evaluating their own learning, both formatively and summatively. A program that emphasizes self-direction also embraces choice for students in clinical courses, as they choose the setting for clinical practice and the particular learning goals to be met, keeping in mind the guidelines and expected learning outcomes of the particular course.

So we return to the definition of Knowles and conclude that the self-directed component of the problem-based model being presented in this book is indeed congruent with the dimensions of that definition, namely, students take initiative, diagnose their individual learning needs, formulate learning goals, identify and use learning resources, and evaluate learning outcomes.

CHALLENGES IN BECOMING A SELF-DIRECTED LEARNER

Although the self-directed nature of the PBL Model is identified repeatedly as a strength, (Barrows, 1988; Barrows and Tamblyn, 1980; Rideout, 1998; Walton and Matthews, 1989), it is clearly not without its challenges (Lunyk-Child et al., 2000; Stinson and Milter, 1996; von Döblen, 1996). In the beginning, students frequently express frustration when they are asked to make decisions and to determine how they will undertake learning experiences and how evaluation should occur. They often have little or no experience in controlling their learning and have no insight into its construction. They have not had to articulate their thinking process publicly and are challenged and threatened in having to do so. During this phase of a self-directed process, students may also feel mistrust, suspicion, anxiety, doubt, and anger (Lunyk-Child et al., 2000). These negative feelings are often aimed at the faculty tutor for not being directive and the anxiety stems from their own fear and lack of confidence with new learning expectations. Statements such as these are not uncommon: What am I supposed to do? If only you would tell me what you want me to do. During this time faculty tutors adopt a strong, facilitative role. They ask students to examine their experiences and feelings about specific situations. They might ask, "What did you get out of this experience?" or point out gains that are less obvious to students. Providing clear statements of expected course outcomes and complete descriptions of student evaluation methods is also helpful in alleviating anxiety.

As students progress in their education, they soon learn to trust their own abilities, and in time, to work with their group, to make decisions about learning, to become responsible and accountable for learning, and finally, to expand their world view. It generally takes one or two terms for the majority of students to understand the process of SDL and to cease to plea for explicit teacher direction about how they should approach problems being explored (Rideout, 1998). By their senior years, students direct their own inquiry about the problems presented, and assist one another in general hypothesis generation, data collection, and intervention. Research involves exploring the full range of resources (text books, journal articles, multiple data bases) and identifying human resources. By expanding their knowledge base there is a greater appreciation for the interrelationship among basic sciences, humanities, and nursing science in the cases under discussion. Their critical appraisal skills develop simultaneously with their expanding ability to explore knowledge which improves the quality of information brought back to the group. By the end of a program using the PBL Model, students become proficient at self-direction, and graduate with skills that help them continue to learn and take control of that learning over their lifetime. SDL is a process, and our individual makeup and abilities limit or extend our progress through that process.

The gradual change from feelings of uncertainty and anxiety to feelings of confidence and security are supported by the SDL literature. Kasworm (1983) describes a similar process, comprised of five components that depict change over time: (1) from learner dependence on "authority" to independence; (2) from extrinsic to intrinsic motivators for learning; (3) from passive acceptance of information to proactive inquiry and self-evaluation of intellectual development; (4) from authority designated learning structures to learner-selected ones; and (5) from unidimensional to multidimensional strategies for planning and conducting personal and group learning activities. Kasworm also contends that this process requires direction and assistance as the learner develops the actions required for change.

Taylor (1986) describes SDL as a connected, chronological flow of events over time, consisting of four phases, namely, disorientation, exploration, reorientation, and equilibrium. In the first phase, learners question why previous patterns are no longer working. They challenge previously held assumptions about the roles and responsibilities of both students and teachers in the process of learning. Exploration of approaches to learning and reflection on activities lead to a philosophical shift in the meaning of education and the re-establishment of equilibrium.

COMPETENCIES FOR SELF-DIRECTION IN LEARNING

There are specific competencies required to be an effective self-directed learner and, as we have described above, these competencies are developed over time. SDL does not usually develop naturally, and students require guidance in understanding the principles of self-direction. This is an important development in their educational experience since students who are proactive learn more effectively than reactive students. Knowles (1975) states that "self-directed learning is more in tune with our natural processes of psychological development" (p. 14), and goes on to suggest that an important phase of an individual's maturation is to take responsibility for his/her life—"to become increasingly self-directing" (p. 15).

Knowles (1975) identified seven competencies for being a self-directed student:

1. Understanding the differences between teacher-directed and self-directed learning
2. Determining one's concept as a self-directed being
3. Relating to peers collaboratively and as resources for learning
4. Diagnosing learning needs and formulating objectives
5. Viewing teachers as facilitators
6. Identifying other resources
7. Collecting and validating evidence of accomplishments

The process of PBL is designed to facilitate those competencies, by focusing on the following skills and dispositions:

- Self-assessment of learning gaps within a specific learning context
- Self-evaluation
- Reflection
- Critical thinking
- Information management
- Group skills

These skills and abilities are not mutually exclusive; they are interrelated so that students simultaneously use all, or a combination of them, to direct and control their learning experience. In addition, specific personal attributes—empathy, collegiality, communication, flexibility, negotiation skills, and insight—need to be developed or fostered for students to take charge of their learning in a positive way and to share it within a group setting. Since self-assessment of learning gaps and self-evaluation are intrinsic to SDL, they will be explored in detail in this chapter. The other skills and abilities listed above are discussed briefly here but explored in detail in specific chapters of this book, with Chapter 4 focusing on group skills, Chapter 5 on information management, and Chapter 6 on the development of critical reflection and reflective practice.

Self-Assessment of Learning Gaps

Self-assessment of learning gaps is an important part of the PBL process and a starting point for developing SDL skills. Assessment occurs when the students explore their specific interests and evaluate their present state of knowledge and skills in relation to course requirements during exploration of a problem. In order to help students develop self-assessment skills, the faculty tutor may use several strategies. For example, the faculty tutor may begin by helping them to assess their current level of self-direction and reflect on past experiences to identify what helped or hindered learning (Brockett and Hiemstra, 1991; Guglielmino and Guglielmino, 1992). The tutor might pose specific questions for students to gain an understanding of their present knowledge base and learning goals:

- What do I want to get out of this (learning situation)?
- Where do I want to get to?
- What will it look like when I get there?
- What do I need to get there?
- What limits are there?
- What am I able to do?
- What should I do in this situation?
- What will I do?
- Where does this all fit in? (p. 33)

Beginning students may have only limited awareness of the complexity of the problem, and a limited volume of knowledge and skills required to address a situation. It is important that they be guided to identify their learning gaps and how to seek resources and strategies to fill these gaps in a logical and meaningful way. For this reason, students need to be led through the process of becoming aware of *what they know* and *what they do not know.* The faculty member must be clear about the outcomes of learning and guide students to appropriate resources that may include the community at large.

As students gain skills and knowledge, they will have developed a logical means to assess their learning needs and the faculty role becomes one of support and clarification. Faculty need to continue to be involved throughout the learning process to ensure that students integrate self-assessment into daily practice.

Self-evaluation

In addition to self-assessment of learning gaps, students are required to take a more objective and comprehensive view of their progress. Mann and Kaufmann (1995) suggest that accurate and valid self-evaluation is a critical feature of lifelong learning and professional education. Two characteristics conducive to valid self-evaluation have been documented. First, students should be familiar with the evaluative standards and criteria, and systematically gather and interpret data on their own performance. Second, the level of threat related to the reception and processing of feedback about oneself must be minimized. Self-evaluation requires an assessment of the knowledge, skills, and attitudes as well as the professional, technical, and ethical behaviors appropriate to the experience.

Individually, students begin by examining their own comforts and discomforts with SDL and self-evaluation. In fact, they may find it uncomfortable to openly explore their own method of learning, to communicate their anxieties about their strengths and weaknesses in learning, and to explore their frustrations with the different approaches that occur. Students who have learned privately and shared little, except on examinations or papers submitted to teachers, may find it difficult to discuss their ideas and have them challenged publicly in group. However, public evaluation brings to light their strengths as others see them and offers strategies for improvement, further study, and added practice. What students see as limitations may be perceived by others as strengths within the group context. In response to challenges, students develop more confidence in supporting their position as they become more aware of their strengths and limitations.

In order to minimize confusion around evaluation, the teacher must be explicit in clarifying the standards, expectations, and outcomes. The responsibility of students in a self-directed program is to gather and provide evidences of learning. Faculty provide feedback to students within a framework of critical and objective thought, which fosters higher levels of self-esteem and lower levels of anxiety (Brown and Gallagher, 1992; Brown and Mankowski, 1993; Frey, Stahlberg, and Fries, 1986).

Farnill, Hayes, and Todisco (1997) suggest that self-evaluation exercises should be ongoing and formative rather than summative. By building upon previous assessments of peers, self, and tutor in both private and public contexts, the student is reminded of how the self-directed capacities he or she has developed are progressing. While some students find this anxiety provoking, most students use the feedback to construct learning plans that address areas of concern identified by self, tutor, or group.

Reflection

Reflection is integral to the process of SDL and helps students to attribute meaning in the learning experience. Reflection promotes introspection into group and individual experiences. In the literature, it has been described as an active, deliberate, and conscious activity (Boud, Keough, and Walker, 1985; Mezirow, 1990) of intellect and affect (Andrusyszyn and Davie, 1995). Three key stages characterize the reflective process: students revisit and describe an experience retrospectively; they attend to feelings that may help or hinder learning; and finally, they validate previous learning and arrive at new learning (Boud et al., 1985). According to Schön (1983), reflection needs to be made explicit; it can be both integral to an activity (reflection *in* action) or undertaken after the event (reflection *on* action).

The skills for reflection have been described as self-awareness, critical analysis, openness to new perspectives, and an ability to evaluate the learning process. Reflection, like other skills, requires a developmental approach which moves from relatively simple and undemanding strategies to more complex processes at later stages of education. The outcome of reflection is to explore learning experiences and develop new understandings.

Students may be unaware of how they reflect on their learning and the means they use to engage in the process. Conscious and periodic examination of learning is required to develop the necessary skills for autonomous reflection. Faculty can begin to stimulate reflection through activities designed to develop the students' abilities. They might begin by simply asking the learner to look at an experience and to describe their feelings, and determine the source and reasons for the feelings. Where the learner needs to go next to challenge him or herself may be an outcome of this reflective process. Values and beliefs play a significant role in attitudes to learning and success in achieving desired outcomes. Students must address beliefs that hinder their progress and plan to minimize or eliminate these blocks. Similarly, they need to understand what it is about a situation that makes them uncomfortable or unable to progress. When they are able to examine situations objectively, they are more apt to identify any prejudices or biases.

Critical Thinking

Critical thinking is defined as an intellectually disciplined process. Richard Paul (1992) states that critical thinking is "thinking about your thinking while you are thinking, in order to make your thinking better" (p. 7). Critical thinking requires both discipline and restraint. Discipline is needed to actively and skillfully conceptualize, apply, analyse, synthesize, and/or evaluate information gathered from, or generated by, observation, experience, reflection, reasoning, or communication. Restraint relates to systematic reasoning, testing of inferences, and weighing of evidence. Critical thinking, then, allows the learner to think fairly, explore, and appreciate the adequacy and cohesion of their own beliefs and opinions, as well as those of others. In essence, critical thinkers suspend judgment until all the evidence is weighed and tested.

The student who employs critical thinking displays recognizable behaviors that might also be used to describe a self-directed learner engaged in the PBL process.

- The purpose of learning is clearly stated, significant, and realistic.
- The issue or question to be addressed is stated, every angle is considered and possible reasoning strategies are explored openly.
- Assumptions carried to the problem are identified, justified, or discarded.
- Point of view is openly examined against alternative points of view for strengths and weaknesses in dealing with the problem or question.

- Data are sufficient to support claims, and alternative data are considered that contradict claims.
- Key concepts are identified, explained, explored, and used with precision.
- Inferences develop from evidence and consistency among and between assumptions, and inferences are constantly checked.
- The process of reasoning itself is examined to determine how it leads to implications and consequences (Alfaro-Le Fevre, 1995; Brookfield, 1987; Paul, 1992).

Students who have integrated the skills of critical thinking will also exhibit such attitudes and behaviors as: confidence, independence, fairness, responsibility, risk taking, discipline, perseverance, creativity, curiosity, integrity, and humility in exploring and developing critical thinking skills (Kataoka-Yohiro and Saylor, 1996).

Information Management

Information management refers to the skills of searching, retrieving, and filing information. Self-directed students must develop a method for information management that allows them to gain competence in the use of computers and the appraisal of large volumes of information. When students enter a self-directed program and are required to extend their research to more current resources, they often experience difficulty. In part, this is due to previous reliance on text as "truth." Texts usually present a unified point of view so the attitude is understandable. By learning how to use up-to-date resources including journals and the Internet, students see many different points of view and a range of good and bad science. They require information management skills, which are learned best when they are integrated into their educational program, and this is particularly relevant when the curriculum uses the PBL Model.

Group Process and SDL

Most PBL curricula utilize small groups so that interactions with peers and faculty will allow students to explore their learning related to both content and process. The information students are exploring within the group is challenged, developed, enriched, and manipulated through group interactions. Groups are powerful vehicles for fostering individual responsibility and accountability for learning, as well as for acknowledging learning outcomes (Brundage and MacKeracher, 1980). Many educational experiences occur in groups, and SDL activities may emanate from the individual or the collective. Brundage and MacKeracher (1980) examined the developmental process of SDL in a group context. They defined the entry stage as a time when students are faced with novel or uncertain situations. Uncertainty creates personal stress; students seek out and tend to rely on external standards to guide behavior. In the proactive stage, students feel confident and accepted by peers. They have respect for the uniqueness of other students in their group who may have different learning styles and backgrounds. Successful SDL is marked by an integration of the perspective of others with one's own, and a balance in individual and group goals. In a group situation, competition is discouraged while collaboration is encouraged and rewarded.

RESOURCES FOR DEVELOPING SELF-DIRECTED LEARNING COMPETENCIES

The tools and resources used to facilitate development of SDL competencies are numerous. The following section is a small sampling of those used commonly by educators where some evidence of validity and effectiveness has been established.

The Learning Styles Inventory

Although there are a number of learning style or learning preference inventories cited in the literature, the most commonly referenced is that of Kolb (1984). The appeal for faculty facilitating the development of self-directed skill is the congruence between beliefs fundamental to SDL and Kolb's experiential learning theory, with its emphasis on active involvement of the learner in the personal transformation of experience (Carpio et al., 1999; Massee and Thomas, 1988). Kolb postulates a four stage, sequential theory of learning in which affect and experience play an equal role with cognition and reflection. Students move through the learning cycle in the following manner: after exposure to a "concrete experience" the learner reflects on the experience and creates abstractions; these abstractions and their implications are then tested in new situations; learning increases in scope and depth over time; and cumulative experiences contribute to this sequential process of learning (Kolb, 1984).

It became clear to Kolb that students require specific abilities to be effective (Kolb, 1984; Laschinger and Boss, 1989; Massee and Thomas, 1988; Remington and Kroll, 1990):

- Students must involve themselves without bias in a new learning situation.
- Students must possess the ability to observe phenomena from a number of perspectives and reflect on each view.
- Students must be able to create concepts and coherent theory about the relationships of concepts from observation and reflection.
- Students must have the ability to use theories as a basis for decision making and problem solving.

The difficulty, as Kolb acknowledges, is that people emphasize or prefer two modes or styles of learning over others. In order to be effective students, the challenge then becomes the need to develop skills in all styles. Learners preferring to work from "concrete experience" to "reflective observation" are termed *divergers,* whose predominant modes of learning are feeling and observing (Kolb, 1984; Laschinger, 1990; Remington and Kroll, 1990). They tend to be sensitive to feelings and values and listen with an open mind to gather information. Their strength is in imagining the implications of the information they gather and in their relationships with people.

Assimilators, working from "reflective observation" to "abstract conceptu-alization," are logical and perceptual, able to organize and synthesize material, create models, test theories, design experiments, and analyse quan-titative data. Their strength is in independent analysis and completeness of thought. In comparison, *convergers* are both symbolic and practical, working from "abstract conceptualization" to "active experimentation." Their partic-ular strength is in making theories and ideas useful in problem solving. They are creative in ways of thinking and doing, selecting best solutions to a problem, setting goals, and making decisions.

The *accommodator* blends "active experimentation" and enthusiasm to seek out new experiences and take risks. Accommodators are impulsive but adapt to new situations readily with intense personal involvement as they prefer change over routine.

Learning how one prefers to learn is examined through a learning styles inventory, which was developed by Kolb (1984). There is evidence that understanding of one's preferred learning style has been correlated with increased academic success (Lenehan, Dunn, Ingham, Murray, and Singer, 1994; Nelson et al., 1993). Other advantages for students knowing their preferred style are the understanding gained about the strengths and limita-tions of that style, and second, the opportunity to expand strengths in complimentary or opposing styles. Balance is essential in order for mature learning to take place (Kolb, 1984). Awareness of learning preferences allows students to see how they presently structure learning and in time, with reflec-tion and self-appraisal, allows them to expand learning skills and viewpoints. Proficient students are recognized as individuals who select an appropriate learning style from a range of styles, according to the demands of the situation and their own learning capacity. The ability of students to actively select from a range of styles is clearly a component of SDL. By understanding how one learns, and how others learn, students also tend to approach SDL with increased self-confidence and understanding of the diversity of learning styles and strategies available to them.

The Learning Plan

The use of a learning plan is a strategy for developing SDL skills that was originally proposed by Malcolm Knowles (1974) for individual use to assist in personalizing learning according to learning needs. Since then it has been used as an integral part of problem-based, self-directed learning programs (Tompkins and McGraw, 1988).

Within the PBL process, students are required to prioritize learning needs, set learning goals and objectives, and determine resources to be consulted (Chapter 2). A learning plan is useful to organize these tasks since it allows students to work systematically through each of the components of the task. The sharing of learning plans also enhances group process by allowing group members to be self-directing in identifying collective learning needs, and focusing learning on group objectives. However, students must remember that they are developing their learning plan with the course objectives in mind. All learning and activity in problem-based class must in some way meet one or more of the course objectives.

In clinical courses, the learning plan functions as a blueprint for learning since it allows the student to consider personal learning needs within the context of the clinical setting and learning opportunities available to the student. The principles of humanism and determinism clearly emerge during the development of a learning plan. Learning plans allow students to individualize the learning process; promote autonomy/independence or self-directedness; promote goal-directed learning with specific outcomes; and assist in the development of habits related to lifelong learning. Active student participation in designing clinical learning experiences that are tailored to their learning needs and interests also increases confidence in their abilities as independent practitioners. In turn, increased confidence facilitates students' transition to the role of practicing nurses.

There are also potential disadvantages to the use of learning plans. Students who are conditioned to traditional teaching strategies may experience anxiety and frustration when asked to define their own learning goals, and particularly, when they must describe how they wish their learning to be evaluated. Learning plans may increase faculty workload in the facilitation and development phases. As well, faculty may experience anxiety as they relinquish control and use student-centered approaches.

The course expectations function as the framework or "givens" within which the student assesses learning needs and develops a plan. The clinical behaviors outlined constitute the minimal course expectations. Students assess their learning gaps in relation to these course expectations and the chosen clinical setting. They develop learning objectives that reflect the uniqueness of the clinical setting as well as the course objectives, all of which must be met to pass the course.

The relationship between student and faculty is of prime importance in self-directed learning and in particular, in the use of learning plans. The relationship should be one of mutual trust, responsibility, and decision making. The use of learning plans calls upon four key faculty roles that emerge consistently in the literature about SDL—those of facilitator, advisor/counselor, negotiator, and evaluator (Boyd, 1979; Clark, 1981). The last role is often in

Table 3.1 *Components of a learning plan*

Learning Goal	Learning Questions	Learning Resources / Strategies	Evidences	Criteria for Evaluation
What do I want or need to learn? • knowledge • skills • attitudes/values	What specific questions/issues will I address?	What or who can help me learn what I want to learn? What will I do to meet my objectives?	How will I demonstrate what I have learned?	Who will evaluate my evidence? What criteria? What deadline?

conflict or contradictory to the others and may diminish teacher effectiveness. However, as the students' exposure to, and experience with, SDL increases and their ability for self-evaluation develops, the students may begin to perceive evaluation as a shared responsibility between student and teacher.

Donaldson (1992) found that students writing learning plans need assistance in three major areas: writing objectives, limiting scope and size of learning plan, and accessing resources. In our experience, we have found that students also need assistance in specifying the criteria to be used in evaluating evidence of learning. The purpose of evaluation is to determine if learning objectives and course expectations have been met, hence the need for students to specify the criteria against which they wish to be evaluated. Guidelines that outline the components of the learning plan are helpful to students as they develop the skill of writing and clear a descriptive plan (Table 3.1).

Care must be taken by faculty to ensure that the student maintains control over his or her learning plan, while at the same time confirming that the stated outcomes are within the parameters of the course objectives and the clinical setting. It is incumbent upon the student to be a self-directed learner and negotiate with faculty tutor to be sure their learning plan reflects course expectations, that learning needs relate to course objectives, that the opportunities are available in the clinical setting and that individual learning style is accounted for. Some questions that are helpful for both students and faculty when reviewing a learning plan are presented in Table 3.2.

An example of a learning plan that was developed by a beginning student in the Bachelor of Science of Nursing program is presented in Table 3.3.

Critical Incident Questionnaire

Stephen Brookfield (1995) proposes a method to identify "how students are experiencing their learning and your teaching" (p. 114). He suggests that students be asked to reflect on critical incidents that occurred during class. Critical incidents can be defined as significant, concrete happenings that

Table 3.2 *Questions to consider in reviewing a learning plan*

Learning Objectives

• Are the learning objectives clear, understandable, and realistic?

• Do the learning objectives describe what you propose to learn?

• Are there other objectives you might consider?

• Do your learning objectives meet all course expectations?

Learning Resources and Strategies

• Do the learning activities seem reasonable, appropriate, and effective tools with which to meet the objectives?

• Are resources current?

• Are there other activities you might consider?

Evidence

• Does the evidence seem relevant to the various objectives?

• Is it a valid way to provide evidence of learning?

• Do the evidences demonstrate variety and creativity?

• Is your time line realistic? Are the due dates specified?

• Are there other evidences you might consider?

Criteria for Evaluation of Evidences

• Are the criteria/means for validating evidences clear, relevant, understandable, and convincing?

• Are the criteria congruent with learning objectives?

• Are there other ways that you might consider to validate the evidence?

people remember (Tripp, 1993; Woods, 1993). Each class contains such events, and knowing what they are can be helpful in revealing how your teaching affects students and in identifying the "emotional highs and lows of their learning" (Brookfield, 1995, p. 114). The latter is particularly important in a SDL program since it can give the teacher insight into the process students are experiencing as they adapt to this learning and teaching style.

At the end of each class, students are asked to complete a questionnaire with five questions, each of which asks them to focus on specific occurrences in class. Students record when they felt "most engaged" or "most distanced" during the class; what actions were "most affirming and helpful" or "most puzzling and confusing"; and what was "most surprising" (Brookfield, 1995, p. 115). Students are given five to ten minutes to answer the questions. To ensure anonymity students are asked not to sign the questionnaires.

The tutor then reviews each questionnaire for common themes, looking in particular for problems or confusions. The comments are summarized and form the basis of a debriefing session at the beginning of the next class, thus providing the opportunity to address concerns publicly. At this time, the

Table 3.3. *Example of a Problem-Based Learning Plan*

Learning Goal	Learning Questions	Learning Resources and Strategies	Evidences	Criteria for Evaluation
To develop skills in communicating with patients and in group settings using the concepts and principles of communication theory.	What are the elements of the communication process? What are different styles of communication? What is active listening? What does advocacy, confidentiality, mutuality, diversity, and empathy mean? What are the stages of the interview?	Canadian Fundamentals of Nursing Interpersonal Relationships: Professional Communication Skills for Nurses Perform and receive feedback on two interviews Review video of an interview with a standardized patient	Perform an interview in tutorial and receive feedback from tutor and peers	Follow steps of the communication process: **Orientation** • identify role and name • state duration and purpose of interview • address confidentiality • build trust • identify problems and goals **Working** • client-centered • use a variety of therapeutic communication strategies • relevant questions • organized in my approach to asking questions • allow the patient freedom to discuss issues **Termination** • summarize information • clarify • encourage further information • evaluate goals

tutor can report and discuss criticisms of his or her actions; acknowledge any changes he or she plans to make as a result of the responses; clarify actions, course requirements, or assignments that may be confusing to the students; and negotiate and resolve contentious issues that have emerged in class.

There are numerous advantages to using the Critical Incident Questionnaire (CIQ). In developing competencies for SDL, the CIQ encourages students to become reflective and evaluative. It is a formal, yet anonymous and nonthreatening technique to help students reflect and give feedback on critical events in the class. Responses to the questionnaire can alert the teacher to problems occurring in the group and provide direction for tutor development. Finally, the CIQ encourages teachers to be reflective as they continue to develop personally and professionally as educators.

An example of a CIQ completed by an intermediate level PBL group is presented in Table 3.4. The students' comments indicated they felt most engaged during brainstorming activities related to issue identification and when their research was applied to the patient scenario. They felt most distanced during planning activities, such as deciding how tasks would be assigned. By recognizing this and discussing it openly, suggestions can be made about how to do things differently in the group. The CIQ is not only helpful in identifying present or potential problems, but also is very useful in highlighting behaviors that acknowledge and facilitate growth and development of the group (e.g., the amount of direction given by the tutor and the flexibility within the group). Certainly the theme of surprise and pleasure at how productive, prepared, and positive the group experience was at Week Five would be gratifying to the tutor and the students. This example demonstrates that the CIQ can be used to diagnose problems, find solutions, and share rewards during PBL.

Cognitive Mind Maps

Cognitive mind mapping is an educational strategy that is used to facilitate meaningful learning in many educational programs. It is particularly useful in problem-based self-directed programs, since it is a creative method of displaying

Table 3.4 *CIQ from a level 3 problem-based class*

Question	Week 2	Week 5
Most Engaged	Group role discussion	Questions after presentation
	Generating issues for the paper problem; brainstorming process	During my presentation
		Presentations
	Sorting out issues for research	Discussing agenda
	Figuring out group objectives	No one thing
	Selection of topics for next week	When people were relating topics
	Discussing agenda	of research to the case study
	Entire time	

continued

Table 3.4 *CIQ from a level 3 problem-based class, continued*

Question	Week 2	Week 5
Most Distanced	Never When writing issues on the board Nursing theory discussion at beginning, talk about models—not sure at first what to do When discussing format for assessing/taking history of SP Tired—so not attentive When trying to pick interviewer	During evaluations When assigning group roles No one thing Before and after my presentation—I was too nervous beforehand to focus and afterward there was very little comment (positive or negative) from group members During some presentations
Most Affirming	Some clarifying Tutor gave direction when group lost Tutor summarized key points Clarification from peers re: group roles and issues for next week Tutor's clarification on how to incorporate theory Others listened when I talked When we examined the way to do the standardized patient	Clarification by group Direction given by group Less direction needed by tutor Positive feedback for presentation A good "passing" around of ideas and communication Group organizing ahead of time Group willing to change class time to accommodate student's needs
Most Puzzling or Confusing	Nothing How to direct the interview and choose the model during decision to split up roles Discussion about the various models we needed to use Amount of ideas generated about the case was at first a little overwhelming	When trying to decide what to do in class next week About how we are going to interpret this sort of evaluation Switching gears from presentations to research topics although the break helped Group roles Did not have an agenda from beginning of class "No information found"
Surprised	Nothing Everyone had input and participated How well group communicated Group dynamics considering it was only the second week Problem case confusing to organize	The high degree of preparedness of most of the people who presented research topics Group works well together How much preparation one student had done—it was great! PBL is actually productive Nothing really

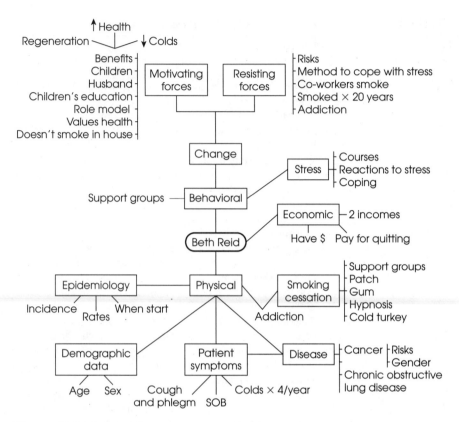

Figure 3.1 Mind Map of a Tutorial Problem

the links among key concepts that deal with a specific topic, and demonstrating new meaning based on prior knowledge (All and Havens, 1997). In both clinical and problem-based courses, students add breadth and depth to the content under study, generating increasingly complex mind maps.

Students can be encouraged to use mind maps during note taking from books, lectures, essays, projects, and reports, or for planning schedules (Buzan and Buzan, 1993). One of the most powerful ways to use mind maps is in small group tutorials. An example of a mind map for a beginning level course is presented in Figure 3.1. This graphic representation evolved from the Beth Reid scenario (Box 3.1), after the group had identified and researched generic learning issues and interviewed the standardized patient.

They constructed the map as an aid to reviewing what they knew, what they did not know, and what they needed to know, in order to work therapeutically with Ms. Reid. In other words, the mind map helped the group in the processes of self- and group assessment of learning issues.

Box 3.1   Beth Reid Scenario

Beth is a 34-year-old woman who comes to your health care clinic because she wants to stop smoking.

Her husband does not smoke and since her two children started to receive heath education about the dangers of smoking all three "bug" her about her habit.

She has noticed that she has a productive morning cough, gets frequent colds, and sometimes is short of breath when she climbs stairs.

SELF-DIRECTED LEARNING IN DIVERSE LEARNER POPULATIONS

One unique population of students who present particular challenges are post-diploma registered nurses returning to school to complete their baccalaureate degree. These students have learned and worked in settings where clear direction is the norm and specific outcomes have been expected. These students often feel that the faculty tutor is withholding vital pieces of information that will determine their success or failure. When information is perceived to be withheld, they experience frustration. Most have worked, some for many years, and faculty must acknowledge this expertise and build on it in a way that links theory to reality. It is imperative that faculty assess the skills and knowledge base of each student and foster self-direction at a pace the learner can accept and digest. Once post-diploma students realize that their previous learning is acknowledged and the present experience will build on it, they are more comfortable entering the self-directed zone.

Self-evaluation and open peer evaluation are particularly difficult for all students initially. Post-diploma students have often been exposed to punitive evaluation in the work setting and objective testing in previous educational activities. This former evaluative climate creates expectations for a negative experience, while limited objective testing within self-directed programs fails to provide the usual bench marks through which progress has been judged. Midterm evaluation is generally honest but very general and superficial regarding learning and the educational experience. By the end of the first term in a self-directed program, however, the evaluation generally demonstrates more depth in reflection, introspection, awareness of the principles of self-directed education, and an ability to assess personal progress with plans for change. Toward the end of the program, post-diploma students have caught up and sometimes surpassed the basic/generic students who have had more experience with SDL and are more able to approach learning situations with clear goals, outcomes, and creative strategies.

Learners coming from diverse cultures also create challenges for faculty in self-directed programs. SDL in the context of problem-based tutorials brings the expectation that knowledge will be shared openly with eight to ten peers. Students from different cultures may have difficulty entering group discussions, describing or discussing research, arguing points, negotiating goals, and directing learning. While in the North American culture these activities are considered the norm, other cultures may not value these behaviors which, in fact, may be contradictory to their values and beliefs.

The challenge for teachers is to be culturally sensitive, maintain the tenets of the PBL Model, and assist students to develop self-directed behaviors. Students may be encouraged to use hand outs or charts to facilitate discussion and decrease anxiety about speaking up in group. Ultimately, the learner must engage in the learning process in a visible way, and demonstrate the self-directed skills of reflection, critical thinking, critical appraisal, and evaluation within the group in order to succeed in the program. An ethical dilemma for teachers lies in socializing students to become self-directed, reflective thinkers when they may be returning to their native cultures in which those characteristics fundamental to self-direction may be unacceptable.

RESOURCES FOR SELF-DIRECTED LEARNING

Self-directed students require specific resources in order to develop knowledge and skills. In addition to teachers and peers, these include a skills laboratory that is well-equipped and supervised. A clinical skills specialist on site to guide students requesting help and to provide feedback on progress is an excellent resource. A well-stocked library with texts, journals, computer databases, and resource librarians is essential as students are developing their information management skills. In addition, there should be access to computers for Internet searching, word processing, and database management.

Curriculum development must be logical with each level building on the previous one, with the expectations for the development of self-directed skills outlined clearly. In order to maintain currency, extensive orientation, yearly retreats and small group meetings are important for faculty to attain, and maintain their skills. A multipronged approach is costly in time but necessary for development of the program, faculty, and students.

Use of the PBL Model with its emphasis on self-directed learning requires that students are exposed to situations that present multiple perspectives and expand the learner's world view. Evaluation measures must also be congruent with the approach to education. Multiple methods are used, which provide both summative and formative evaluation, from an array of options that includes essays, presentations, oral exams, Objective Structured Clinical Exam (OSCE), double and triple jumps, seminars, health fairs, and portfolios (See Chapter 9 for details on these various methods). All of these resources are costly to maintain but we believe them to be essential to learning in a self-directed program.

CONCLUSION

Promotion of self-directed strategies is important for the development of lifelong students. In this era of rapidly changing technologies and environments, individuals must quickly acquire, integrate, and apply new knowledge and skills. Individuals need to constantly reflect and determine the types of educational activities that will build a relevant skill set for this dynamic environment.

Educators play a major role in assisting students to obtain the necessary self-directed learning skills to ensure success in their future endeavors. However, as with any educational method, there are challenges. For students, the transformative process students undergo as they adapt to self-directed learning can be stressful and confusing. The awareness of variation in learning styles among their peers can hinder or stimulate personal growth. Students struggle to outline their specific learning objectives within a course having broad objectives that can be met in a variety of ways. For basic, mature, and post-basic students who have experienced with only teacher-centered learning, the transition to SDL can be especially difficult. They are forced to challenge all previous beliefs about learning. For the learner and teacher, cultural diversity adds another dimension of difficulty to the process of becoming a self-directed learner. Each is challenged to acknowledge and accept differences in approach, behavior, and learning style that may be culturally based.

Faculty must ensure that students meet all course objectives; however, they must balance this goal with a level of objectivity and flexibility that is congruent with this style of learning. Faculty development is essential for assisting teachers to explore new and effective approaches to facilitating SDL. Inherent in this educational methodology is the need for administrative support for increased workloads and resource management issues.

REFERENCES

Alfaro-LeFevre, R. (1995). *Critical Thinking in Nursing.* Philadelphia: W.B. Saunders.

All, A. C. and Havens, R. L. (1997). Cognitive/concept mapping: A teaching strategy for nursing. *Journal of Advanced Nursing, 25,* 1210–1219.

Andrusyszyn, M. and Davie, L. (1995). Reflection as a design tool in computer mediated education. Distance Education Conference, San Antonio, Texas, January 26, 1995. From http://www.oise.utoronto.ca/~ldavie/reflect.html.

Barrows, H. (1988). *The Tutorial Process.* Springfield IL: Southern Illinois University School of Medicine.

Barrows, H. S. and Tamblyn, R. (1980). *Problem Based Learning.* New York: PS Springer-Verlag.

Blais, D. (1988). Constructivism: A theoretical revolution in teaching. *Journal of Developmental Education, 11*(3), 2–7.

Boud, D., Keough R., and Walker, D. (1985). *Reflection: Turning Experience into Learning.* London: Kogan Page.

Boyd, J. (1979). The advisor is the key. *Scholastic Editor* 59(2), 6–7.

Brockett, R. G. and Hiemstra, R. (1991). *Self-direction in Learning: Perspectives on Theory, Research, and Practice.* New York: Routledge.

Brookfield, S. (1987). *Developing Critical Thinkers.* San Francisco: Jossey-Bass.

Brookfield, S. D. (1995). *Becoming a Critically Reflective Teacher.* San Francisco: Jossey-Bass.

Brown, J. D. and Gallagher, F. M. (1992). Coming to terms with failure: Private self-enhancement & public self-effacement. *Journal of Experimental Social Psychology, 28,* 3–22.

Brown, J. D. and Mankowski, T. A. (1993). Self esteem, mood and self evaluation: Changes in mood and the way you see you. *Journal of Personality & Social Psychology, 64,* 421–430.

Brundage, D. H. and MacKeracher, D. (1980). *Adult Learning Principles and Their Application to Programme Planning.* Toronto, ON: Ministry of Education.

Buzan, T. and Buzan, B. (1993). *The Mind Map Book.* London: BBC Books.

Candy, P. (1991). *Self-direction for Lifelong Learning.* San Francisco: Jossey Bass.

Carpio, B., Illesca, M., Ellis, P., Crooks, D., Droghetti, J., Tompkins, C., and Noesgaard, C. (1999). Student and faculty learning styles in a Canadian and a Chilean self-directed, problem-based nursing program. *Canadian Journal of Nursing Research, 31*(3), 31–50.

Clark, D. (1981). Handbook for co-operative planning and co-operative arrangements in Adult Basic Education, Springfield VA: ERIC Document Reproduction Service.

Creedy, D., Horsfall, J., and Hand, B. (1992). Problem based learning in nursing education. *Journal of Advanced Nursing, 17,* 727–733.

Donaldson, I. (1992). The use of learning contracts in the clinical area. *Nurse Educator, 12,* 431–436.

DeCoux, V. (1990). Kolb's learning styles inventory: A review of its application in nursing research. *Journal of Nursing Education, 29*(5), 202–207.

Farnill, D., Hayes, S., and Todisco, J. (1997). Interviewing skills: self evaluation by medical students. *Medical Education, 31,* 122–127.

Frey, D., Stahlberg, D., and Fries, A. (1986). Information seeking of high and low anxiety subjects after receiving positive and negative self relevant feedback. *Journal of Personality, 54,* 694–703.

Garrison, D. R. (1992). Critical thinking and self-directed learning in adult education: An analysis of responsibility and control issues. *Adult Education Quarterly, 42*(3), 136–148.

Guglielmino, P. and Guglielmino, L. (1992). The self-directed learner: A valued human resource of the 21st century. *Sundridge Park Management Review, 5*(4), 32–39.

Kasworm, C. (1983). Self-directed learning and lifespan development. *International Journal of Lifelong Education, 2*(1), 26–46.

Kataoka-Yahiro, M. and Saylor, C. (1995). A critical thinking model for nursing judgment. *Journal of Nursing Education, 33*(8), 351–356.

Knowles, M. (1975). *Self-directed Learning: A Guide for Students and Teachers.* New Jersey: Prentice Hall.

Knowles, M. (1986). *Using Learning Contracts.* San Francisco: Jossey-Bass.

Kolb, D. (1984). *Experiential Learning: Experience as a Source of Learning and Development.* New Jersey: Prentice Hall.

Laschinger, H. (1990). Review of experiential learning theory research in the nursing profession. *Journal of Advanced Nursing, 15,* 985–993.

Laschinger, H. and Boss, M. (1989). Learning styles of Baccalaureate nursing students and attitudes to theory-based nursing. *Journal of Professional Nursing, 5*(4), 215–223.

Lenehan, M. C., Dunn, R., Ingham, J., Murray, W., and Singer, B. (1994). Learning style: Necessary know-how for academic success in college. *Journal of College Student Development, 35,* 461–466.

Lunyk-Child, O., Crooks, D., Ellis, P., Ofosu, C., O'Mara, L., and Rideout, E. (2000). Self-directed learning: Faculty and student perceptions. *Journal of Nursing Education,* in press.

Mann, K. V. and Kaufman, D. M. (1995). A response to the ACME-TRI Report: The Dalhousie problem-based learning curriculum. *Medical Education, 29,* 12–21.

Massee, C. and Thomas, K. (1988). Toward whole brain education in nursing. *Nurse Educator, 13*(1), 30–34.

McMillan, M. and Dwyer, J. (1990). Facilitating a match between teaching and learning styles. *Nurse Education Today, 10,* 186–192.

Mezirow, J. (1985). A critical theory of self-directed learning. In S. Brookfield (Ed.). *Self-directed Learning: From Theory to Practice.* San Francisco: Jossey-Bass.

Mezirow, J. (1990). *Fostering Critical Reflection in Adulthood.* San Fransisco: Jossey-Bass.

Mezirow, J. (1991). *Transformative Dimensions of Adult Learning.* San Francisco: Jossey-Bass.

Nelson, B., Dunn, R., Griggs, S. A., Primavera, L., Fitzpatrick, M., and Miller, R. (1993). Effects of learning style intervention on college students' retention and achievement. *Journal of College Student Development, 34* (5), 364–369.

Norman, G. R. (2000). The adult learner: A mythological species. *Academic Medicine, 74*(8), 886–889.

Paul, R. (1992). *Critical Thinking* (2nd ed.). Santa Rosa, California: Foundation for Critical Thinking.

Remington, M. and Kroll, C. (1990). The "high risk" nursing learner: Identifying their characteristics and learning style preferences. *Nurse Education Today, 10,* 31–37.

Rideout, E. (1998). *The Experience of Learning and Teaching in a Non-Conventional Nursing Curriculum.* Unpublished Doctoral Dissertation, University of Toronto.

Schön, D. A. (1983). *The Reflective Practitioner.* New York: Basic Books.

Starr, M. and Krajeik, J. (1990). Concept maps as a heuristic for science curriculum development: Toward improvement in process and product. *Journal of Research in Science Teaching, 27,* 987–1000.

Stinson, J. and Milter, R. (1996). Problem-Based Learning in Business Education: Curriculum Design and Implementation issues. *New Directions for Teaching and Learning, 68,* 33–42.

Taylor, M. (1986). Learning for Self-direction in the classroom: The pattern of a transition process. *Studies in Higher Education, 11*(1), 55–72.

Tompkins, C. and McGraw, M. L. (1988). Enhancing autonomy: The Negotiated Learning Centers. In D. Boud (Ed.). *Developing Student Autonomy in Learning.* (2nd Ed.) pp. 172–191. London: Kagar.

Tripp, D. (1993). *Critical Incidents in Teaching: Developing Professional Judgement.* New York: Routledge, 1989.

von Döblen, G. (1996). Four years of problem-based learning: A students' perspective. *Postgraduate Medical Journal, 72,* 95–98.

Walton, H. J. and Matthews, M. B. (1989). Essentials of problem-based learning. *Medical Education, 23,* 542–558.

Woods, P. (1993). *Critical Events in Teaching and Learning.* Bristol, PA: Falmer Press.

Facilitating Small Group Learning

Gerry Benson, Charlotte Noesgaard, and Michele Drummond-Young

Although problem-based learning (PBL) sometimes takes place in large groups where both critical inquiry and self-directed learning can be fostered (Allen, Duch, and Groh, 1996; Barrows, 1988; Woods, 1996), it is generally acknowledged that the development of communication skills, self-knowledge, and collaboration are best learned through membership in a small learning group. Active involvement, inherent in all small group learning, nurtures skills that enable graduates of professional programs to be well-prepared for entering the workforce (Davis and Harden, 1999; Westberg and Jason, 1996). This chapter will explore the relevance of small groups to the use of the PBL Model in nursing, the challenges and advantages of small group learning, and the structure and process issues associated with group learning. Incorporated within the chapter are strategies for novice and experienced tutors and students to facilitate and evaluate small groups.

SMALL GROUP LEARNING IN PBL

First and foremost, small group PBL puts students at the center of the learning experience by giving them a framework to find and evaluate information, discuss and debate it, and determine its applicability to the problem situation. Although small group learning in PBL is not dissimilar to small group learning in any other educational model, it is within the PBL Model that the small group is used consciously and conscientiously to achieve particular learning outcomes, since it is an integral part of the approach. Group learning allows students to examine meaningful, real-world situations, with five to ten other learners and a faculty tutor. Neufeld and Barrows (1974) state that learning in a small group "represents a laboratory for group problem solving, which allows learners to:

- compare learning performance with peers,
- develop a sense of responsibility for their learning progress,
- learn about human interaction, develop interpersonal skills, and become aware of one's own emotional reactions, and
- learn how to listen, receive criticism, and give accurate and candid feedback to each other; and facilitate self-evaluation" (p. 1044).

THE RELEVANCE OF SMALL GROUP LEARNING TO NURSING

Nurses' roles have changed and health care issues that nurses are facing are also changing. Working collaboratively, identifying and resolving conflicts, and expressing a well-supported point of view in an assertive manner are just some of the skills that students learn, practice, and develop in small group PBL. These skills are much in demand by employers of new nursing graduates.

Learning to work collaboratively has long been described as an outcome of PBL. Barrows and Tamblyn (1980) describe the small group as a "potent format" for learning in the health sciences. Patients and their health issues provide the organizing structure in the PBL Model from which students develop an understanding of their profession, and the skills required for a team approach. This strategy helps nursing students work effectively in multi-disciplinary teams, as they, in essence, "try-on" their nursing professional role. The group process skills learned within the small group are valued in the work of professional nurses within multidisciplinary teams, organizations, and community groups (Watkins and Marsick, 1993).

In recent years, learners from different health disciplines, including medicine, physiotherapy, occupational therapy, and midwifery, have come together to learn within small groups (Adler, Bryk, Cesta, and McEachen, 1995). The current approach to health care, including managing health care outcomes, requires nurses and all health care professionals to work effectively within and between groups. The teamwork skills such as communication, negotiation, conflict resolution, and critical thinking result from exposure to small group learning. Applying principles of group dynamics to their interactions with families and community groups during care is also a part of the everyday work of nurses. Experiencing small group learning is particularly advantageous given the nursing role in patient education groups such as support groups, pre- and post-natal classes, and/or parent education groups (Nasmith and Daigle, 1996).

In its drive to limit costs, the health care industry has reduced access to professional nurses and has employed less educated and less costly nonregulated workers. Nurses are now expected to teach and supervise co-workers, to delegate tasks, and to negotiate resources because of changes in the health care system, and again the skills associated with collaborative practice are valued.

THE IMPORTANCE OF GROUP PROCESS TO LEARNING OUTCOMES IN THE PBL MODEL

The importance, as well as the challenges, of incorporating small group learning as a part of the PBL Model have been well-articulated. Herbert and Bravo (1996) developed an instrument for evaluating student performance in small group learning, and identified four factors that are important to learning: group effectiveness, communication and leadership, scientific curiosity, and respect for colleagues. Of these, group effectiveness accounted for 61 percent of the variance in learning outcomes.

The importance of group dynamics to effective PBL was also identified by Tipping, Freeman, and Rachlis (1995) in their study to determine the essential content of a faculty development program. Like Herbert and Bravo (1996) group dynamics were noted by faculty and students as crucial to the PBL experience. Furthermore, they found both groups reported limited awareness of effective group dynamics and analyses, including the ability to deal with or redirect a "dysfunctional" group. They concluded that schools adopting PBL need to "develop comprehensive training programs to teach group members to evaluate group performance and engage in open discussion of effective and ineffective group behaviours" (p. 1050). In another study, Kalain and Mullen (1996) explored students' perceptions of PBL in four domains: tutor effectiveness, learning materials, small group process, and academic support. Group process accounted for 16 percent of the variance in response to the PBL Model, indicating again the importance of the small group experience to overall perceptions of the PBL approach.

The centrality of an effective group to learning was also evident in the work of Rideout (1998) who investigated the perceptions of nursing students enrolled in a four-year Bachelor of Science in Nursing program. Students made comments such as: "The group makes or breaks it," "If you have a group that doesn't work well together you are not going to accomplish everything that you should accomplish," and " . . . (learning) the content is sometimes overshadowed by our frustration with the group." The students also described what they perceived to be the drawbacks to effective group function, including too much or too little direction from the tutor, and a reluctance on the part of members to discuss issues openly.

Finally, Thomas (1997) concurs that issues of group dynamics are crucial to learning within the PBL Model, but concludes that there is a paucity of research on how best to develop group skills for students as well as faculty.

Challenges for Students

Students new to learning in small groups are faced with a variety of challenges. The small group tutorial, with its implicit pressures to perform within the obligatory group discussions, can be threatening to students (Moore-West, Harrington, Mennin, Kaufman, and Skipper, 1989; Reinders, 1993; Rideout, 1999). Students who are introverts, or those who need time for reflective analysis before speaking, may find the pace of conversation in tutorial intimidating (Brookfield, 1995). In fact, Berkson (1993) questions whether, for some individuals, the group situation is a stimulus or an interference to learning, since levels of individual commitment, personality differences, and lack of progress towards accomplishing group tasks are all issues for groups. "Having to contribute to the group, to perform and react to group process, and to facilitate the learning of others" were "group-related" pressures that physiotherapy students cited as being stressors in a study of their adjustment to small group PBL (Solomon and Finch, 1999, pp. 7–8). Other difficult issues for some students include taking on different group roles and evaluating others by providing feedback on their performance within the group (Townsend, 1990).

Culture also influences communication and interactional styles, since cultural norms govern the conditions and circumstances under which various messages may or may not be sent, noticed, or interpreted, such as who talks to whom, about what, how, when, and for how long. Students from cultures where a hierarchical social order is valued often have a difficult time with spontaneous discussion in tutorial, challenging peer-presented information, and being self-directed. Students, whose second language is English, might feel threatened by the expectations to speak spontaneously in tutorial (Hodne, 1997). Since these cultural influences present dilemmas for the tutor and may create conflict within the group, they must be acknowledged and dealt with in the tutorial for effective group function to occur. Working with culturally diverse groups compels group members to gain heightened cultural sensitivity and awareness of the skills needed to effectively manage diversity issues (Corey and Corey, 1997).

The new challenges with which students are confronted in small group tutorials require transformative behaviors if small group collaborative learning is to succeed. Students must change from:

- Passive observer and record taker to active listener and engaged discussant
- Minimal pre-class preparation to greater self-preparation
- Being only an attendee to being a risk taker
- Personal choice for attendance to a class to group norm expectations for attendance to a group
- Competition to cooperation with peers
- Self-motivated learning to interdependent learning
- Perceiving knowledge authority as texts and teachers to accepting self and peers as relevant learning resources.

These changes are facilitated by a number of actions and actors including, among others, reflection, self-evaluation, and the interventions of skilled faculty.

Challenges for Faculty

Faculty members also acknowledge that the change in role to small group facilitator is ultimately rewarding but always challenging. A lack of knowledge about group process, lack of clarity about course content, inadequate facilitation skills, and a tendency to maintain rather than share control over the groups activities are all potential limitations for faculty adopting the PBL tutor role (Tipping et al., 1995; Davis and Harden, 1999; Miller, Trimbur, and Wilkes, 1994; Wilkerson, 1996). A need for orientation, ongoing development, and evaluation to attain and maintain skills has been identified (Rideout, 1998), and faculty development programs are recommended that address such issues as:

- The components of group structure
- The aspects of group process
- Creating a context for open discussion
- Encouraging creativity in discussion
- Acknowledging and managing group conflict
- Evaluating the level of skills and abilities of faculty and students (Davis and Harden, 1999; Preston-Whyte, McCulloch, and Fraser, 1996; Schmidt, 1994).

Since the importance of a sound knowledge base around small group learning and its particular application within the PBL Model is professed by many writers and researchers, the following sections provide an overview of the key issues to consider when implementing and maintaining a small group PBL approach.

STRUCTURAL ISSUES AND GROUP FUNCTION

Students and faculty new to learning in small groups need to apply group theory while gaining knowledge related to course objectives. Structural factors such as group size, physical environment, and course design all affect small group learning.

Group Size

Group size influences whether or not all learners can participate in the intended activities. The optimal size suggested for most PBL groups is five to ten members, since a group of this size is more likely to be cohesive, more interactive, and allow for more mutual caring, which affects relationship-building, (Johnson and Johnson, 1991; Dimock and Devine, 1996; Westberg and Jason, 1996; Hare, Blumberg, Davies, and Kent, 1994). If the group is too small, there may be insufficient diversity of ideas, which tends to foster a dependency on the tutor and results in too few students being available to complete group tasks (Westberg and Jason, 1996).

The most significant effect of group size lies in the complexity of member interrelationships in the group. As the membership increases, complexity increases exponentially, making it difficult for learners to have sufficient opportunity for meaningful participation. For example, Hare et al. (1994) suggest that meaningful participation decreases since only the bolder or more aggressive members speak when groups become larger than seven.

Members in groups over seven also have difficulty observing and evaluating individuals. However, the resources in larger groups are potentially greater for problem solving (Johnson and Johnson, 1991). Tiberius (1990) states that optimal "size" may vary with the length of time the group has been together, believing that group members who know one another are more comfortable with each other and interact more, allowing for larger groups to still be productive and supportive (Tiberius, 1990).

Hare et al. (1994) provide another description of optimal group size, when they state that a group is "small, if after a session of face-to-face interaction, each member can remember something about the contributions of every other member. As well, small groups are less likely to contain subgroups, more easily share common resources, are more cohesive, and have a more democratic leadership" (p. 1).

Physical Environment

It is recommended that classrooms be structured to promote nondominant face-to-face interaction and opportunities for equal participation. A number of factors within the environment can influence learning. Bright glaring colors, too dim or too bright lighting in a room, external noise, temperature that is too hot or too cold, and inadequate air flow all influence the degree of participation of some group members, and can hinder or facilitate group dialogue (Johnson and Johnson, 1991). Ergonomic design of the furniture may also influence student's comfort and ability to learn. The physical positioning of group members, including the faculty member, impacts on group dynamics. Equity of membership could be promoted by a circle arrangement, since rectangular group formation tends to reinforce the hierarchal relationship between members and facilitator, and to interfere with equality of discussion among peers.

Course Design Factors

Course design factors to consider are the length of the term, the frequency of sessions, the duration of each session, and the experience of the tutor. Miller et al. (1994) recommend that the composition of groups remain stable as: "the growing together process takes time; if members are too frequently shuffled, they can become more dependent on the tutor." Keeping students in a single group over two terms, for an entire year, facilitates incremental acquisition of knowledge and group development skills.

Students need a timetable that allows time for information searching and analysis. There is a tendency in nursing programs to commit each hour of the school day to class time, which of course does not allow time for self-study. Similarly, there must be a minimum of one day between PBL classes for students to pursue their learning issues and prepare for their next session.

ISSUES IN GROUP PROCESS

The term "group process" applies to a number of issues, among them: how relationships emerge within a group, how they grow and develop over time, how they are maintained at a relatively stable or steady state, and how they are transformed or changed (Sampson and Marthas, 1990). To learn about these issues requires us to look at group roles, group function, and group development.

Roles and Responsibilities of Group Members

Roles in groups, like those in society, can be prescribed, subjective, or enacted (Turner, 1982). *Prescribed roles* refer to the statuses of the group members, either as student member or faculty tutor. For faculty, the challenge in small group learning is to decrease the use of the didactic model and shift into a model that values the principles of adult learning in which the tutor is a facilitator, coach, guide, and navigator (Kaufmann, Day, and Mensink, 1996) who enables group members to learn content and process from each other. In addition, the tutor has a monitoring role (Barrows and Tamblyn, 1980). For students, the challenge is to determine the expectations associated with the student role and to develop their individual style within those expectations.

Subjective roles depend on the perceptions and interpretations of the group members, since they become apparent to members in sessions that include peer to peer feedback (Turner, 1982). Developing an awareness of subjective roles requires that group members can describe their own behavior in group, and learn to respond to compliments and criticisms of peers. As members describe their behaviors, then listen and interpret feedback from others, the roles they play in the group become more clear to themselves and to their peers.

Last, the *enacted roles* evolve as each member undergoes adjustments in his/her group role performance (Turner, 1982). As peers give each other feedback about their ability to advance individual and group knowledge in an effective way, they increase understanding of their enacted roles. Ineffective or nonproductive behaviors are also identified and group members develop strategies to clarify and transform undesired behaviors. Group evaluations, where feedback about group roles is shared, may be seen as a growth opportunity or may escalate tensions within the group.

A common typology of group roles differentiates between two categories of functional roles in groups—task roles and maintenance roles (Sampson and Marthas, 1990; Dimock and Devine, 1996). Observation and understanding of the roles that group members play, and their predominant modes of communication and interaction provide the tutor with information cues that the tutor uses for analysing the group's activities and relationships. Knowledge of the various roles provides students with the language they can use to describe their own subjective and enacted roles and to give feedback to peers and to faculty members.

Task roles include initiating, clarifying, informing or sharing information, and evaluating or assessing if goals are being achieved. A common task role of small groups is agenda setting, which helps to provide structure to class sessions (Uys and Gwele, 1999). *Maintenance roles* foster emotional support among members, and act to strengthen and perpetuate the group. Maintenance group activities include keeping communication channels open, compromising as needed, and offering encouragement and support to other members in the group. A balance between task and maintenance roles is a hallmark of a productive and enjoyable group.

Self-oriented roles, or blocking roles, can also be observed in groups. Members tend to use these roles to meet their own needs and they are not helpful toward accomplishing the group's tasks. Some examples include dominating or monopolizing the group, being apathetic and uninvolved, or demonstrating emotionality (Sampson and Marthas, 1990; Dimock, 1985).

It is through developing awareness of the various roles, both productive and nonproductive, that individuals (both students and tutors) play in groups that positive and productive behaviors can be reinforced and action taken to deal with the less effective and perhaps deleterious ones. As Antai-Otong (1997) suggests, nurses need knowledge of group roles and expertise in group process to be prepared for the future challenges facing nurses and the nursing profession.

Group Functions

Sampson and Marthas (1990) describe a number of group functions that have particular relevance for student nurses, and that are congruent with the cognitive and constructivist philosophy underlying the PBL Model. They include:

- The *socialization* function facilitates learning about the culture of the new group, work environment, and community; and acquiring new knowledge, techniques, and ways to operate. This function is particularly significant in the early stages of a new group.
- The *support and camaraderie* function contributes toward the maintenance of a healthy group, since it provides problem-related and self-help support, collegiality, and a general level of acceptance.
- Goal-orientation and co-operative *task completion* functions use specialized skills of individualized team members. Inherent in this function is the *informational function* that helps members define attitudes, beliefs, and social behaviors. These functions are relevant in PBL since it is the small group that provides the forum for not only learning the content of nursing but also the skills and abilities associated with being a member of a group. The dynamic process of

PBL is most effective when opinions and information of group members are shared and debated.

- The *empowerment function* motivates the group to organize and seek change. This is an essential function if students are to learn to challenge the status quo and take on issues of inequality and diversity. The group should provide a safe place to begin to grapple with these complex but necessary issues.
- A *normative function* in which groups identify the rules and procedures by which members comply with groups standards, combined with a *governance function* as members meet to make decisions and recommendations within their areas of responsibility. By learning how and when to comply and when to challenge standards, students are encouraged to become critical in their thinking and assertive in their presentation of self.

Stages of Group Development

There is a variety of terminology to describe the stages of a group. Tuckman and Jensen (1977) describe six developmental stages of a group: orientation, forming, storming, norming, performing, and terminating. Dimock (1985) suggests the TORI framework which has four phases: trust, openness, realization, and independence. Although different group theorists use different terms to describe the stages of group development, they all incorporate three essential phases: initiating, accomplishing the work of the group, and terminating. There is consensus that every working group should progress effectively through these stages so that members can gain knowledge and develop effective team and leadership skills. The developmental process of any group is not necessarily steady and progressive, and may be quite variable within groups.

In the initial stage of group development, members get to know one another. They begin to establish communication patterns, but tend to work in a more individual rather than a team style. Role expectations are unclear and there is a higher dependency on the faculty tutor. Members are very reluctant to challenge each other's ideas, or take responsibility for decision making. In this early stage, learners need considerable guidance, and the tutor may need to be quite directive initially, and model various group task and/or maintenance roles. This will assist students in their transition to group learners and help to alleviate some of the challenges facing new group learners. For a group to advance beyond the initiating phase, the members must be willing to challenge the status quo and manage the discomfort that accompanies advanced group development.

In the early intermediate portion of the working stage, groups take on an identity, have more structure, and clearer role expectations. Conflicts within groups occur frequently during this stage, since it is the stage of storming (Tuckman and Jenson, 1977). Facilitator skills are most challenged at this stage. Later on in the working stage of group development, there is a move toward responsible goal accomplishment and greater productivity. The group is quite self-sufficient and is able to work independently; there is minimal need for tutor-directed facilitation (Dimock, 1985; Wass, 2000; Westberg and Jason, 1996). It is at this stage that the tutor must find an effective balance of involvement in the group, to assist it in its productivity while not deterring it in any way.

Although the termination phase should begin before the final group meeting, there are particular activities that should be a part of the concluding meeting of the group. It is important to summarize achievements and unresolved issues, and to decide "where to go from here." It is useful to have the group explore what the group has meant to them, how they have grown personally and professionally, and what factors were most effective in facilitating change. Some members may experience feelings of sadness and loss, and have difficulty disengaging from their group. Some may even continue to participate in other activities with group members, after the formal group has ended. Many groups plan an end-of-group activity, such as having a meal together, to celebrate their time together, and their achievements. Groups use this time to discuss how they will utilize what they have learned, to form new directions, and to construct new meanings from their experiences. Sharing the gains from the group as well as sharing perceptions of growth in their colleagues is particularly meaningful (Corey and Corey, 1997; Wass, 2000).

COMMON GROUP ISSUES AT VARIOUS GROUP STAGES

Groups confront a variety of issues as they progress through the various stages of group development. Although there is variation in the ways in which groups respond, there are also commonalities among the responses. We will address a number of these issues and describe some possible strategies to deal with them in this next section.

Adapting to a New Group Environment

Three opening issues confront all new groups at their initial meeting: *Who is here? What are our goals and purpose? How shall we go about working together?* (Sampson and Marthas, 1990). A successful beginning for any new group requires that these issues be addressed.

Who Is Here?

Learning who the other group members are is essential to build the trust and rapport required for the group to work well together. Historically, the majority of learners in an undergraduate baccalaureate nursing program come directly from high school, are single, and female. A minority of students will have had some other educational and life experiences; perhaps up to 10 percent will be male; and the students will generally be a microcosm of the larger community which is often multicultural, so a number of students will bring different cultural norms and realities to the group. Some will have a first language other than English.

The socialization function (Sampson and Marthas, 1990) becomes paramount as each individual is required to both influence and adjust to the culture of the group. Consequently, it is important that, at the initial meeting, individuals become acquainted with the backgrounds of each of the group members. A variety of ice-breakers (Crosby, 1996) can be used to promote the sense of knowing each other. A useful example is the use of dyads in which each student interviews another student, then introduces them to the whole group using four key characteristics, such as a brief description of their family, their summer job, the areas of nursing that most excite and interest them, and what they like best and least about PBL. These questions provide a range of information about a student and begin to pinpoint their particular interests and enthusiasms and allow students to gain a more holistic view of the variety among the individuals within the group. Another example might be for each student to develop a pictorial representation of themselves and share it with the group. The intent of these exercises is to increase the familiarity of group members with each other, which should lessen the anxiety that exists at the beginning of any new learning group (Kozier, Erb, and Blais, 1997).

What Are Our Goals and Purpose?

During Tuckman and Jensen's beginning phases (1977) of orienting and forming, groups have to attain some comfort with the socialization and normative functions of the group. In addition, the group needs to address how individuals will meet the goals of the course and how individual learning objectives will be managed. Although the overall "why" of a PBL group is to learning about nursing, it is important for new groups to understand why PBL is the educational approach chosen, and the process issues in implementation of PBL. There are a number of strategies that are helpful as students learn about working in groups within the PBL Model. Wallis and Mitchell (1995) outline a program devised for their medical curriculum at Newcastle University, Australia, which consists of eight sessions designed to develop group process skills of students. Brookfield and Preskill (1999) suggest that faculty role play a typical PBL session for new students, to demonstrate the process, expectations, and some of the common issues. Readings about PBL and group function are useful, as are videotapes that portray common issues for groups at various stages of their development. An assignment that asks students to write a short paper on one of the components of the PBL Model, such as small group learning, can also be a useful orientation. An example of the purpose and guidelines for such a paper, for beginning students, is presented in Figure 4.1.

SCHOLARLY PAPER

Purpose: To learn about specific topic areas and relate these to nursing. To provide practice in writing a scholarly paper using appropriate research of library resources and correct APA format.

Length: Six to eight pages (1500 to 2,000 words)

Weight: 20% of the Final Grade

Topics: 1. Self-directed learning   2. Problem-based learning
              3. Small group learning   4. Learning styles
              5. Professional portfolios   6. Reflective practice

Evaluation Criteria:

Rating & Comments
(0 = low; 4 = high)

A. Format

1. The paper is about one topic only.   0 — 2 — 3 — 4
2. The writer relates the topic to nursing.   0 — 2 — 3 — 4
3. The writer has made a sufficiently thorough review   0 — 2 — 3 — 4
   of the literature.
4. Primary sources are used throughout the paper.   0 — 2 — 3 — 4
5. Resources used are current and/or relevant to   0 — 2 — 3 — 4
   the topic.
6. Six or more references are used including journal   0 — 2 — 3 — 4
   articles on course references lists.

B. Organization

1. The topic and scope of the paper are introduced in   0 — 2 — 3 — 4
   the first paragraph.
2. The main topic is clearly presented.   0 — 2 — 3 — 4
3. Parts of the paper relate to one another and follow   0 — 2 — 3 — 4
   a logical sequence.
4. Each paragraph presents one idea and the   0 — 2 — 3 — 4
   sentences flow.
5. Transitions are smooth throughout the paper.   0 — 2 — 3 — 4
6. The closing paragraph summarizes the ideas   0 — 2 — 3 — 4
   discussed in the paper

Figure 4.1 Scholarly Paper for Beginning Students in a PBL Program

---

C. Style and Mechanics

1. The vocabulary is extensive, accurate, and appropriate for a scholarly paper.
   0 — 2 — 3 — 4

2. Correct grammar is used.
   0 — 2 — 3 — 4

3. Correct spelling is used.
   0 — 2 — 3 — 4

4. Correct punctuation is used.
   0 — 2 — 3 — 4

5. Sentences are varied in structure and length for readability.
   0 — 2 — 3 — 4

6. The paper is within the page limit.
   0 — 2 — 3 — 4

7. The paper is neatly presented.
   0 — 2 — 3 — 4

8. Sources of information and ideas of others are documented using APA format.
   0 — 2 — 3 — 4

Overall Comments

Grading Scheme

Grade A All of the above criteria are met *consistently* with evidence of creative thinking, depth of presentation, and mastery of writing skills.

Grade B The above criteria are met *consistently.*

Grade C The above criteria are met *generally* with evidence of inconsistency in some areas.

Grade D The above criteria are not adequately met, with major problems in five to eight of the criteria stated.

Grade F Major problems are noted in more than eight of the criteria stated.

Letter Grade: _____ **Marker:** _____

© School of Nursing, McMaster University.

How Shall We Go about Working Together?

The governance group function of Sampson and Marthas (1990) describes how members develop strategies to make decisions and recommendations that facilitate group growth and advance the group's knowledge and critical thinking. Exploration of how the group will operate influences the development of norms, which in turn affect how groups build knowledge and develop group skills (Sampson and Marthas, 1990). In the first few meetings, groups develop ground rules on time management, how decisions will be made, mutual expectations, use of resources, confidentiality, management of tensions, and a format for feedback.

Because norms lessen anxiety within a group, beginning groups need to have multiple procedural rules, and begin to describe some process and content ground rules. Intermediate groups reduce procedural rules and emphasize either content or process rules based on course objectives. Intermediate students also try to establish norms or ground rules that have worked in previous groups and often focus on what not to do and lobby the new group members to create a norm that will resolve a prior group's difficulties. Senior groups usually begin the course with fewer norms overall, and are more open to modifying and refining their norms throughout the semester.

Other norms guide what information is to be shared among group members, and how information is presented. Beginning students use narrowly defined topic areas to research and sometimes present information as mini-lectures based on their high school experiences. Consequently, time management becomes an issue if all students do not get time to present their information. As frustrations rise about who presents what and concerns are raised about the effectiveness of the mini-lecture format, the group recognizes that other strategies are necessary. This often leads two, or perhaps all group members, to choose to research the same learning issues and then to share the information in a discussion or debate format. Sometimes students will choose to develop a game, where they test each others knowledge of background information, as well as the topic under discussion. For example, if the problem they are exploring concerns a patient with Adult Onset Diabetes Mellitus, and a learning issue is achieving a balance between exercise and nutrition, they might want to first review metabolism and digestion in some experiential format.

Typical Group Issues

Almost any writing on small group learning, and discussion with any faculty member who has been a small group PBL tutor, will reveal a number of typical issues that groups face, such as developing an approach to decision making, establishing group leadership, and learning how to deal with conflict.

Decision Making/Achieving Consensus

Groups need to develop procedures that regulate the process of decision making and the role performances of group members (Sampson and Marthas, 1990). Beginning groups require assistance in exploring the options for decision making. Intermediate groups have an increased capacity to outline management practices, but members may continue to need some tutor assistance in developing negotiation and consensual decision making skills as agendas broaden. Negotiation of positive ground rules to achieve group goals needs to be articulated clearly and agreed upon (Wilkinson and Wilkinson, 1996). Goal setting and decision making require group members to develop skills of negotiation, prioritization, and collaboration. Embedded within goal setting is the expectation that all members will be responsible and accountable for achieving common goals.

Consensus implies a commitment by group members to be active listeners, to tolerate diversity, and promote collegiality. Recognizing that listening to each other, and incorporating the ideas of many members, has advantages over solo problem solving requires a paradigm shift from the competitive learning model to a co-operative learning model. Consensus is achieved when all group members support a decision, related to the content or process of the group. Sequential and incremental goal setting should link prior and current learning to promote retention (Woods, 1994; Dolmans and Schmidt, 1996).

Group Leadership

In an effective group, participation and leadership are equally distributed among members so that decision making is flexible and conflicts are managed constructively. All groups have to contend with the issues of power and power sharing (Johnson and Johnson, 1991). Influence can be acquired informally through personal prestige or by being more dominant verbally (Dimock, 1985). Influence or power within a group may also be acquired through formal recognition of status through the title of tutor or student facilitator. Many PBL groups choose to have a rotating student facilitator, since it provides an effective way for group members to develop the mind set and skills set of a facilitator. Students often choose to develop a personal learning objective around the facilitator role, indicating on their learning plan that they will review the purpose and process of the role, enact the role, reflect on their performance in the role, and receive feedback from others, according to predetermined criteria.

To assist students to develop the knowledge and skills of group process, including the issue of leadership, it is useful to specify course outcomes that guide students to explore the group process in depth, both theoretically and experientially. Since student evaluation methods guide the energy students put into learning activities, one way to ensure a commitment to learning about groups is to develop a graded assignment related to the many components of group process (Figure 4.2).

In this assignment, each student group videotapes one PBL session. The intent is for the student to use knowledge of group theory to present and evaluate process issues such as group roles, functions, leadership, and group development at a set point in time. This assignment enables the student to understand her/his own group behavior in greater depth as well as the

This is an individual assignment designed to provide the student with an opportunity to use concepts and theories of group functioning to assess and analyze group process. The intent is for the student to use knowledge of group theory to present and evaluate group structure (roles, functions, etc.) and group development at a set point in time.

Weight: 35% of final grade **Length:** 7 - 10 pages typewritten, double-spaced

Guidelines	Weighting
1. The paper will present an analysis of a group session which has been videotaped on an agreed upon date.	
2. The group situation on the day of videotaping should be described briefly.	.............5%
3. The framework selected to organize and analyze the data should be described briefly.	.............15%
4. The student will select a framework to organize and analyze the data. While the entire tape must be viewed, the observations should be organized and summarized according to the framework and interpretive conclusions about group process reached.	.............30%
5. Group process will be analyzed by examining: • the developmental stage of the group • the various roles within the group • strengths of the group • issues/problems with individual roles • strengths/problems with individual roles	.............40%
6. Based on the analysis, the student will identify personal learning objectives related to group performance and describe strategies to be used to meet these objectives.	.............10%

The paper will be evaluated using the "Guidelines for Grading a Scholarly Paper" in the BScN Programme Handbook. The overall grade is a global rating (using a letter grade, i.e., A, B+, etc.) and encompasses the use of APA scholarly format.

Scholarly format includes the use of the following: correct grammar, spelling, syntax, writing style, and smooth flow of ideas. A variety of current, relevant resources is to be included.

Figure 4.2   Group Process Assignment

Revised: June/99, © McMaster University School of Nursing.

behavior of others. Based on their analysis, students identify personal learning objectives related to their taped performance and describe strategies to be used to meet these objectives. As a result of this exercise, students develop a heightened awareness that the group has a life of its own. They learn about the complex nature of groups, the role of the tutor, the impact of each member's behavior on group function. Since this assignment is independent and confidential, the student's analysis is not encumbered by the need to be diplomatic as is the case when students give peer feedback during evaluation sessions. This frees them up to explore a more risky range of interpretations of the dynamics of their group.

The heightened awareness of group functioning that results from the assignment should also be shared through group discussion by explicitly drawing the connections between theory and the lived experience; norms can be revisited and concerns related to individual performance are voiced.

Managing Differences, Tensions, and Conflict Within a Group

Tutors have a pivotal influence on moderating tensions within groups, although some variables such as issues within a student's personal life, the need to work and study, program course timetable demands, and adequacy of tutorial rooms for effective group learning, are not within the tutor's control. Variables over which tutors do have some influence include orienting new members to group life, allowing individual choice in group assignments, establishing a climate conducive to motivating learners, taking a personal interest in the learners, and influencing group work activities (Miller et al., 1994, Schmidt and Moust, 1995; Wilkerson, 1996).

With beginning students it is important that the tutor conscientiously promote a safe climate which supports uncertainty, ambiguity, and experimentation. One strategy that encourages experimentation is brainstorming (Crosby, 1996). Brainstorming in consecutively larger groups, such as dyads and quads, enables the hesitant or quiet student to share knowledge and gain the respect of another peer for the knowledge each contributes. This enables everyone some "air time" for their ideas and lessens the initial risk taking for quieter students. Strategies that encourage interactive communication will facilitate the group to develop trust and awareness of each others' learning needs.

As facilitators and coaches for beginning level groups, tutors need to discuss the different group roles and how each contributes or hinders achievement of learning goals. The tutor should also model the task and maintenance roles for students to observe. One strategy to increase students' awareness of behaviors exhibited when performing the different roles is to use a strategy called *time-out*. This was first developed as a way in which to enter and exit from an interaction in which one group member interviews a standardized patient (Barrows and Tamblyn, 1980). Time-out enables the tutor and other group members to halt the discussion, thereby capturing the moment of an event or interactive dialogue. This enables students to gain a clearer understanding of how their own behaviors and those of their peers influence the group as a whole. Uys and Gwele (1999) describe this as the diagnostic role of the tutor, as students get feedback immediately about their faulty reasoning or nonparticipation. Strategies to influence group dynamics are continuously evolving to help group participants to be open, creative, and engaged in learning. Innovative strategies and time-tested approaches are required to expand the ways that small group learners interact.

Conflict is a normal stage of group development, and so all conflict should not necessarily be eliminated. According to Sampson and Marthas (1990), conflict is often indicative of liveliness and innovation in a group. The essential thing for faculty and students is to monitor the level and sources of conflict, so action can be taken if it becomes detrimental to learning, since it must always be remembered that the purpose of small PBL groups is to learn.

EVALUATION OF PERFORMANCE IN GROUP

It is recommended that evaluation of the group takes place on a regular basis. Discussing the stage of development of the group, the functions being performed, and issues such as the process used for decision making are all useful, since the focus of evaluation should be on the process and effectiveness of the group as a whole, as well as the performance of individual group members within the group. Group cohesion can be measured by:

- How a group monitors its progress toward goal achievement
- Whether or not the group enjoys what they are doing
- Group harmony
- Whether members assume responsibility for the group's work (Westberg and Jason, 1994)

Feedback concerning each person's actions within the group may be done at each meeting, once a month or at formal specific course-scheduled evaluation times. Barrows (1988) recommends that evaluation occurs within each tutorial so that students initiate evaluation of themselves, reflecting on their performance of problem-solving skills, self-directed study skills, and group support skills. These reviews may be guided by Dimock's categories of task and maintenance roles, and individual or nonfunctioning roles. Members need to develop sensitivity in giving and responding to feedback. A tutor should encourage the group to be self-reflective, making its own discoveries as well as providing feedback. In order to promote openness and minimize defensive behavior, the feedback should be both descriptive and evaluative (Westberg and Jason, 1996). Descriptive feedback should be nonjudgmental; spoken in a caring, supportive way; focused on behavior; and given in a way to avoid embarrassment. When providing evaluative feedback, a few principles might be helpful: link the evaluative statement to the description of the event or behavior; use an hypothesis-type of format such as beginning with "I wonder if"; do not treat your observations as if they are facts (you could be wrong and lose credibility or an immature group may not be ready to deal with the problem, resulting in a defensive reaction); be overt about the subjectivity of your own perceptions and encourage this in your students; and, make it a norm to use "I" statements such as "I think" or "I feel."

Review of group maintenance functions may be fostered by weekly debriefing—a technique to monitor the progress of the group and how the group needs to change (Peterson, 1997). If done frequently enough, the group can de-escalate tensions that arise when tasks are not achieved or potential interpersonal conflicts loom. Most students are comfortable with demonstrating and appraising their ideas, less comfortable receiving peer feedback about interactions with others, and sometimes more uncomfortable about discussing their social and emotional attitudes (Gerlach, 1994). Ideally the group should become a safe place for students to learn self-appraisal and seek and give constructive feedback.

Formal scheduled evaluations usually begin with self-evaluation, followed by peer and tutor feedback. By providing systematic feedback to peers about the content each brings and about the ways in which each member interacts with the group, each group member has the potential to advance to a higher level of performance. Criteria that specify the desired group behaviors are useful for students and faculty as they evaluate their own contributions to the group as well as those of others (see Figure 4.3).

Most often, in the formal midterm and end-of-term evaluations, group members will use these or similar criteria to conduct their self-evaluation and to prepare feedback for other group members. Other approaches to formal evaluation include the use of cards that have the various group roles written on them. The students shuffle the deck, choose a card, and then give feedback to the person on their right (or left or across the table) about that person's performance in relation to the criteria on the card. In another variation for an evaluation session, each member randomly selects another group member to whom she/he will give feedback, either through drawing a picture, making up a poem, or devising an anagram. The other group members also add their comments about the individual being evaluated. Whatever technique is used, the importance of self, peer, and tutor evaluation remains paramount to effective small group learning.

SUMMARY OF BENEFITS OF SMALL GROUP LEARNING

The work of Westburg and Jason (1996) provides a useful summary of the ideas presented in this chapter, and highlights several reasons for using the small group approach to PBL:

Group Process

1. Contributes to the development of group objectives.

   Never Almost Sometimes Often Almost Always Always

2. Helps to keep the group task-oriented.

   Never Almost Sometimes Often Almost Always Always

3. Completes tasks as negotiated within the group.

   Never Almost Sometimes Often Almost Always Always

4. Communicates ideas and information effectively.

   Never Almost Sometimes Often Almost Always Always

5. Listens and responds to others.

   Never Almost Sometimes Often Almost Always Always

6. Encourages participation by others.

   Never Almost Sometimes Often Almost Always Always

7. Assists other group members in their learning.

   Never Almost Sometimes Often Almost Always Always

8. Respects the rights of group members to express their values and opinions.

   Never Almost Sometimes Often Almost Always Always

9. Gives constructive feedback.

   Never Almost Sometimes Often Almost Always Always

10. Takes constructive actions to deal with group conflict.

    Never Almost Sometimes Often Almost Always Always

Figure 4.3 Criteria for Evaluation of Individual Performance in Tutorial - Group Process

© School of Nursing, McMaster University.

- *Group process and team-building skills:* Small group learning has intrapersonal, interpersonal, and intragroup benefits. By sharing ideas with their peers, group members learn to value different perspectives and capabilities which they translate into their work with other groups, and transfer later into their professional worklife (Dimock, 1986; Corey and Corey, 1997; Westberg and Jason, 1996). Learning in small groups creates issues for members such as how to work together, how to be supportive, how to deal with apathy, tension, conflict, control, and competition. Learning team-building skills enables students to practice the development of a cohesive, effective, and efficient team, built on trust, productivity, and clearly determined goals and mutual decision making (Dimock, 1985; Corey and Corey, 1997; Woods, 1994).
- *Peer-to-peer learning:* Individuals in a small group tutorial gain the benefits of peer learning. Peers facilitate, clarify knowledge gaps, explore and examine concepts, and share resources and relevant personal experiences. Through discussion with each other, students can broaden their own views within the context of their peers' opinions, learn effective interpersonal skills, and identify their own and peers' strengths and areas for growth. Repetition of this approach to learning assists learners to gain confidence and competence in building their ongoing knowledge and group process skills (Bosworth and Hamilton, 1994; Westberg and Jason, 1996; Wilkinson and Wilkinson, 1996; Cranton, 1998).
- *Learning is active and individualized:* Within the small group context that emphasizes collaboration, individuals are actively involved in the process of learning, as they personally identify their learning needs, goals, and styles of learning. Individualizing one's learning within the small group can enhance self-concept, enthusiasm, confidence, and motivation to learn. Since learning is active and personal, it is more likely to be meaningful and easily recalled.
- *Learning is incremental:* Learning groups act as an anchor upon which to create and construct progressive knowledge (Gijselaers, 1996; Cranton, 1998; Brookfield and Preskill, 1999). Students can be assisted to link new information to existing knowledge, develop their problem solving skills, elaborate on ideas, seek a deeper understanding of learning issues, set learning goals, develop strategies to achieve them, and monitor and evaluate their learning progress (Gijselaers, 1996; Kleffner & Dadian, 1997; Cranton, 1998; Brookfield and Preskill, 1999). As members learn about each other through discussion and critical reflection, they begin to analytically examine their own beliefs, values, and assumptions and widen their perspectives and understandings.
- *Evaluative/growth oriented:* Evaluative feedback is essential to facilitate individual and group growth. Critical self-reflection and feedback

from others is fundamental to enhance individual learning and professional growth. Feedback helps students understand the process and stages of group development. Together, with constructive feedback from others, and strategies such as self-reflection, students learn to know what they are doing satisfactorily and what still needs work.

- *Testing ground for professional development:* Small group learning provides a safe environment and testing ground to learn and apply knowledge and skills that will be transferable to work situations. In the small group, students can experiment and model different roles with their peers and tutor.
- *Learning to learn:* The problem acts as a springboard for the exploration of learning issues. Discussion of the problem challenges students to explore all possible explanations, to recall what they know, to identify learning gaps, and then to arrive at a solution. The inquisitive style of learning is stimulating, motivating, and fosters competence in learners, as they learn to work together in groups to achieve their learning tasks. "Group-think" gives meaning to student's learning, aids retention of learned material, and can be a powerful motivator for further learning (Barrows, 1988; Woods, 1994; Dolmans and Schmidt, 1996; Wilkinson and Wilkinson, 1996; Cranton, 1998). Vernon and Blake (1993) conclude that students in PBL programs are consistently more positive about their program, and learned to gain more in-depth understanding, as opposed to memorization.

DRAWBACKS OF SMALL GROUP LEARNING

Drawbacks to small group PBL can be grouped under six headings: changing roles and relationships; intrapersonal, intragroup, and interpersonal problems; tutor skills and expectations; incongruence with students' learning style; incongruence with educational environment; and dependency on groups.

- *Changing roles and relationships:* Small group learning does not appeal to all learners. Students initially may find small group learning intimidating. The appearance of lack of structured content may be an issue for some students. Some students have found the evaluation and feedback processes "intimidating" and "humbling." Many students report that the preparation for small group tutorials is time-consuming, but necessary, as they are committed to their group members who also work equally hard for them. This creates a pressure for individual students to be prepared, to be present at group sessions, and to not let their groups down (Reinders, 1993).
- *Intrapersonal, intragroup, and interpersonal problems:* Intrapersonal, intragroup, and interpersonal problems may occur within groups

and may impede the groups' progress and growth. *Intrapersonal issues* are factors that relate to an individual member but affect the group as a whole, such as personal problems, attitudes toward working in a group, lack of commitment to learning, diverse beliefs, and/or dissimilar cultures. *Intragroup issues* are factors that hinder the development of co-operation, collaboration, and teamwork within the group, such as unclear goals and expectations, dominating or attention-seeking behaviors, competition, or a mid-course change in the group's composition. *Interpersonal issues* are factors that relate to communication issues among group members, such as personality conflicts, ineffective communication, and distrust of others (Dimock and Devine, 1996; Tiberius, 1990).

- *Tutor skills and expectations.* Lack of tutor consistency in expectations and/or being too directive are potentially deleterious actions for groups. Other problems include lack of knowledge about group process, lack of knowledge about course content, and inadequate facilitation skills. Although few studies have addressed how tutors develop, analyze, and manage group behaviors, several researchers have identified a lack of knowledge about group process as an issue for both tutors and learners (Tipping, Freeman, and Rachlis; 1995; Davis and Harden, 1999; Miller, Trimbur, and Wilkes, 1994; Wilkerson, 1996).

- *Incongruence with the student's learning style:* Students who come from traditional curricular programs find the lack of structure and direction a challenge (Townsend, 1990). Students who have difficulty expressing themselves, participating in a group, taking on different group roles, and evaluating others may also find this learning style an uncomfortable experience. Language and culture variables may also impact on the effectiveness of learning within groups. This challenge for group facilitators and members represents an increasingly common phenomenon as student populations become more multicultural. Working with culturally diverse groups compels group members to gain heightened cultural sensitivity and awareness of the skills needed to effectively manage diversity issues (Corey and Corey, 1997, p. 16).

- *Incongruence with the educational environment:* Costs associated with faculty, space, resources, and time required for curriculum revisions are possible program issues. It is suggested by Albanese and Mitchell (1993) and Berkson (1993) that these costs are particularly high in schools with classes of more than 100 students.

Small group learning in an integrated curriculum may have some disadvantages that are still unknown. More educational research needs to augment current knowledge on small group learning in order to better understand the benefits and limitations that may emerge as the twenty-first century unfolds.

CONCLUSION

Shifting small group learning into mainstream teaching–learning environments will require a transition not only by students but also by faculty. Small PBL groups are an exemplar for other groups in society. Corey and Corey (1997) reflect that small group learners are group members who grow personally and professionally through sharing common problems, struggles and conflicts, giving and receiving feedback from peers and tutors, trying new approaches and broader attitudes, and developing better interpersonal skills. As students move beyond their educational programs, they move into professional learning communities as twenty-first century knowledge workers.

Desirable attributes of professional learning communities are "shared leadership, collective creativity, shared values and vision, supportive conditions and shared personal practice" (Hord, 1997, p. 2). These attributes are congruent with the benefits accrued when small group learners achieve their goals. Inquiry within the small group builds a collective creativity that continues to grow as graduates foster innovations within health care services. This expanded creativity is sometimes associated with collective critical thinking in which creative solutions evolve as change occurs. Effective problem solvers must be committed to a vision that fosters caring, trust, and open dialogue. Small group learning requires support from educational institutions. Last, small group learning has embedded within its core the philosophy that "peers help peers" which is how learning becomes meaningful and applicable.

REFERENCES

Adler, S. L., Bryk, E., Cesta, T. G., and McEachen, I. (1995). Collaboration: The solution to multidisciplinary care planning. *Orthopedic Nursing, 14*(2), 21–29.

Albanese, M. A. and Mitchell, S. (1993). Problem-based learning: A review of literature on its outcomes and implementation issues. *Academic Medicine, 68*(1), 52–58.

Allen, D. E., Duch, B. J., and Groh, S. E. (1996). The power of problem-based learning in teaching introductory science courses. In L. Wilkerson and W. M. Gijselaers (Eds.). *Bringing Problem Based Learning to Higher Education: Theory and Practice.* San Francisco: Jossey-Bass.

Antai-Otong, D. (1997). Team building in a health care setting. *American Journal of Nursing, 97*(7), 48–51.

Barrows, H. S. (1988). *The Tutorial Process.* Springfield: Southern Illinois University.

Barrows, H. S. and Tamblyn, R. M. (1980). *Problem-based Learning: An Approach to Medical Education.* New York: Springer.

Berkson, L. (1993). Problem based learning: Have the expectations been met? *Academic Medicine, 68*(10), S79–S88.

Bosworth, K. and Hamilton, S. J. (Ed.). (1994). *Collaborative Learning: Underlying Processes and Effective Techniques.* San Francisco: Jossey-Bass.

Brookfield, S. D. (1986). *Understanding and Facilitating Adult Learning.* San Francisco: Jossey-Bass.

Brookfield, S. D. (1995). *Becoming a Critically Reflective Teacher.* San Francisco: Jossey-Bass.

Brookfield, S. D. and Preskill, S. (1999). *Discussion as a Way of Teaching: Tools and Techniques for Democratic Classrooms.* San Francisco: Jossey-Bass.

Corey, M. S. and Corey, G. (1997). *Groups: Process and Practice.* Pacific Grove, CA: Brooks/Cole.

Cranton, P. (1998). *No One Way: Teaching and Learning in Higher Education.* Toronto, ON: Wall and Emerson.

Crosby, J. (1996). AMEE Medical Education Guide No. 8: Learning in small groups. *Medical Teacher, 18*(3), 189–202.

Davis, M. H. and Harden, R. M. (1999). AMEE Medical Education Guide No. 15: Problem-based learning: A practical guide. *Medical Teacher, 21*(2), 130–138.

Dimock, H. G. (1985). *How to Observe Your Group* (2nd ed.). Guelph, ON: University of Guelph.

Dimock, H. G. (1986). *Planning Group Development* (2nd ed.). Guelph, ON: University of Guelph.

Dimock, H. G. and Devine, I. (1996). *Managing Dynamic Groups.* North York, ON: Captus Press.

Dolmans, D. and Schmidt, H. (1996). Advantages of problem-based curricula. *Postgraduate Medical Journal, 72,* 535–538.

Gerlach, J. M. (1994). Is this collaboration? In K. Bosworth and S. J. Hamilton (Eds.). *Collaborative Learning: Underlying Processes and Effective Techniques.* San Francisco: Jossey-Bass.

Gijselaers, W. H. (1996). Connecting problem-based practices with educational theory. In L. Wilkerson and W. H. Gijselaers (Eds.). *Bringing Problem-based Learning to Higher Education: Theory and Practice.* San Francisco: Jossey-Bass.

Hare, A. P., Blumberg, H. H., Davies, M. F., and Kent, M. V. (1994). *Small Group Research: A Handbook.* Norwood, NJ: Ablex Publishing.

Herbert, R. and Bravo, G. (1996). Development and validation of an evaluation instrument for medical students in tutorials. *Academic Medicine, 71*(5), 488–494.

Hodne, B. D. (1997). Please speak up: Asian immigrant students in American college classrooms. In D. L. Sigsbee, B. W. Speck, and B. Maytlath (Eds.). *New Directions for Teaching and Learning,* Vol. 70. San Francisco: Jossey-Bass.

Hord, S. M. (1997). Professional Learning Communities: What are they and why are they important? *Issues . . . about Change,* 6(1). Austin, Texas: Southwest Educational Development Laboratory [SEDL].

Johnson, D. W. and Johnson, F. P. (1991). *Joining Together: Group Theory and Groups Skills.* Englewood Cliffs, NJ: Prentice-Hall.

Kalain, H. A. and Mullen, P. B. (1996). Exploratory factor analysis of students' ratings of a problem-based learning curriculum. *Academic Medicine, 71*(4), 390–392.

Kaufman, D., Day, V., and Mensink, D. (1996). Stressors in first-year medical school: Comparison of conventional and problem-based curriculum. *Teaching and Learning in Medicine, 8*(4), 188–194.

Kleffner, J. H. and Dadian, T. (1997). Using collaborative learning in dental education. *Journal of Dental Education, 61*(1), 66–72.

Kozier, B., Erb, G., and Blais, K. (1997). *Professional Nursing Practice: Concepts and Perspectives.* New York: Addison-Wesley.

McAllister, M. and Osborne, Y. (1997). Peer review: A strategy to enhance cooperative student learning. *Nurse Educator, 22*(1), 40–44.

Mezirow, J. (1990). How critical reflection triggers transformative learning. In J. Mezirow and Associates (Ed.). *Fostering Critical Reflection in Adulthood: A Guide to Transformative and Emancipatory Learning.* San Francisco: Jossey-Bass.

Miller, J. E., Trimbur, J., and Wilkes, J. M. (1994). Group dynamics: Understanding group success and failure in collaborative learning. In K. Bosworth and S. J. Hamilton (Eds.). *Collaborative Learning: Underlying Processes and Effective Techniques.* San Francisco: Jossey-Bass.

Moore-West, M., Harrington, D. L., Mennin, S. P., Kaufman, A., and Skipper, B. J. (1989). Distress and attitudes toward the learning environment: Effects of a curriculum innovation. *Teaching and Learning Medicine, 1*(3), 151–157.

Nasmith, L. and Daigle, N. (1996). Small group teaching in patient education. *Medical Teacher, 18*(3), 209–211.

Neufeld, V. and Barrows, H. (1974). The "McMaster philosophy": An approach to medical education. *Journal of Medical Education, 49*(11), 1040–1051.

Peterson, M. (1997). Skills to enhance problem-based learning, *Med Educ Online* [serial on-line];2,3. Available from URL *http://www.Med-Ed-Online.*

Preston-Whyte, M. E., McCulloch, R., and Fraser, R. C. (1996). Establishing the face validity of the criteria of teaching competence in the Leicester package for the assessment of teaching skills (L-PAST) for tutor-led, task-oriented, small-group teaching. *Medical Teacher, 18*(2), 135–139.

Reinders, S. (1993). Problem-based learning from a student's point of view. In P. Bouhuijs, H. Schmidt, and H. Van Berkel (Eds.). *Problem-based Learning as an Educational Strategy.* Maastricht, The Netherlands: Network Publications, pp. 151–154.

Rideout, E. (1998). The experience of learning and teaching in a nonconventional nursing curriculum. Unpublished doctoral dissertation, University of Toronto.

Rideout, E. (1999). Like ducks to water? Learning to learn in a small group, self-directed, problem-based undergraduate nursing curriculum. *Pedagogue, 9,* 9–11.

Sampson, E. E. and Marthas, M. (1990). *Group process for the health professions.* Albany, NY: Delmar.

Schmidt, H. G. (1994). Resolving inconsistencies in tutor expertise research: Does lack of structure cause students to seek tutor guidance? *Academic Medicine, 69,* 656–62.

Schmidt, H. G. and Moust, J. H. C. (1995). What makes the tutor effective? A structural-equations modeling approach to learning and problem-based curricula. *Academic Medicine, 70,* 708–714.

Solomon, P. and Finch, E. (1998). A qualitative study identifying stressors associated with adapting to problem-based learning. *Teaching and learning in medicine, 10*(2), 58–64.

Solomon, P. and Finch, E. (1999). Adapting to problem-based learning. *Pedagogue, 9,* 6–9.

Tiberius, R. G. (1990). *Small Group Teaching: A Troubleshooting Guide.* Toronto, ON: OISE Press.

Tipping, J., Freeman, R., and Rachlis, A. (1995). Using faculty and student perceptions of group dynamics to develop recommendations for PBL training. *Academic Medicine, 70*(11), 1050–1052.

Thomas, R. E. (1997). Problem-based learning: Measurable outcomes. *Medical Education, 31,* 320–329.

Townsend, J. (1990). Teaching/learning strategies. *Nursing Times, 86*(23), 66–68.

Tuckman, B. W. and Jensen, M. A. (1977). Stages of small group development revisited. *Group and Group Organizational Studies, 2,* 419–427.

Turner, J. (1982). *The structure of sociological theory.* Homewood, IL: Dorsey Press.

Uys, L. R. and Gwele, N. S. (1999). A descriptive analysis of the process of problem-based teaching/learning. In J. Conway and A. Williams (Eds.). *Themes and variations in PBL.* Callaghan, Australia: PROBLARC.

Vernon, D. T. A. and Blake, R. L. (1993). Does problem-based learning work? A meta-analysis of evaluative research. *Academic Medicine, 68*(7), 550–563.

Wallis, B. and Mitchell, K. (1995). The teaching of small group skills as a basis for problem-based learning in small task-oriented groups. In D. Boud (Ed.). Problem-based Learning in Education for the Professions. Sydney, Australia: HERDSA.

Wass, A. (2000). *Promoting Health: The Primary Health Care Approach.* Sydney, Australia: Harcourt Saunders.

Watkins, K. and Marsick, V. (1993). *Sculpting the Learning Organizations: Lessons in the Art and Science of Systematic Change.* San Francisco: Jossey-Bass.

Westberg, J. and Jason, H. (1994). Fostering learners' reflection and self assessment. *Family Medicine, 26*(5), 278–282.

Westberg, J. and Jason, H. (1996). *Fostering Learning in Small Groups: A Practical Guide.* New York: Springer.

Wilkinson, J. and Wilkinson, C. (1996). Group discussions in nursing education: A learning process. *Nursing Standard, 10*(44), 46–47.

Wilkerson, L. (1996). Tutors and small groups in problem-based learning: Lessons from the literature. In L. Wilkerson and W. H. Gijselaers (Ed.).

Bringing Problem-based Learning to Higher Education: Theory and Practice. San Francisco: Jossey-Bass.

Woods, D. R. (1994). *Problem-based learning: How to gain the most from PBL.* Waterdown, ON: Donald R. Woods.

Woods, D. R. (1996). Problem-based learning for large group classes in chemical engineering. In L. Wilkerson and W. H. Gijselaers (Ed.). *Bringing Problem-based Learning to Higher Education: Theory and Practice.* San Francisco: Jossey-Bass.

Facilitating Information Management Skills and Dispositions

Liz Bayley, Neera Bhatnagar, and Patricia Ellis

Information management is an integral part of problem-based learning (PBL). As the steps of the PBL process outlined in Chapter 2 indicate, the initial analysis of the problem is followed by identification of learning issues, self-directed gathering of information, and application of the new knowledge to the problem scenario. To take these actions requires a number of information management skills, which include: recognizing the need for information; searching for and evaluating the information obtained; applying that information to clinical decision making; organizing and communicating information; and increasingly, participating in the creation of information and assisting patients to become information literate.

This chapter begins with an overview of information management and makes the case for its inclusion as a desired and required outcome of nursing education. The chapter will then present specific strategies for incorporating information management into a PBL curriculum, to ensure that students become effective in identifying, evaluating, and applying relevant information.

COMPONENTS OF INFORMATION MANAGEMENT SKILLS

By mastering information management skills, one becomes information literate. Breivik (1985) defines information literacy as "the ability to effectively access and evaluate information for a given need" (p. 723), which requires the following approaches and abilities:

- The use of an integrated set of skills and knowledge
  - skills (research strategy, evaluation)
  - knowledge of tools and resources
- Which are developed through the acquisition of attitudes
  - persistence
  - attention to detail
  - caution in accepting printed work and single sources

- Which are in turn
  - time and labor intensive
  - need driven (a problem-solving activity)
  - distinct but relevant to literacy and computer literacy

In a later article, Breivik provides a description of information literacy developed by the American Library Association Presidential Committee on Information Literacy:

> The report defines information-literate people as those who know when they have a need for information, can identify information needed to address a given problem or issue, can find needed information, and can evaluate and organize it to address effectively the problem or issue at hand. Information literacy is, in fact, the first component on the continuum of critical thinking skills. In this information age, it does not matter how well people can analyse or synthesize; if they do not start with an adequate, accurate and up-to-date body of information, they will not come up with a good answer." (Breivik, 1991, p. 226)

Cheek and Doskatsch (1988) recognize that information literacy is a "complex and constantly changing mosaic of skills, knowledge and attitudes" (p. 245), and they define it in terms of the characteristics and attributes of an information literate person. Being information literate "empower[s] and enable[s] individuals to effectively access, evaluate and use the appropriate and relevant information regardless of how the information is packaged" (Cheek and Doskatsch, 1998, p. 245).

Both Breivik and Gee (1989) and Cheek and Doskatsch (1998) emphasize that computer literacy is not to be equated with information literacy. Computers are powerful tools for the storage and organization of and access to information. However, they are a means to an end rather than the end themselves, and technical skills in using computers and information technology need to be complemented by expertise to select accurate, current, authoritative, and relevant information (Cheek and Doskatsch, 1998). With the increasing pervasiveness of the Internet, this latter expertise becomes even more essential.

A related component of information management is nursing informatics, which Grobe (1988) defines as "the application of the principles of information science and theory to the study and scientific analysis of nursing information for the purposes of establishing a body of nursing knowledge" (p. 29). Sibbald (1998) adds to our understanding by pointing out that "[n]ursing informatics is not about computers or the Internet. It is about using information technology to improve patient care, something that lies at the heart of nursing" (p. 22).

THE NEED FOR INFORMATION MANAGEMENT SKILLS IN NURSING

It is estimated that information pertaining to the nursing profession doubles every five years (Weaver, 1993). If nurses are to take advantage of this wealth of knowledge, they must acquire the necessary skills, knowledge, and attitudes to retrieve the relevant information, and the ability to do this must begin when they are students. Several studies have shown that the lack of these skills results in nurses not using the nursing literature in their daily practice (Blythe and Royle, 1993; Blythe, Royle, Oolup, Potvin, and Smith, 1995).

Nursing is moving towards complex evidence-based practice, and the amount and type of information nurses will have to process in order to support this is ever increasing. Information technologies can help nurses meet these challenges by identifying and locating vital health care information. As Bachman and Panzarine (1998) point out, telecommunication applications such as telemedicine, telehealth, telenursing, telehome health care, teleradiology, telepsychiatry, and virtual medical centers are emerging as methods to deliver health care and health information to patients and health professionals in remote locations and at major medical centers. In their practice, nurses will encounter many computerized devices such as microprocessor implants and electronic monitoring devices, and the future will rely more on automated imaging systems, telecomputing, and robotics (Travis and Brennan, 1998). Thus, it is imperative that students have an understanding of these technologies when they graduate.

As noted above, evidence-based practice is a significant trend in health care, and nursing is a part of that trend. Flemming (1998) describes the five stages of evidence-based nursing, which bear a striking resemblance to the approach of an information literate person:

- Information needs from practice are converted into focused, structured questions.
- The focused questions are used as a basis for literature searching in order to identify relevant external evidence from research.
- The research evidence is critically appraised for validity and generalizability.
- The best available evidence is used alongside clinical expertise and the patient's perspective to plan care.
- Performance is evaluated through a process of self-reflection, audit, or peer assessment (p. 36).

Increasingly, the informed use of research in clinical practice is becoming an essential requirement for professional credentialing and competency assessment. Lenburg (1999) speaks of the need to redesign expectations for initial and continuing competence to meet the escalating complexities of health care delivery systems, and lists eight core practice competencies, including critical thinking and knowledge integration. The regulating body for nursing practice in Ontario, the College of Nurses of Ontario (1999), has acknowledged the importance of the informed use of research in its entry to practice competencies that include several references to information management.

Professional Standard #2: Knowledge

K-1 Reads and critiques research in nursing, health sciences, and related disciplines.

K-2 Integrates research findings from nursing, health sciences, and related disciplines into own nursing practice.

Professional Standard #3: Application of Knowledge

A-1 Applies critical thinking skills in all practice activities.

A-2 Contributes to health or nursing research.

A-6 Consults with the literature, colleagues, and other sources in selecting appropriate assessment tools and techniques.

A-13 Uses evidence-based knowledge from nursing, health sciences, and related disciplines to select and individualize nursing interventions.

A-43 Critically appraises research evidence and applies relevant findings to the care of clients.

A-51 Incorporates relevant research findings in health promotion activities.

Altogether there is considerable evidence that nursing practice has particular requirements for information management skills. As well, lifelong learning is now recognized as an important aspect of today's nursing practice and information management provides the framework to be able to continue to access and use information. Educators are aware that nursing graduates must have these skills if they are to be evidence-based practitioners and to continue learning in their professional careers (Cheek and Doskatasch, 1998; Weaver, 1993).

To accomplish this it is necessary for schools of nursing to integrate information management content and practice into their curricula. Some institutions have recognized this need and have developed such programs, integrating them into their particular educational curriculum and philosophy. For example, the University of Colorado School of Nursing developed the Pathways to Information Literacy Program (Fox, Richter, and White, 1996) while the San Francisco State University School of Nursing developed an integrated program to teach information literacy in their undergraduate curriculum (Verhey, 1999). Allegri (1995) states that course integrated instruction must meet three of the following four criteria: faculty outside the library are involved in the design, execution, and evaluation of the program; the instruction is directly related to the students' course work or assignments; students are required to participate; and the students' work is graded or credit is received for participation.

As has been demonstrated in earlier chapters of this book, PBL is particularly well-suited to the development of information management skills, since it is an explicit expectation of the PBL process. The strategies to integrate these skills into a PBL program, to ensure that graduates are indeed information literate, will be discussed next.

INFORMATION MANAGEMENT WITHIN A PBL CURRICULUM

Any plan to incorporate information management should be designed to ensure students develop the necessary skills, and that they acquire the confidence to apply the skills. Several elements must be in place to implement a successful information management program (see Table 5.1).

Table 5.1   *Elements of an Information Management Program in a PBL Setting*

- Development of clearly defined outcomes
- Integration of computer literacy skills
- Phased introduction of information management skills
- Strategies for active engagement
- Evaluation in an information management program
- Faculty role in information management
- Faculty–library collaboration

DEVELOPMENT OF CLEARLY DEFINED OUTCOMES

Any plan of study should begin with defined outcomes or objectives, and an information management program is no exception. Redman, Lenburg, and Walker (1999) list ten competencies that students must develop in order to fulfill provider roles, including the ability to "[p]ractice nursing reflectively, guided by theory, based on best evidence, and integrating creative and critical thinking" and to "[i]ntegrate the ethical use of technology, and information systems to augment the human capacity for health, facilitate decision-making, support collaboration, and foster communication." Such competencies as these might form the basis for stating the desired outcomes of information management program.

The terminal objectives and goals of the information literacy program of the School of Nursing at the University of Northern Colorado (Fox et al., 1989, p. 423) provide another example:

- Assist the student in understanding library organization and services
- Promote student skills in locating and evaluating the accuracy of information for academic use and for lifelong learning
- Help students understand information-seeking strategies and the appropriate use of those strategies
- Give students the skills and knowledge to emulate scholarly activities of professional nurses

Program outcomes might be developed that are a restatement of the information management and evidence-based process (Table 5.2).

Integration of Computer Literacy Skills

As stated earlier, computer literacy skills are a key component of an information management program. Students entering undergraduate nursing programs generally have a positive attitude toward computers, since they have been exposed to them in their everyday lives and are comfortable using them to access information. An information program in nursing

Table 5.2 *An Example of Outcomes of an Information Management Program*

- Frame a question
- Analyse the question into key components
- Identify appropriate resources to answer the question
- Carry out the search by
  - identifying the appropriate terminology used in the resource
  - mapping the question components to the terminology
- Retrieve the information
- Evaluate the search process
- Evaluate the information found
- Apply the information to the question

education must focus on exposing students to the various information systems relevant to nursing and making the links between information searching and the nursing profession; so it should be designed to build on the strengths that students bring to their learning. As Travis and Brennan (1995) state: "Nurse educators face a challenge not only to make nurses more technologically competent but also to produce a new type of graduate who will excel in acute care clinical practice through the effective use of computer technologies" (p. 162).

PHASED INTRODUCTION OF INFORMATION MANAGEMENT SKILLS

Another principle of education that has particular relevance for the design of an information management program involves introducing new learning in a sequential manner. The specific outcomes that students are expected to work towards in each course within the program of study should be identified, and these should be geared to the level of the student. For example, a beginning student might be expected to become familiar with the library and its resources, and to begin to evaluate their information seeking strategies and the information found (Table 5.3).

In PBL, the information management skills can be phased in so they build exponentially with each successive problem. The following examples come from the four-year Bachelor of Science of Nursing (BScN) program at McMaster University, which uses PBL as the educational approach for all nursing courses. In the first course for beginning students, a total of five problems are explored, and the Information Management (IM) component of the course is integrated with the problems as presented in Table 5.4.

Table 5.3   *Information Management Outcomes Beginning Level Course*

By the end of the course, the student will be able to:

1. Identify their information needs and *key concepts* to be investigated.

2. Identify *appropriate types of resources* to answer the information need, for example, textbooks, journal articles, drug directories, videotapes, Web sites.

3. Master the *tools available* to locate specific resources, in particular MORRIS (the Library's online catalogue), Cumulative Index to Nursing and Allied Health Literature, and the CINAHL database.

4. Choose appropriate *terminology,* in particular, the Medical Subject Headings (MeSH) to use MORRIS, and CINAHL subject headings to search for journal articles.

5. Understand the *arrangement of resources,* for example, the National Library of Medicine classification scheme, journal shelving order.

6. *Locate resources,* in particular, the collections of the Health Sciences Library, and the resources available at other libraries on campus.

7. *Evaluate resources,* following the criteria provided in the Information Seeking Survival Skills handouts.

8. *Cite resources* according to the *Publication Manual of the American Psychological Association,* 4th edition.

© School of Nursing, McMaster University.

Table 5.4   *Integration of Information Management and Problem-based Learning Course for Beginning Students*

Problem #1

Resources to be used:

• Books

• Audiovisual resources

Skills to be developed:

• Using the library catalogue

• Understanding subject headings

• Locating materials

• Understanding a library classification system

• Evaluating the resources

• Citing the resources in a bibliography according to a set standard, for example, *Publication of the American Psychological Association,* 4th edition.

continued

Table 5.4 *Integration of Information Management and Problem-based Learning Course for Beginning Students   continued*

Problem #2

Resources to be used:

• Journal articles

Skills to be developed:

• Using a printed journal index, for example, Cumulative Index to Nursing and Allied Health Literature (CINAHL)

• Evaluating the articles

• Citing the articles in a bibliography

Problem #3

Resources to be used:

• Bibliographic databases, for example, Nursing and Allied Health

Skills to be developed:

 • Formulating a search strategy

 • Carrying out a search

 • Evaluating the search strategy

Problem #4

Resources to be used:

 • Web resources

Skills to be developed:

• Using a Web browser

• Using a Web search engine

• Evaluating Web resources

• Citing Web resources in a bibliography

Problem #5

Resources to be used:

• Integration of all of the types of resources

Skills to be developed:

• Identifying which type of resource should be used for which information need

• Evaluating each type of resource for its usefulness to answer the information need

With each successive course taken in the BScN program, students use more advanced IM skills. For example, second-year students at the end of their first semester are expected to:

1. Continue to evaluate resources according to specific criteria
2. Develop a personal filing system to organize collected information sources so they are quickly retrievable
3. Expand searching to include MEDLINE
4. Analyze learning resources, search strategies, and the usefulness of information obtained (in the PBL component)

At the end of the second semester, the students are required to:

1. Analyze learning resources, search strategies, and the usefulness of information obtained (in the clinical component)
2. Develop a beginning understanding of nursing research and its application to nursing practice
3. Analyze research-based evidence and its application to clinical questions (in the PBL component).

Courses in research methodologies and critical appraisal are introduced in the third year. Throughout this process, students are encouraged to transfer the information management skills from the problem-based setting to the clinical component of their education. By the final year, senior students should integrate information management within the clinical setting on a regular basis, refine their skills to adapt to the time and resource requirements of a practice setting, and meet the goals and objectives set out by the credentialing body.

The School of Nursing at San Francisco State University has also integrated information literacy throughout its undergraduate curriculum, choosing learner empowerment and the enhancement of critical thinking as its two primary constructs. Verhey (1999) outlines the information literacy strand both in the theory and the practicum courses and describes a variety of instructional strategies which are used over five semesters. Careful phasing of information management skills based on student readiness and needs allows learners to build and practice their skills to meet identified learning issues.

STRATEGIES FOR ACTIVE ENGAGEMENT

Many schools offer a course in information management, with regular assignments and tests. However, a main feature of PBL is the development of knowledge in context, in an active rather than a passive learning environment. As we have noted before, information management is an integral part of the PBL process. By having students seeking information related to a specific problem, students can acquire and practice skills directly applicable to their learning. Skills training can be identified as a learning issue and resource sessions planned. The faculty tutor could arrange to have a librarian come to class as a guest speaker or could organize a library tour for the students. If there is a learning laboratory in the library, a session that coincides with the skills related to the problem being studied could be proposed.

Although the application of these skills may need to be explicit at first, with specific activities and expectations, as the students become more proficient, the efficient and effective identification of information becomes an integral part of their learning process.

Methods should be developed that allow students to demonstrate their skills. These can be planned to assess ongoing learning and identify learning needs and they may also be used to measure achievement through summative evaluation. One way to identify learning needs related to the individual student's information management skills is to request that each student identify a topic for the problem being studied and then find two or three references, based on the selection, which are used to generate a reference list to be shared among class members. At the same time the faculty tutor is able to see the quality, quantity, and variety of references the student has selected. Given this information, students who are using a limited selection of references can be identified and assistance to expand resource selection can be provided by other group members and the faculty tutor. For instance, if a student continues to use texts when he or she should be expanding the search to include journals, the tutor may identify that the student has not yet developed the skill of using indexes to help with the search.

Another approach is to use preset worksheets. Since developing effective search strategies is integral to becoming information literate, a worksheet to assist students with their search strategies has proven useful. In their preparation for class, students search for and select references relevant to the problem being studied. For each reference, the student completes a worksheet in which they demonstrate their ability to identify a specific learning issue, the relevant search terms, and the references identified and retrieved. They also evaluate their search process and the usefulness of the resources found. An example of this worksheet is presented in Figure 5.1.

This process can be taken a step further by having students critique the resources selected using more specific criteria, summarize briefly their search strategy and the information obtained, and reflect on the relevance of the learning to the problem being studied. (See Chapter 6 for detail on the integration of critical reflection and PBL). A sample worksheet for evaluation of information searching is found in Figure 5.2. Initially the worksheets are reviewed by the faculty tutor (and student peers if the review takes place within a PBL group) and feedback is provided. The worksheets can also be used as part of the summative evaluation of student performance.

EVALUATION IN AN INFORMATION MANAGEMENT PROGRAM

Student motivation to learn is enhanced when their learning is formally evaluated and they receive credit or grades for work done. It is important to plan assignments that will be used to demonstrate the achievement of information management skills and reward students for this achievement. The worksheets described above can be used to provide evidence of the students' learning. They can be submitted in a binder at the end of the course. Examples of criteria to evaluate these assignments include: (1) evidence of consistent preparation for class; (2) a selection of relevant resources including books, journals, Web sites, and people resources; and (3) evidence of critical analysis of the resources selected. Actual contributions in class

---

Student Name: **Date:**

Student Number:

Question to be answered:

_____

1. Source(s) searched: (e.g., databases, Web, MORRIS)

_____

2. Time spent:

_____

3. Breakdown of the question into concepts:

_____

4. Possible search terms for the concepts: (e.g., CINAHL subject headings, subheadings, limits, text words, words for Web search tools)

_____

5. Resources found: (list 3-5 in APA format)

_____

6. Evaluation of the search:

_____

7. Analysis of resources found and their usefulness to answer the question:

Figure 5.1   Information seeking exercise
© School of Nursing, McMaster University.

related to information management skills can be included in tutorial performance evaluation for which the student either receives a pass/fail or receives a percentage of the course grade.

As well as evaluating student skill development, it is important to measure the IM program as a whole. Verhey (1999) describes a self-report

Student name: **Date:**

Student #:

Resource (complete reference using APA format)

Type of Source: ☐ General Textbook   ☐ Specialized Textbook

☐ Book   ☐ Encyclopedia   ☐ Dictionary   ☐ Directory

☐ Journal article: Type of article   ☐ Web page(s): URL

☐ Other (please specify):

1. Authority, for example: • Who wrote it? published it? mounted it on the Web? • What are their credentials?	
2. Content, for example: • Is it at an appropriate level? • What audience is it aimed at? • How detailed is it? • Is it an appropriate type of resource?	
3. Currency, for example: • When was it published? mounted or revised? • Is this a rapidly changing subject area?	
4. Objectivity/disclosure, for example: • Who published it? mounted it? • Who funded it? sponsored it? • What was the aim of the author? • Does the author or sponsor have a vested interest or possible bias?	
5. Organization/layout, for example: • Is the order of the material clear and logical? • Is there a good index? table of contents? search tool? • Is material easy to find?	

Learning question:

Brief summary of the information found:

Reflection: What did I learn? How does this relate to the problem/objective? Did this resource help me answer my learning question? Why or why not? What further learning questions has this resource stimulated?

Figure 5.2   Worksheet for the evaluation of information resources
© School of Nursing, McMaster University.

instrument used to evaluate the information literacy curriculum strand at the San Francisco State University School of Nursing. Six primary content areas are addressed:

- Information resources used to complete assignments
- Use of bibliographic databases
- Use of libraries and the School of Nursing's learning resource center
- Comfort level in accessing information resources
- Barriers encountered in accessing information resources
- Plans for accessing current information after graduation (p. 255)

A useful standard against which to measure an information management program is the set of competencies for higher education established by the Association of College and Research Libraries (2000), which include performance indicators and outcomes for the following standards:

Standard One   The information literate student determines the nature and extent of the information needed.

Standard Two   The information literate student accesses information effectively and efficiently.

Standard Three   The information literate student evaluates information and its sources critically and incorporates selected information into his or her knowledge base and value system.

Standard Four   The information literate student, individually or as a member of a group, uses information effectively to accomplish a specific purpose.

Standard Five   The information literate student understands many of the economic, legal, and social concerns surrounding the use of information and accesses and uses information ethically and legally.

FACULTY ROLE IN INFORMATION MANAGEMENT

It is important that all faculty involved in implementing the IM program have a common understanding of the desired outcomes and the planned strategies for the program. Initial orientation of faculty to the goals of the IM program and how it fits into the PBL curriculum is essential, as is ongoing communication and support. In order to do this, faculty need to be very comfortable with the skills themselves. Role modeling of the skills is a powerful tool, not only in the educational but also in the clinical and research settings. Particularly in the entry-level courses, faculty should play a major role in identifying the need for skills training and the evaluation of the students' progress. By assisting students to set focused learning objectives, to identify sources of information, to evaluate search strategies and the information found, and to relate the information back to the problem scenario, faculty can challenge the students to enhance their skills and broaden their range of information sources.

The faculty tutor could become a mentor to the students by demonstrating the skills at the appropriate time based on the students' learning needs. For instance, if the faculty tutor has access to the Internet, she or he could spend part of class time with the students searching the Web using the identified learning question. The problem-based, self-directed, small group class lends itself to these activities.

In order to provide these kinds of support to students, faculty need to develop the skills themselves. This can be done concurrently as students are learning the skills, or some faculty may chose to attend the introductory sessions on information searching which are usually available in the library. Wherever possible, hands-on training should be offered. If the tutor or students identify particular problems or learning issues around their skill development, special resource sessions should be arranged. This "on demand" training is a much more successful way to introduce and reinforce skills, since students (and faculty) are motivated to practice the skills immediately in response to their identified needs.

Training is particularly important for the development of informatics skills. Saranto and Tallberg (1998) found that although nursing informatics is acknowledged to be important, relatively few undergraduate nursing programs have actually implemented and integrated it into the curriculum. Their study concluded nurse educators are often unfamiliar with the software available for nursing education purposes and they lack the confidence in their abilities. Educators themselves indicated they would need regular training to maintain their skills.

FACULTY–LIBRARY COLLABORATION

Librarians and nursing faculty should work together closely when developing a program to incorporate information management skills into the nursing curriculum. The involvement of a librarian will help to ensure the inclusion of essential information management concepts (Layton and Hahn, 1995; Weaver, 1993). Librarians have the education and experience and libraries have the resources needed to support a program. However, to make the most productive use of the library and its staff, faculty must work with them, since they know the particular requirements of the nursing curriculum. Librarians can and should serve on curriculum committees, helping to set objectives, develop evaluation tools, and organize support structures. If at all possible, they should also take on roles as co-tutors in PBL and critical appraisal of research literature courses.

Faculty tutors and librarians also work together to develop resources that will assist students in learning information management skills. Examples include worksheets (described earlier in the chapter), a workbook on setting up a filing system, and overviews of how to search and retrieve information resources. These should be included in the course manual or student handbook, along with the information management objectives. As students become ever more comfortable and dependent on the World Wide Web, consideration should be given to setting up Web pages including links to recommended online resources.

A core element for a successful program is ready access to information resources, including an appropriately established library and computer lab. The mutual respect for skill sets and the open exchange of ideas between two professions, nursing and librarianship, strengthens the learning environment, and has proven to be a powerful combination (Ellis, Carpio, and Bayley, 1999).

CONCLUSION

Professional nursing practice requires nurses to have skills in assessing, critiquing, and using information in order to provide effective and current care to their patients. It is essential that nursing education includes outcomes and course requirements that enable students to develop these skills. PBL, with its emphasis on identifying learning issues and finding information to address those issues, is ideally suited to the integration of information management skills into the curriculum.

REFERENCES

Association of College and Research Libraries. Task Force on Information Literacy Competency Standards. (2000). Information literacy competency standards for higher education. *College & Research Libraries News, 61*(3), 207–215.

Allegri, F. (1995). Course integrated instruction: metamorphosis for the twenty-first century. *Medical Reference Services Quarterly, 4*(4), 47–66.

Bachman, J. A. and Panzarine, S. (1998). Enabling student nurses to use the information superhighway. *Journal of Nursing Education, 37*(4), 155–161.

Blythe, J. and Royle, J. A. (1993). Assessing nurses' information needs in the work environment. *Bulletin of the Medical Library Association, 81*(4), 433–435.

Blythe, J., Royle, J. A., Oolup, P., Potvin, C., and Smith, S. D. (1995). Linking the professional literature to nursing practice: challenges and opportunities. *AAOHN Journal, 43*(6), 342–345.

Breivik, P. S. (1991). Information literacy. *Bulletin of the Medical Library Association, 79*(2), 226–229.

Breivik, P. (1985). Putting libraries back into the Information Society. *American Library, 16,* 723.

Breivik, P. and Gee, E. G. (1989). *Information Literacy: Revolution in the Library.* New York: American Council on Education: Macmillan.

Cheek, J. and Doskatsch, I. (1998). Information literacy: A resource for nurses as lifelong learners. *Nurse Education Today, 18*(3), 243–250.

College of Nurses of Ontario. (1999). *Entry to practice competencies for Ontario Registered Nurses as of January 1, 2005.*

Ellis, P., Carpio, B., and Bayley, L. (1999). Faculty informatics mentorship: A pilot project. Paper presented at the 19th Annual Lilly Conference on College Teaching, November 19–21, 1999, Oxford, Ohio. <http://www.muohio.edu/lillycon/99ProposalBook.htm#z17a> [2000, July 21]

Flemming, K. (1998). EBN notebook. Asking answerable questions. *Evidence-Based Nursing, 1*(2), 36–37.

Fox, L. M., Richter, J. M., and White, N. (1989). Pathways to information literacy. *Journal of Nursing Education, 28*(9), 422–425.

Fox, L. M., Richter, J. M., and White, N. E. (1996). A multidimensional evaluation of a nursing information-literacy program. *Bulletin of the Medical Library Association, 84*(2), 182–190.

Grobe, S. J. (1988). Nursing informatics competencies for nurse educators and researchers. In *Preparing nurses for using information systems: Recommended informatics competencies.* National League for Nursing Publications. NAN PUB. #14-2234.

Layton, B. and Hahn, K. (1995). The librarian as a partner in nursing education. *Bulletin of the Medical Library Association, 83*(4), 499–502.

Lenburg, C. B. (1999). Redesigning expectations for initial and continuing competence for contemporary nursing practice. *Online Journal of Issues in Nursing. Sept. 30, 1999.* <http://www.nursingworld.org/ojin/topic10/tpc10_1.htm> [2000, June 18]

Redman, R. W., Lenburg, C. B., and Walker, P. H. (1999). Competency assessment: Methods for development and implementation in nursing education. *Online Journal of Issues in Nursing. Sept. 30,1999.* <http://www.nursingworld.org/ojin/topic10/tpc10_3.htm> [2000, June 18]

Saranto, K. and Tallberg, M. (1998). Nursing informatics in nursing education: A challenge to nurse teachers. *Nurse Education Today, 18*(1), 79–87.

Sibbald, B. (1998). Nursing informatics for beginners. *Canadian Nurse, 94*(4), 22–30.

Travis, L. and Brennan, P. F. (1998). Information science for the future: An innovative nursing informatics curriculum. *Journal of Nursing Education, 37*(4), 162–168.

Verhey, M. P. (1999). Information literacy in an undergraduate nursing curriculum: Development, implementation, and evaluation. *Journal of Nursing Education, 38*(6), 252–259.

Weaver, S. M. (1993). Information literacy: Educating for life-long learning. *Nurse Educator, 18*(4), 30–32.

Fostering Reflection and Reflective Practice

Barbara Brown, Nancy Matthew-Maich, and Joan Royle

A competent professional nurse, in a quality setting, will practice according to standards, and engage in reflective practice and on-going learning, to provide appropriate, effective and ethical care, that contributes to the best possible health outcome for the client. (CNO, 1996)

PREPARING FOR THE FUTURE: THE CHALLENGE FOR REFLECTION IN NURSING EDUCATION

If professional practice is about change, development and meaningful conscious action, the art of reflection, becomes a prerequisite. (Burrows, 1995, p. 347)

Mezirow (1990) claims that as we move into the post-modern era, changes in old sources of authority, taken-for-granted norms, and culturally dictated power and privilege force us to critically reflect on the paradigms that we were previously taught to understand our everyday experiences. This in turn holds the potential to profoundly influence our lives; how we interpret our experiences, relationships, work, organizations, and the entire socioeconomic system. In a time of unprecedented social, technical, and professional change, nursing graduates must be equipped with skills of problem solving and ongoing learning, plus critical, innovative, and creative thinking. They must continuously learn from their experiences, apply relevant theory, and develop new practice-based theories as the context evolves (Brookfield, 1995; Cranton, 1992; Mezirow, 1991; Schön, 1987). Educators can no longer make "deposits" of knowledge into students and adequately prepare them for a professional future. Consequently, educational theorists have embraced reflection to prepare professionals for the future.

The modern nursing profession is committed to reflective practice. The United Kingdom Central Council for Nursing (UKCC) and the College of Nurses of Ontario, Canada (CNO) have adopted reflection as a mandatory and essential component of nursing practice and registration. The future nurse will be required to present evidence of a personal philosophy, goals, and objectives and exhibit knowledge and skills based on established standards and competencies (Ryan and Carlton, 1997). This is a present reality for nurses in Canada and the United Kingdom and reflection is the thread enabling this process (Alsop, 1995; Matthew-Maich, Brown, and Royle, 2000).

Problem-based learning (PBL) is also a thread that is woven through the rationale for the changes required in nursing education, to foster the qualities of decision making, autonomy of practice, creativity, inquiry, and effective team membership expected in post-modern nursing practice. As noted in Chapter 2, PBL is purported to develop these qualitites through the process of self-directed study, small group work and the application of learning to the understanding and/or resolution of patient issues. Inherent in PBL is the self-evaluation of learning which Cranton (1992) suggests occurs through critical reflection. While Woods (1994) identifies reflection as one step in PBL, we suggest that reflection permeates the entire PBL process. Reflective deliberation is required not only to assess the need for new knowledge, the possible approaches to problem resolution and what needs to be done next, but also in the recall and analysis of the effectiveness of the actions and processes used. Through self-evaluation and self-monitoring, students are expected to evaluate their own strengths and areas for improvement, to determine their future learning needs and proceed to meet these needs.

In PBL the faculty act as facilitators with the expectation that they, along with their students, become active participants in the learning, collaboration, and evaluation process. Thus reflection can be seen as a central and integral component of PBL. Using a reflective approach to nursing practice both personally and professionally is one of the hallmarks of a PBL nursing graduate (Wolff, 2000). Consequently, the purpose of this chapter is to explore: What is reflection? What are the pitfalls? How can reflection be facilitated? How is it integrated into PBL? How can it be assessed? What successes and struggles can be shared? What are future directions?

EXPLORING REFLECTION AND REFLECTIVE PRACTICE: IN QUEST OF A DEFINITION

No need is more fundamentally human than our need to understand the meaning of our experience. Free, full participation in critical and reflective discourse may be interpreted as a basic human right (Mezirow, 1990, p. 11).

Contemporary work involving reflection and reflective practice is strongly influenced by Dewey (1933) who described reflection as, "a better way of thinking" and "the active, persistent and careful consideration of any belief or supposed form of knowledge in the light of the grounds that support it and the further conclusions to which it leads—it includes a conscious involuntary effort to establish belief upon a firm basis of evidence and rationality"

(p. 9). Numerous writers have contributed definitions of reflection and reflective practice, among them Boud, Keogh, and Walker (1985); Boyd and Fayles (1983); Glen, Clarke, and Nichol (1995); Jarvis (1992); Reid (1993); Reed and Proctor (1993); and Wong, Kember, Chung, and Yan (1995). Hancock (1998) reviews the numerous definitions that exist, and concludes that they contain the following common characteristics that define effective reflective practice:

> . . . be based in practice; be capable of developing new knowledge; be consciousness raising; help turn experience into learning; raise self awareness; develop intellectual skills; liberate individuals from conventional, traditional ways of thinking; be creative; and be both an adult and experiential learning technique." (p. 38)

OFFERING CRITICAL REFLECTION PROCESSES: THE ROAD TO EMANCIPATORY EDUCATION

> Learning . . . is defined in terms of not merely acquiring knowledge or gathering and correlating facts, but in seeing the significance of life as a whole, discovering lasting values, relating learning to personal reality experiences, and being aware of social injustices. (Bevis and Murray, 1990, p. 330)

In exploring processes of reflection, various levels, stages, cycles, models, and frameworks have been identified by numerous authors (Atkins and Murphy, 1993; Boyd and Fayles, 1983; Boud et al., 1985; Dewey, 1933; Goodman, 1984; Mezirow, 1981, 1990; Schön, 1991; Van Manen, 1977). While a detailed description and analysis is beyond the scope of this chapter, and the reader is encouraged to seek out the original sources in the listed references, it is important to address to some degree the philosophical and theoretical underpinnings associated with the process of reflection as they lead us to understand the nature and practice of reflection in nursing and the PBL process.

Dewey's (1933) seminal work on reflective thinking serves as a foundation for this chapter section. Building on his definition of reflection, Dewey offers a reflective process model which briefly includes: (1) pre-reflection or the "state of doubt" that sets thinking in motion; (2) reflection, which is akin to problem solving and characterized by five phases including suggestions, problem, hypothesis, reasoning, and testing; and (3) post-reflection in which, having solved the problem, there is a feeling of "mastery, satisfaction, enjoyment" and "restored stability." He suggests that this sequence is not fixed, a phase can be expanded, left out, or overlap and persist for a period of time.

Reflection is also purported by Van Manen (1977) to consist of three levels, where the first and second levels of reflection include technical aspects and understanding practice while the third level involves exploration of the underpinnings of practice including the moral–ethical aspects.

Goodman (1984) supports Van Manen's (1977) reflective levels and describes the three levels as: reflection with techniques to reach a given objective; reflection on the relationship between principles and practice; and reflection building on the above through incorporation of ethical and political concerns. James and Clarke (1992, 1994) have added a fourth level or domain of nursing knowledge in which reflection can take place, where the focus of reflection for the nurse is "knowledge of herself" which entails an exploration of personal qualities and attributes along with experiences. This domain also serves the cognitive interests of emancipation and liberation (James and Clarke, 1994). Ultimately nurses who are "genuinely critical of their own practice" will use all four levels and only then will they "come to fully understand their own practice" (p. 86). Herein lies the attraction of reflection to nursing.

In looking at the process of reflection from the viewpoint of the learner, Boud et al. (1985) start with the premise that any useful model of reflection must indicate the processes that need to be considered, draw attention to the importance of reflective activity, and plan for the reflective stage of the learning process. To meet this end, they too propose a three-stage model. Stage 1 is Returning to Experience(s), which is recollecting thoughts, feelings, and actions in order to reconstruct a particular experience, which Bolt and Powell (1993) contend is not as straightforward as might be suggested since memory and personal constructs influence perceptions. Boud et al. (1985) label Stage 2 as Attending to Feelings, which involves "focussing on positive feelings about learning and the experience which is subject to reflection" (p. 26) and removing obstructive feelings in order to "facilitate continued support for future learners" (p. 30). Re-evaluating Experiences is the third and most important stage and involves association, interpretation, validation, and appropriation. The latter is similar to Boyd and Fayle's (1983) concept of "change in self, which can be accelerated by the level of support, encouragement and facilitative interventions from teachers" and, perhaps most important, by alerting learners "to the nature of reflection in the learning process" (Boud et al., 1985, p. 38).

In light of the varied descriptions and processes of reflection that exist in the literature, Atkins and Murphy (1993) conducted an exhaustive review to identify shared meanings. They concluded that the differences in accounts of the reflective process are largely due to "terminology, detail and the extent to which the processes are arranged in a hierarchy" (p. 1189). Essentially, Atkins and Murphy determined three common phases in the reflective process which Scanlan and Chernomas (1997) suggest are the most useful for nursing education (Figure 6.1).

The first stage of the process is triggered by an awareness of uncomfortable feelings and thoughts, which provides insights that present knowledge is insufficient to explain or deal with the situation at hand. Schön (1983) describes this as a feeling of surprise, while Boyd and Fayles (1983) label it as inner discomfort. During the second stage, a critical analysis of the situation

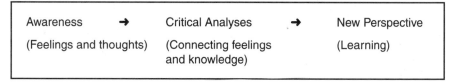

Figure 6.1 The Reflective Process
Atkins, S. M. and Murphy, K. (1993). Reflection: A review of the literature. *Journal of Advanced Nursing, 18,* 1188–1192. Reprinted with permission.

occurs that is constructive and involves an examination of one's feelings and knowledge base. The practitioner may analyse existing knowledge, apply other knowledge, and may examine or generate new knowledge. Finally, a new perspective results that may include new attitudes, values, beliefs, and/or behaviors. Mezirow (1990) identifies this stage as *perspective transformation* while Schön (1983) labels it as *action.*

PBL tutorials set the stage for the process of reflection and reflective practice to be played out over the course of the nursing program. The stages of reflection described by Atkins and Murphy (1993) bear a distinct resemblance to aspects of PBL. A problem scenario is introduced without previous preparation or study. In generating a number of possible hypotheses, students recognize that existing knowledge is insufficient to explain the problem that gives rise to an inner discomfort which leads to identifying learning issues and gathering information. As Rideout and Carpio point out in Chapter 2, it is within the group that acquired knowledge is discussed and debated and applied back to the presenting patient scenario. The second stage of reflection calls for this type of critical analysis. The final step consists of summarizing and integrating the learning that has occurred through processing the patient scenario. This creates the third stage of reflection in which a changed perspective results in new cognitive and affective outcomes. In turn, the self-directed learning element promotes reflection in the form of evaluation of self and group progress in the context of achieving identified learning objectives (Wolff, 2000). If this reflective stage does not happen, Wolff contends that the impact of PBL is lost.

BECOMING A CRITICALLY REFLECTIVE STUDENT: THE NECESSARY SKILLS

> . . . [C]ertain cognitive and affective skills are necessary to engage in reflection" (Atkins and Murphy, 1993, p. 1190)

The acceptance of reflection in nursing education must come with the caveat that the development of reflective practice is complex and that a number of factors influence this process. If nurse educators are to facilitate reflective practice in their students, they must first be aware of these factors and secondly foster skills that promote reflective practitioners. Mezirow (1990) believes that critical reflection is the hallmark of adult learning, yet Burrows (1995) is concerned that most university students are not ready for this level of reflection. In their seven-stage developmental reflective judgment model, Kitchener and King (1990) suggest that while reflective judgment begins in pre-teen years, critical reflective judgment or the seventh stage does not develop until the late twenties or early thirties. With the majority of nursing students ranging from 18 to 23 years of age, their cognitive readiness for reflective thinking needs to be considered (Burrows, 1995). Kitchener and King (1990) support this based on their discovery that older students recognized the value of reflection and thus more thoroughly maintained their journals, while younger students frequently cited excuses for not completing their reflections such as lack of time, boredom, and not seeing the usefulness of the task.

Burrows (1995) suggests that since reflective judgment has only begun to develop in the early undergraduate years, it is prudent to introduce students to the concepts of reflection and the skills and practice needed just as students are introduced to other needed learning skills, such as SDL skills. Atkins and Murphy (1993) recognize an assumption inherent in the reflection literature that certain cognitive and affective skills are necessary for reflection including self-awareness, description, critical analysis, synthesis, and evaluation (Table 6.1). Certainly, few students are going to start out with these skills; they need to be nurtured and developed over time as students learn to use reflection and reflective practice. Reflection should be a natural outcome of the PBL process, since the cognitive and affective skills summarized above are an integral part of the PBL process. Woods (1994) points out that, in the context of personal growth through SDL and self-evaluation, reflection amounts to the students "deliberately taking time to recall and analyse the actions you took and the processes you used" (pp. 1–19).

DEVELOPING THE CRITICALLY REFLECTIVE TEACHER: AUTHENTIC VOICES

We teach to change the world. (Brookfield, 1995, p. 1)

Scanlan and Chernomas (1997) contend that "to teach reflectively, we must be reflective ourselves" (p. 1141). They go on to suggest that this means thinking about ourselves as teachers; modeling reflective strategies and, in turn, using specific teaching strategies to encourage students to become reflective. Ultimately, assisting students to adopt reflection requires nurse educators to evaluate their own teaching. The need for faculty engaging in

Table 6.1   *Skills Required to Promote Reflection*

Skill	Definition
Self-awareness	An honest examination of feelings
	• How did this experience affect me?
	• Why is this experience important to me?
Description	Accurate recall of experiences in detail
	• What happened including thoughts and feelings?
Critical analysis	Examining all aspects of the experience including:
	• challenging assumptions
	• identifying current knowledge
	• seeking alternatives
	• What sense can I make of this experience?
	• What are the significant aspects of this experience?
	• How is this like other experiences?
Synthesis	Integration of new and current knowledge to creatively solve problems and predict consequences.
	• How will I apply this to another experience?
	• What will I change or complement in my nursing care?
Evaluation	Making value judgments using criteria and standards.
	• How has this experience changed my values, by beliefs?
	• How do I think about others?

Adapted from Atkins, S. and Murphy, K. (1993). Reflection: A review of the literature. *Journal of Advanced Nursing, 18,* 1188–1192.

PBL to reflect on their philosophy of education, and their values as educators is acknowledged as the first step in making the transition from conventional to problem-based teacher, and faculty development programs to foster this transition are described in Chapter 8.

Brookfield (1995) suggests reflective teaching can best be achieved by accessing data from four sources: (1) through our autobiography as teachers; (2) through the eyes of our students; (3) through interaction with colleagues; and (4) through continual learning about educational theory and practice (Table 6.2).

The *value of autobiography* is widely supported and can be achieved in several ways, including self-assessment, keeping a reflective journal, having annual career reviews (Scanlan and Chernomas, 1997) and developing a teaching portfolio (Jensen and Saylor, 1994). In courses that use the PBL Model, faculty self-evaluation, done weekly after each tutorial and upon completion of the course, is suggested by Wolff (2000), so that reflection on areas of strength as well as those for improvement can occur. A teaching

Table 6.2 *Strategies to Promote Reflective Teaching*

Autobiographies as Teachers/Learners

Teaching Logs	• weekly record of critical incidents
Teacher Learner Audits	• recently developed skills, knowledge, and insights
Role Model Profiles	• choice and description of role models
Survival Advice Memos	• best advice memo to successor
Videotaping	• see yourself as others see you
Peer Observation	• observations of teaching practice
Ideology Critique	• critical incidents to explore embedded ideologies and alternatives

Students' Eyes

Student Learning Journals	• regularly compiled summaries of learning experiences
Troubleshooting	• class time devoted to process issues
Participant Learning Portfolios	• cumulative document of learning and reflection for assessment
Letters to Successors	• survival strategies for new students
Survival Keynote Exercise	• five minute survival skills introduction to new students
Critical Incident Questionnaire	• information about student learning, emotional sphere and effects of teaching
Communicating Rationale	• teaching philosophy as part of course outline

Colleagues' Experiences

Critical Conversation	• respective, inclusive, and democratic structured discussions
	• can use a variety of strategies
Good Practice Audit	• three-phase process to find good responses to common problems

Reading Theory Critically

Asking Epistemological Questions	• search for assertions of truth
Asking Experiential Questions	• view written descriptions of teaching from our own experiences
Asking Communicative Questions	• become aware of power and control in educational writing
Asking Political Questions	• make own values and preferences clear

Summarized from Brookfield (1995). *Becoming a Critically Reflective Teacher.* San Francisco: Jossey-Bass.

portfolio also incorporates that level of analysis, since it usually begins with reflective statements of beliefs about nursing and teaching philosophy and goals. A number of other evidences about teaching are provided, and the portfolio concludes with a reflective summary based on a critical self-reflection of teaching (Brown et al., 1995).

Seeing ourselves as teachers *through our students' eyes* is what Brookfield (1995) considers "the most fundamental meta-criterion for judging whether or not good teaching is happening" (p. 35). End-of-course evaluations provide one opportunity to learn about students' perceptions of a course and how they were taught (Scanlan and Chernomas, 1997), although Brookfield cautions these can be viewed as mere satisfaction indexes. Students should also give verbal feedback and complete faculty evaluations during and at the end of term since students can provide helpful and meaningful feedback. Interestingly, Wolff (2000) points out that tutors "are more likely to be motivated to improve when a discrepancy exists between their perceptions of themselves and the students' perceptions" (p. C-9).

While developing critical reflection usually begins from the autobiographical perspective, only when others are involved can it reach fruition (Brookfield, 1995). *Our peers* can act as reflective mirrors by observing our teaching and engaging in critical discussions which in turn helps us "to check, reframe and broaden our own theories of practice" (p. 35). Scanlan and Chernoma (1997) encourage "coaching each other" in reflective teaching through formal and informal situations such as talking at coffee, having teaching seminars, sharing teaching stories, discussions and including teaching in year-end curriculum reviews. Cranton (1996) suggests keeping a shared journal with a colleague; discussing the reflective component of your teaching portfolio with a colleague; justifying your teaching practice with a colleague; analysing videotapes of your teaching with a colleague or writing a description of a favourite educator's philosophy.

The final strategy for assisting faculty on their journey to being critically reflective is involvement in *ongoing learning*, whether it is through formal or informal means (Brookfield, 1995). The importance of this strategy is evident in the courses and workshops available as part of faculty development programs where the PBL Model is being implemented (see Chapter 8 for more detail).

Scanlan and Chernomas (1997) reiterate the importance of reflection on teaching if we are to assist students to become critically reflective: "[it is] through reflection that the teacher is able to come to a personal understanding of his/her/our practice, developing a framework of practice which facilitates further development of professional expertise" (p. 1143). It seems imperative that some combination of the strategies outlined above becomes a part of each nursing faculty members' practice if they are to be the role models, mentors, and guides to reflective practice required now and into the future.

STRATEGIES FOR FACILITATING REFLECTION

As the discussion above indicates, educators have a significant role in the development of reflection and reflective skills in their students. What processes facilitate the development of reflective practitioners? In the following sections of this chapter a number of specific faculty interventions are described that will assist students to become critically reflective of their learning *and* their nursing practice.

Facilitating Reflection: Being Available

> Reflective practice, as a concept, cannot be given but rather needs to be shared (Reid, 1993, p. 309).

The process begins within ourselves as educators and the relationship we hold with our students. Andrews (1996a) suggests the best method available to becoming reflective is to learn with an experienced, committed mentor, who is a credible, effective, and reflective practitioner (Reid, 1993). As discussed previously, the more we understand our own experiences, the better prepared we will be to facilitate reflection with our students through role modeling, dialogue, and facilitation of reflective strategies.

To optimally facilitate reflection, a positive, collaborative, valued relationship with the teacher and reflector must occur within an equal power base (John, 1997; Kim, 1999). There is a consensus in the literature that educators/mentors cannot facilitate reflection with students without giving up their authoritative power position, so that teachers and students work together to discover meanings through a collaborative partnership. Pierson (1998) claims that teachers must feel as vulnerable as students by sharing their thoughts, feelings, and experiences openly with students. This shared vulnerability leads to shared trust, open and honest sharing of thoughts, feelings, and experiences. Trust is a critical element of this relationship, since it enables and uncovers shared meaning and understanding between students and teachers (Heinrich, 1992; Paterson, 1995; Tryssenaar, 1995). Such a relationship develops slowly within an atmosphere of mutual respect and care, through interactive and participatory shared dialogue (Pierson 1998).

Johns (1998) has developed a "Being Available" framework (Table 6.3) that depicts the desired relationship between the mentor and reflector to optimally facilitate reflection. This relationship offers a "transformative milieu" that enhances the responsibility of the student or practitioner to monitor her own practice to ensure its effectiveness.

The faculty role in the PBL Model emphasizes these same qualities and behaviors that are required to facilitate the development of critical reflection. Wolff (2000) provides a useful summary of the PBL faculty roles and responsibilities that are analogous with "being available." In the role of "creator," the faculty tutor helps to foster a safe learning environment so that

Table 6.3 *"Being Available" Framework*

Clinical Context		Guided Reflection Context
Concern		Positive regard
		• Practitioner commitment
Knowing the person	Being available to work with the client/practitioner	Knowing the practitioner
		• Creating a climate for disclosure of experiences
		• Knowing their practice
Responding with appropriate ethical, informed, and skilled interventions	Shared vision	Responding with an appropriate helping style
		• Balance of challenge and support
		• Framing perspectives
Knowing and managing self within a relationship		Knowing and managing self within a relationship
		• Controlling the agenda
		• Managing own concerns
Creating and sustaining an environment where being available is possible		Creating and sustaining an environment where being available is possible
		• Practicalities of ensuring frequent continuity supervision
		• Conducive environment

Johns, C. and McCormack, B. (1998). Unfolding the conditions where the transformative potential of guided reflection (Clinical Supervision) might flourish or flounder. In C. Johns and D. Freshwater (Eds.), *Transforming Nursing Through Reflective Practice* (p. 65). Oxford: Blackwell Science. Reprinted with permission.

students will explore and reflect without demeaning personal integrity and self-confidence. As a "facilitator," the faculty tutor guides the students through their thinking and reflections. Faculty need to be "designers" in that they design learning situations that will generate appropriate learning objectives by the students. As a "challenger" the faculty tutor encourages students to be reflective in exploring their attitudes and beliefs, and the role of "negotiator" is essential as the faculty member "negotiates meaning and probes the limits of the students' understanding" (Wolff, 2000, A-26). Students appreciate seeing the faculty member as a "learner" as well, and this can be demonstrated during formative and summative tutorial evaluations, when the faculty tutor models the same performance that he/she expects of students, offering constructive feedback to students but also emulating critical reflection through their self evaluations. As Woods (1994) states "trust is the glue that builds relationships" (p. S-5) and faculty should facilitate trusting relationships that enhance being reflective.

Facilitating Reflection: Setting the Stage

> Psychiatric patients are just like you and me. (Year III Student)

Nurse educators must clearly articulate to their students the purpose and aims of reflection, their expectations, and also the limits or boundaries. The literature consistently suggests that we provide clear guidelines; an early introduction to reflection and reflective practice; a clear, thorough orientation to self-reflection; and specific strategies such as journaling, portfolio development, and reflective dialogue (Alsop, 1995; Burrows, 1995; Glen and Hight, 1992; Mitchell, 1994; Paterson, 1995; Snowball, Ross, and Murphy, 1994; Walker, 1985; Witmer, 1996).

A set of concepts that can guide facilitating reflection were developed by Durgahee (1998) with the acronym, PACTS: Purposeful; Action; Collaboration; Thinking, Critical Thinking; and Support and Confrontation summarizes these concepts. First, "students must experience reflection as a purposeful activity centred towards clarification and discovery of knowledge" (p. 161). They want to know the aim of the reflective session(s), their role, boundaries, ground rules, and how it will be done. This "knowing" reduces insecurities and hastens trust and open sharing. Second, since reflection is an active process, the faculty member must enable students to become active participants by working together on practice-based issues. Third, fostering collaboration assists the students to participate more actively, and serves as a mechanism to take risks in learning. Fourth, encouragement of critical thinking is part of the faculty role. "The strategy is to put clinical situations under the microscope and dissect them into smaller components to identify the various issues which form the situation" (p. 162). Fifth, there must be a continuous balance between confrontation and support. Consequently, Durgahee (1998) suggests that, in using these concepts to facilitate reflection, the role of the faculty member moves "from a sage on the stage to a guide on the side" (p. 158) as the students tap into their own "reservoirs of knowledge and untapped potential."

Using Critical Reflection Frameworks: A Window to Look Inside

> . . . [A]s people reflect on themselves and their performance in some setting, they open themselves up to the possibility of change. (Boud et al., 1985, p. 115)

There is considerable support for the use of frameworks to assist beginning students to develop their skills, which can be adjusted as the practitioner becomes skilled with reflection (Foster and Greenwood, 1998; Johns, 1998). Although some critics oppose the use of frameworks claiming that they may be too rigid, too compartmentalized and may cause the practitioner to lose the "uniqueness of the experience" (Heath, 1998), it is generally recognized that a framework is not intended to imply how the practitioner "should" reflect, but rather it serves as a guide to get the practitioner started. In time, the questions will fuse with the practitioner's context and personal self and be adapted to the individuals' uniqueness (Johns, 1998).

There are numerous reflective frameworks available and a sampling of them will be used to demonstrate the progression of facilitating critical reflection in nursing students from simple to complex or, in the terminology of Argyris and Schön (1974), from single- to double-loop learning, or "deep" reflection (Clarke, James, and Kelly, 1996).

Framework for Reflective Action

Burrows' (1995) Framework for Reflective Action (Table 6.4) has been included to represent a framework designed to facilitate single loop learning or simple reflection. She asserts that the cue questions are effective with students who are inexperienced with reflection. She encourages students not to reflect daily but to follow Schön's "element of surprise" and "ad hoc" reflections on both difficult and positive experiences. Once students are comfortable with this format, they can move onto more complex reflective frameworks.

LEARN Framework for Reflection

A more complex framework that is used extensively is the LEARN framework for reflection (CNO, 1996). LEARN (Figure 6.2) is an acronym for the five steps in reflective process: Look back; Elaborate; Analyze; Revise; and New trial. It was developed by the College of Nurses of Ontario (CNO) as part of the Quality Assurance (QA) program for all nurses registered in Ontario, Canada. Reflection is the cornerstone of this QA program.

Table 6.4 *Framework for Reflective Action*

- Describe events as you understand them.
- Describe your feelings about the event.
- What have you learned from this event?
- Given a similar situation in future, how would you behave?
- In what ways do the theories of psychology, sociology, biology, and nursing research underpin the situation you have witnessed?

Adapted from Burrows, D. B. (1995). The nurse teacher's role in the promotion of reflective practice. *Nurse Education Today, 15,* 346–350. Reprinted with permission.

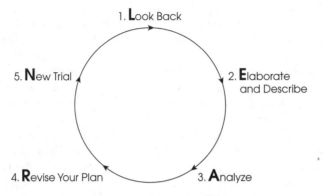

Figure 6.2 LEARN: GUIDELINES FOR REFLECTION
College of Nurses of Ontario. (1996). *Professional profile: A reflective portfolio for contin-uous learning.* Toronto: CNO. Reprinted with permission.

LEARN is unique in that its simplest form can be used by novice reflec-tors and practitioners to facilitate simple, single loop learning. As students mature in practice and reflective ability they can take this tool to different levels to reflect more deeply and critically. As they gain skill and confidence with reflection, students begin to respond more comprehensively to the cue questions (Table 6.5) to facilitate an enhanced depth of reflection; double-loop or critical reflection. Profound personal and professional insights and growth in nursing students and practitioners has resulted from using LEARN to guide their reflections (Witmer, 1997).

Model of Structured Reflection

Johns' (1998) Model of Structured Reflection (MSR) exemplifies a complex framework used to foster double-loop learning and critical reflection (Table 6.6). Johns (1994, 1995, 1998) considers his MSR a "heuristic device to enable practitioners to penetrate the essence of reflection on experience" (Johns, 1998, p. 3). This model is comprised of a set of questions which he calls reflective cues and these guide the nurse into practice in a structured and meaningful way. The reflective cues are built on Carper's (1978) ways of knowing in nursing which include the empirical, ethical, personal, and esthetic, which have been widely acclaimed as providing a way to help nurses "to see, value, embrace and know human caring in deeply personal ways" (Johns, 1995, p. 233).

Categories of Reflective Outcomes

Wong et al. (1995) used Mezirow's three categories of reflection: nonreflec-tors, reflectors, and critical reflectors to classify reflective statements in their

Table 6.5 *The Five Reflective Practice Steps*

Step 1:	**L**ook back at an experience or event that happened in your practice recently. Review it in your mind as if you were watching a video.
Step 2:	**E**laborate and describe, verbally or in writing, what happened during the event. How did you feel and how do you think others felt? What were the outcomes? Were you surprised by what happened during the event or did it turn out as you expected?
Step 3:	**A**nalyze the outcomes. Review why the event turned out the way it did. Why did you feel or react the way you did, and why did others feel/react the way they did? If the event or outcomes were not what you expected, consider how you could improve on them next time. This is an opportunity to really question your beliefs and assumptions, and ask yourself what the experience reveals about what you value. It is also a great time to ask for feedback from others.
Step 4:	**R**evise your approach based on your review of the event and decide how, or if, you will change your approach. This might involve asking others for ideas for dealing with the situation next time or how to work on a learning need. With your new learning, you may decide to try a new approach, learn more about the subject, or decide that you handled the situation very well.
Step 5:	**N**ew trial. Put your new approach into action. This may require anticipating or creating a situation in which you can then try out your new approach.

Together, these steps form the word **LEARN.**

Witmer, D. (1997). Making the choice. What reflective practice option is best for me? *College Communique.* March 15–18. Reprinted with permission.

nursing students' journals. The *nonreflectors* were descriptive and impersonal, tended to report on what was happening, made assumptions without testing their validity or providing supportive evidence, and thinking was concrete with minimal evidence of abstract thinking. *Reflectors* were able to assess how they perceived, thought, felt, or acted. Wong et al. (1995) found, in their study of nursing students, that 75 percent of them could be classified as reflectors since they were able to recognize and describe their use of new knowledge. *Critical reflectors* challenged the validity in pure learning as they explored the "why" of their experiences, not just the "how." Features of critical reflectors were noted by Wong et al. (1995) in 11 percent of the nursing students who adopted a wide multidimensional perspective, pursued alternatives and numerous resources, tended to be courageous, and were able to change.

This framework, Categories of Reflective Outcomes, provides a tool for students, educators, practitioners, and researchers to visualize and have "hands-on criteria" to facilitate, nurture, envision, and progress reflection eventually toward critical reflection. It assists with the assessment of the practitioner's current level of reflection and provides direction to develop

Table 6.6   *Model of Structured Reflection*

Write a description of the experience.

What are the significant issues I need to pay attention to?

Reflective cues:

Aesthetics	What was I trying to achieve?
	Why did I respond as I did?
	What were the consequences of that for:
	• the patient?
	• others?
	• myself?
	How was the person(s) feeling?
	How did I know this?
Personal	How did I feel in this situation?
	What internal factors were influencing me?
Ethics	How did my actions match with my beliefs?
	What factors made me act in incongruent ways?
Empirics	What knowledge did or should have informed me?
Reflexivity	How does this connect with previous experiences?
	Could I handle this better in similar situations?
	What would the consequences be of alternative actions for:
	• the patient?
	• others?
	• myself?
	How do I now feel about this experience?
	Can I support myself and others better as a consequence?
	Has this changed my ways of knowing?

Johns, C. (1998). Opening the doors of perception. In C. Johns and D. Freshwater (Eds.), *Transforming Nursing Through Reflective Practice* (p. 4). Oxford: Blackwell Science. Reprinted with permission.

increasingly deeper, more critical reflections (double-loop learning). This tool is useful within a PBL curriculum to assess student reflections, student progress in developing skills in reflection, and to assist with giving reflective cues and feedback to students. The tool is also useful to assess levels of reflection in journals, portfolios, and dialogue in qualitative research studies (Matthew-Maich et al., 1997). Table 6.7 displays the Categories of Reflection Outcomes, adapted by the authors from the work of Mezirow (1991) and Wong et al. (1995) on identifying levels of reflection.

Table 6.7 *Categories of Reflection Outcomes*

Content Reflection	Process Reflection	Premise Reflection
Nonreflectors	Reflectors	Critical Reflectors
Habitual and Thoughtful Action	Critical Assessment and Problem-solving	Transformation of Meaning
Descriptive	Relate experiences—turn into new learning opportunities	Challenging validity in prior learning
Report on **what's** happening		Concerned with **why**—reasons and consequences
Make assumptions without testing	**How**	Finding a new metaphor that re-orients problem solving
View presented	Identify relationships between prior and new knowledge/feelings	Pursue alternatives
• no supportive evidence	Modify to new situations	Use multidimensional perspectives and resources
• no referencing to experiences	Insight and some originality	Continually examine in critical manner
Straightforward view	How to resolve problems	Critical self-reflection
Concrete "matter of fact"	• reassess strategies	Make knowledge one's own
Minimal abstract thinking	• guide action	Courageous to trying
Little awareness of contextual factors	No effort in	Adaptable to change
Impersonal	• validating assumptions	Learning
Not see learning opportunities	• making knowledge "one's own"	

Summarized from the work of Wong et al. (1995). Assessing the level of student reflection from reflective journals. *Journal of Advanced Nursing, 22,* 48–57, and Mezirow, J. (1991). *Transformative Dimensions of Adult Learning.* San Francisco: Jossey-Bass.

UNDERSTANDING THE ETHICS OF CRITICAL REFLECTION: TO REFLECT OR NOT TO REFLECT?

> Reflective practice is not simply re-examining someone's case, it involves personal interpretation and judgement. The reflector may be recording incidents . . . which would not otherwise be recorded, and may be controversial. This raises questions about the nature and ownership of knowledge, and the responsibilities of people who have such knowledge . . . considerations of rigour, authenticity and informed consent need to be addressed. (Hargreaves, 1997, p. 223)

The very nature of critical reflection—the issues it exposes, the insights it illuminates, and the uninformed clients whose experiences it frequently exposes—renders the process potentially morally and ethically volatile. The literature highlights important warnings yet evidence-based findings and suggestions for practice are lacking. Empirical research in the use of ethically sound techniques to guide reflections are urgently required (Rich and Parker, 1995).

Reflection frequently gives rise to moral dilemmas about situations that students encounter in their clinical practice, particularly if the dilemma reveals unprofessional or dangerous conduct from staff, peers or self. Failure to report this is against nursing's Professional Codes of Conduct, yet as educators we have promised strict confidentiality to the students (Rich and Parker, 1995). These authors cite examples of such revelations including: lack of care, unsafe practice, inappropriate/unprofessional attitudes toward clients and their families, conflict, and truthtelling. An example follows as recorded by a student:

> There was a leaking mask on the ambubag and when it was used for a patient during resuscitation, she died. The nurse in charge promised to replace it because it was faulty. I therefore did not report it to anyone else. Three days later, at another arrest, the same bag was used; this patient also died. I felt so guilty that I found it hard to live with myself. I felt responsible and asked myself repeatedly whether I should have taken any other action by checking up on the bag's replacement. (Rich and Parker, 1995, p. 1054).

The literature frequently describes enhanced vulnerability resulting from reflection (Brookfield, 1995; Kim, 1999; Pierson, 1998). Brookfield claims that becoming critically reflective can be humbling, humiliating, and even damaging. He states that critical reflection can . . . "bring the questions face to face with a power structure whose representatives and beneficiaries are often eager to quell dissension and discourage divergent thinking" (p. 228). He informs us that in some societies, asking critical questions can result in torture or death to deter others or the "critical" person may be labeled a trouble maker who is unwilling to play by the rules. It is important that students returning "home" to various cultures understand the potential consequences of actions.

Hargreaves (1997) emphasizes the ethical questions associated with using client experiences for reflection in written or verbal formats without

Table 6.8 *A Code of Ethics for Reflective Practice in Nurse Education*

- Core elements in any taught program should include ethical issues in reflective practice, for example, using patients, rights and responsibilities, and professional confidentiality.
- Written work submitted for assessment should include a section on the ethical considerations.
- Where reflective practice is being used as a scholarly activity, issues of consent should be considered.

Hargreaves, J. (1997). Using patients: Exploring the ethical dimension of reflective practice in nurse education. *Journal of Advanced Nursing, 25,* 227. Reprinted with permission.

their informed consent. She espouses that the professional relationship is formed on trust, confidentiality, and informed consent and asks, "will patients feel legitimately wronged" if informed that their experience is in the hands of a third party as an academic assignment? If reflections are completed without patient names, does this form of practice development differ significantly from nursing care plans, nursing rounds, medical rounds, or a clinical issue paper? If ethical issues are raised about reflection, it is our opinion that they apply similarly to these other learning formats.

It is essential that we critically reflect on the moral and ethical dimensions of encouraging critical reflection with our nursing students, to enable them to learn and grow within a safe environment. Clearly explicating for students the purpose, aims, guidelines, limits, and potential benefits and risks of critical reflection will augment the creation of this safe environment. Emerging from the moral and ethical concerns inherent in reflection, Hargreaves (1997) developed a Code of Ethics for Reflective Practice in Nursing Education and it is presented in Table 6.8.

ASSESSING REFLECTIVE LEARNING: PROCESS AND OUTCOMES

> If we accept the changing face of nursing practice and education and agree we need to expand our range of assessment tools then we can tackle the complexities of assessing clinical ability in a holistic way. . . (Burns, 1994, p. 22)

Another area of some controversy associated with reflection relates to how, and indeed, whether, reflective learning should be evaluated and graded. Several challenges have been identified. First, students (and faculty) may be uncertain about using this learning approach and therefore reluctant to see it used as part of summative evaluation (Burns, 1994). The "purpose of reflection as part of an assessment of practice" must be very clear to both students and faculty (Getliffe, 1996, p. 369).

Second, faculty members need to be cognizant of the authority and power they exert in both the learning and evaluation process. The contention is that, when there is summative evaluation of reflection, the students will reflect on what faculty want to see and hear rather than what is of interest to the student, which can inhibit true reflection (Wallace, 1996). Differing views of the influence of grading on reflection are evident, with Wellard and Bethune (1996) suggesting that "[T]here is an inherent arrogance in this positioning where the emancipator makes a value judgement on the need of another to be liberated" (p. 1080) while Fitzgerald (1994) counters that it is naive to think that "the degree of control over what nursing students learn is a potential obstruction to radical learning and out of tune with emancipatory pedagogy" (p. 73). Nevertheless, it is imperative that both students and faculty are aware of the strengths and pitfalls of assessing reflective learning.

A third challenge relates to possible inconsistencies in terms of what is expected in reflective learning and in grading. If the decision is made to assess evidence of reflection and assign a grade to it, it is imperative that clear criteria be developed and given to students at the beginning of the course for which they will be used. The work of Van Manan, Mezirow, and Goodman provide the theoretical underpinnings for the grading criteria presented in Table 6.9 that are used in the nursing program at Oxford Brookes University, and that are built on the foundation of valuing and supporting the development of a reflective practitioner (Dearmun, 1997).

Whether or not a grade is assigned to student reflections, providing formative feedback as students learn and master the process is acknowledged as both meaningful and essential. Duke and Copp (1994) point out that we need to remember reflection is a process and while, as faculty, we are responsible for offering support and providing resources "we cannot take away any distress raised by reflection" (p. 107) as this would undermine their experience. In touching on the personal side of reflection, they comment that once students have addressed their initial concerns about reflection, "many students find reflection liberating, enabling them to be in touch with their feelings when caring for others" (p. 107).

Reflection is a significant component of the PBL Model, and it is integrated into assessment measures in various ways. To illustrate, a graded assignment for beginning level students might be to work in small groups and develop a Health Fair display for other university students. Following the Health Fair, students complete a reflective summary on their experience, where the emphasis is "Reflection on Learning" and includes a brief description of the student's experience, the learning that occurred, and, based on this learning, suggestions for what they might have done differently, supported with rationale. Senior students are often expected to complete a learning portfolio containing a negotiated learning plan and evidences demonstrating achievement of the course and student objectives. The portfolio also contains assessments, projects, evaluations, and other

Table 6.9 *Example of Grading Reflective Learning Practice*

Stages in Reflection	Fail	C	B	B+	A
Identification of learning situations	Limited appreciation of module focus.	Some appreciation of module focus. Learning situations not clearly defined.	Obviously constructs experience around the module focus. Learning situations clearly defined.	Consistently recognizes potential of individual situations or critical incidents for learning. Clearly defines situations.	Realizes the potential for exploring individual situations. Highly relevant. Interprets perceptively.
Description of situation, thoughts, and feelings	Relevance of description unclear. Lacks coherence, organization, and clarity.	Lacks focus. Contains irrelevant detail, or relevance not clear.	Comprehensive. Less able to discriminate relevant and irrelevant detail. Coherence, logical organization.	Recognizes and recollects key features of situations, including context, feeling, and thoughts. Clear logical flow, concise.	Consistently captures the essence. Succinct description of relevant features. Fluent expression. Lively stimulating style.
Analysis of feelings	Lacks self-awareness in practice and limited evidence of self-awareness in the contract.	Limited self-awareness. Does not consistently recognize the feelings of others.	Consistently identifies feeling of both self and others.	Constructive exploration of feelings. Shows appreciation of how self and others felt and how that affected the situation.	Consistently demonstrates insight into the situation. Evidence that analysis of feelings has informed practice.

continued

Table 6.9 *Example of Grading Reflective Learning Practice*   continued

Stages in Reflection	Fail	C	B	B+	A
Analysis of knowledge	Very little use of previous knowledge. Very limited reading. Poor referencing.	Appears to use some previous and current knowledge. Reading limited in range and depth. Inaccurate referencing.	Identifies sources of knowledge and their relevance to the situation is evident in discussion. Range of appropriate reading and accurate referencing.	Critically discusses and analyses knowledge and literature and relationship to practice. Explores assumptions in order to question practice.	Consistently utilizes knowledge and literature relevant to the situation. Constructively challenges own and others' assumptions. Demonstrates balanced insight.
Evidence of learning	Minimal evidence.	Evidence only implicit.	Identifies some implications for own practice. Some explicit evidence of learning.	Consistently provides evidence of learning which is explicit. Identifies implications for practice. Integrates new knowledge with previous knowledge.	Evidence of learning always explicit. Consistently integrates new knowledge with previous knowledge to reach original and creative conclusions.
Identification of competency	Relevant/critical competencies not achieved in practice or limited evidence of achievement within the contract.	All relevant competencies achieved and validated. Evidence of reflection on competency only implicit.	All relevant competencies achieved and validated. Evidence of reflection on competency explicit.	All relevant competencies achieved and validated. Evidence of reflection competency explicit.	All relevant competencies achieved and validated. Evidence of reflection competency explicit.

Dearmun, A. K. (1997). Using reflection to assess degree students. *Paediatric Nursing, 9*(1), 25–28. Reprinted with permission.

information that the student wants to submit; weekly journals; and a summary reflective analysis of learning that occurred to meet their personal objectives. The overall portfolio is graded.

STIMULATING REFLECTION: SELECTED STRATEGIES

> In order for experiences to become meaningful, it is necessary for the student to reflect upon and interpret the experience by drawing upon appropriate knowledge. (Reed and Procter, 1993, p. 149)

Numerous innovative strategies are available to stimulate reflection. In selecting strategies, one must remain cognizant of their purpose, goals, context, and student characteristics. Strategies include the use of video (Burnard, 1991); drawing (Cruikshank, 1996); story writing and sharing (Baker, 1991; Heinrich, 1992); myths (Morgan, 1996); metaphors (Heinrich, 1997); peer mentoring (Heinrich and Scherr, 1994; Neville, 1999); and structured reflection (Graham, Waight, and Scammell, 1998; Johns, 1998). Usher, Francis, Owens, and Tollefson (1999) examine a number of reflective writing strategies to foster critical inquiry in nursing students including learning journals, critical incident analysis, written analysis of nursing interactions, and writing workshops. It is beyond the scope of this chapter to discuss each strategy, therefore, we will highlight those we use routinely and successfully within our PBL curriculum, specifically, journals, portfolios, small groups for PBL, and postclinical dialogue as well as self-evaluation. Each of these strategies will be discussed and examples of their application shared.

Journals

> The promise for students: in reflective journaling is to "experience not only an authentic recognition of nursing's purposes and problems, but experience as well the epiphany of feeling empowered to act on those purposes and problems. (Hawks, 1992, p. 616)

Reflective diaries or journals are frequently discussed in the nursing literature as important reflective tools. Since the terms logs, diaries, and journals are all sometimes used interchangeably, some clarification is warranted. Strackbein and Tillman (1987) explain that *logs* facilitate objective, scientific writing; *diaries,* written exclusively for oneself, engage the student in introspection; and *journals* represent diaries written for selected readers—teachers, mentors, peers, and/or colleagues (Heinrich, 1992), which include a reflective component (Landeen, Byrne, and Brown, 1992). Journals include both the objective documentation of logs and the personalized analysis and inquiry of the diary.

The reflective journal can be unstructured, semistructured, or structured (Reed and Procter, 1993). In the unstructured journal, the writer determines what, when, and how much to write. The nurse educator provides general guidelines for the semistructured journal such as important themes or categories for the student to explore in writing. Finally, in the structured journal, the time, context, and focus are completely and specifically determined by teacher guidelines.

For reflective journaling to be most effective, the following considerations are suggested in the literature:

- The experience must be safe, nonthreatening, meaningful, and satisfying (Burnard, 1988; Heinrich, 1992).
- Journaling must be student centered, process oriented, and experientially related (Reed and Procter, 1993).
- The student deserves the same respect from the teacher as is expected of the student when interacting with clients (Kobert, 1995).
- Confidentiality and teacher acceptance of openness and honesty in journal entries must be guaranteed (Burnard, 1988).
- Students need to be ritualistic in setting some time aside each day for reflection and writing (Burnard, 1988; Heinrich, 1992).
- Regularly use creative expression such as colors, pictures, comics, poetry, and jokes (Baker, 1996; Heinrich, 1992).
- Students require different levels of structure; this varies according to individual learning styles and previous experience with reflection and journal writing (Heinrich, 1992). The reflective frameworks provide a valuable resource here.
- Journal assessment should be based on "student defined learning needs" (Brockett and Hiemstra, 1991).
- When English is not the student's first language, encourage the student to write the journal entry in native language first and later translate it into English (Hancock, 1998).

Guidelines must be explicated regarding the use of the journal within the course context; the journal's role, function, the type of data or information to be recorded in the journal, and criteria for analysis and/or grading. An example of journal guidelines for beginning students in a PBL curriculum is presented in Figure 6.3.

Disagreement exists concerning the assessment of journals, just as it does concerning the assessment of reflection in general, with some of the same arguments for and against assessment, and in particular grading, being presented. Some educators feel that journals must not be graded as this may induce "false" entries as well as increase student vulnerability, and that grammar and spelling should not be emphasized to encourage free flowing thoughts and ideas (Paterson, 1995; Reed and Procter, 1993; Walker, 1985; Wellard and Bethune, 1996). Meanwhile, Holly (1989) and Matthew-Maich et al. (2000) claim that students will only invest significant effort if their work

Your journal is meant to provide you with:

a. A tool for your thinking and learning by generating ideas, exploring themes and issues, and developing critical thinking and inquiry skills
b. A channel for two-way communication with your teacher
c. A personal record of your thoughts, attitudes, beliefs, values, and challenges in becoming a nurse
d. A tool for self-evaluation, goal setting and planning in your clinical experiences
e. Preparation to fulfill the College of Nurses of Ontario's Quality Assurance expectations to maintain your Nursing license to practice

In Preparation

Buy a small binder of your favorite color or design. Make sure it feels good to look at it or be around it. You will need to keep adding pages, therefore, a binder is preferable to a notebook.

Journaling is _not_

- A personal diary
- Just a description of activities and situations you were involved in

Journaling is _more_

- It also includes your own reflections, probing, exploration, and critical analysis

Criteria for a Satisfactory Rating

Your journaling must reflect:
- Genuine individual effort
- Self-reflection and appraisal
- A spirit of inquiry
- Critical thinking
- Creative approaches to thinking and learning, integration of literature to clinical practice
- Course content, class and / or clinical experiences
- Use of the **_LEARN_** reflection tool to explore critical incidents or a variation of your choosing

***Make entries after each clinical day. Make it a habit!!!*

When are journals "due"?

- Monday by 1200 hours of Week Four and Friday post-conference in Week Six

continued

Figure 6.3 Guidelines for Journaling

Entries: When, What, and How?

Just write! Don't worry about perfection in grammar, spelling, sentence structure, etc. Entries may be made in point form, using diagrams, jokes, cartoons, pictures, quotes, or whatever. I *must* be able to read your writing.

Make entries in your journal which have meaning to you in this course; to you becoming a nurse as you reflect on your experiences that occur in class, in clinical, in life. . . .

What to Journal? During This Course?

Critical Incidents: These are any incidents which made an emotional impact. It may have been in your interaction with a client, relatives, staff, peers, teacher, etc. It could have been an incident which:

a. Was a positive experience

b. Was particularly demanding emotionally

c. You found difficult to handle, perhaps making you feel anxious or annoyed,

d. You feel that your (or a staff member's) intervention made a significant difference to the outcome of care

Use the following steps (*LEARN*) to explore and learn from experiences and critical incidents as they occur. These steps were adapted from the College of Nurses Professional Portfolio (1996).

1. *Look back:* Recall an event as clearly as possible and try to remember what was going on, almost as if you were replaying the event in your mind as a video. Explore the whole scene using all senses.

2. *Elaborate and describe* the situation in your journal.

3. *Analyze the Outcomes:* Ask yourself the following questions: Was the situation positive or negative? Why did you feel the way you did and others the way they did? What assumptions had you made? How do you feel about your experience now? Were the results of the situation what you expected? Why do you think the results occurred?

   Identify what you learned in this situation by answering the following questions in your journal:
   • What did I do in the situation? What can I now do that I couldn't before?
   • What do I know now that I didn't before?
   • What does this tell me about my attitudes and what I value?

4. *Revise Your Approach:* What do you now realize that you need to know and be able to do? What do you plan to work on and develop? How? What information do you need to gather, research? What will you do differently next time?

Figure 6.3 Guidelines for Journaling *continued*

5. **New Trial:** Consciously plan and practice your new approach and incorporate it into your practice. This may involve obtaining some new information (include this new information or your plans to obtain it). The new information may support your approach.

---

1. Sometimes I will pose questions for your reflection and journaling.
2. Sometimes you will decide to make an entry because a brilliant or challenging thought or question comes to mind. You may strongly agree or disagree with a point or issue posed by a peer, health care professional, teacher, author, etc. Probe these thoughts in your journal.
3. Remember to journal daily, following clinical, in order to maximize your learning from every experience. These reflections will often be linked with A, B, and/or C as described above.

Figure 6.3 Guidelines for Journaling *concluded*

is graded. Hodges (1996) uses journals to develop writing skills, therefore, she insists on grading student journals for content, grammar, spelling, sentence construction, clarity, critical thought, and argument development. Heinrich (1992) suggests another approach, agreeing to grade journals if her students choose this for their course evaluation, and also select the weighting toward their grade, while Wallace (1996) assesses journals based on student-defined learning needs. The best way to prevent students from writing what they think the teacher wants to read is to have peers review and assess the journals according to Cameron and Mitchell (1993). If the decision is made to grade student journals, details on how they will be assessed need to be made explicit to the students. Then, with the purpose, guidelines, and expectations clearly articulated, along with proper supports in place, journaling can offer a simple yet complex strategy to facilitate reflection and PBL.

The literature is rich with accolades for reflective journaling. It is cited as enhancing student ownership and responsibility in learning (Cameron and Mitchell, 1993); critical thinking; self-evaluation; empathy through trying on "different ways of being"; feeling and experiencing; and an understanding of "culture, history, values and beliefs and their influence on self and others" (Kobert, 1995). Heinrich's (1992) experiences with reflective journaling with all levels of nursing education have demonstrated that it fosters self-awareness; shared meaning and genuine collaboration between the teacher and student; integration of theory to practice; assessment of student writing, reading, and reflective abilities; and insight into student problems, successes, and course progress. The reflective journal facilitates the development of writing skills (Hodges, 1996; Heinrich, 1992a), increases students' observational and reporting skills (Callister, 1993), and also strengthens cross-cultural communication (Hancock, 1998). It holds the "potential to be a dynamic, non-threatening, insightful, affirming and powerful tool to make connections" (Cameron and Mitchell, 1993, p. 294), and contribute to summative graded feedback to students.

Professional Portfolios

> Simply put, a professional profile is a comprehensive document completed by the nurse that details the current state of his or her practice, background, skills, expertise and perhaps most important, a working plan for professional growth. (Trossman, 1999, p. 1)

The professional portfolio is a collection of materials that enables the practitioner to reflect on her personal and professional life, offering insight into growth, successes, learning needs, career directions, and validation from both self and others (Alsop, 1995; Budnick and Beaver, 1984; Witmer, 1995, 1996). According to Wenzel, Briggs, and Puryear (1998), a portfolio tells the story of student growth and achievement over time. The literature frequently portrays the professional portfolio as a means to develop an enlightened, holistic, and integrated practitioner. Glen and Hight (1992) suggest that professional portfolios have the potential to facilitate one's cognizance of personal and professional values and norms, self-assessment, self-evaluation skills, and lifelong learning. All of this can be very liberating and empowering for the practitioner.

Walker (1985) identifies three underlying assumptions to portfolio development. First, the learner is in control, and only the learner can learn from and reflect on her experiences. Second, reflection is focused and goal-oriented, not idle daydreaming. Third, reflection involves affective and cognitive processes that are interrelated and interactive. Positive feelings act as catalysts and negative feelings create significant barriers to the process.

The contents of a portfolio depend largely on the model and context within which it is being used. Considering the numerous potential items for inclusion, item selection can be confusing for students.

Stockhausen (1996) elucidates four areas for portfolio inclusion: *artifacts* constructed as part of the learning such as a pamphlet or questionnaire; *reproductions* depicting the developer's experience including essays, photos, drawings, or poetry; *production* documents produced as learning evidence for the portfolio such as learning plans, journal writing extracts, and concept maps; and finally, *attestation* or rather, evaluations of the individual's work including self-evaluations, peer feedback, and staff or teacher reviews or recommendations. Barrow (1993) describes any production documents as the "heart of the portfolio." An important part of most portfolios is the reflective diary, which serves as a vehicle for demonstrating the reflective process (Alsop, 1995; CNO, 1996; Glen, Clark, and Nicol, 1995; Witmer, 1996)—a component of the Professional Profile Portfolio (Profile) as developed by the College of Nurses of Ontario (CNO, 1996). We have used the CNO Profile extensively and successfully in our PBL curriculum and research studies (Matthew-Maich et al., 2000).

There are also identified barriers to portfolio development: individuals lacking writing skills are at a disadvantage for developing portfolios (Budnick and Beaver, 1984; Murray, 1994); portfolio development is frequently cited as very time consuming with the documented time frames between 20 and 50 hours (Murray, 1994; Witmer, 1995, 1996); and the personal nature of some reflections may serve as a deterrent to those perceiving it as an invasion of their privacy (Alsop, 1995; Burnard, 1995; Mitchell, 1994). The issue of assessing and grading portfolios is once again raised, with Walker (1985) informing us that he does not gather and assess student portfolios, but instead asks that students share reflections with the group when they are comfortable. Students he worked with over three years acknowledged that the portfolio would be less personal if it had to be handed in for assessment. However, other students claim that portfolios need to be assessed and graded for them to invest their valued time and energy into their development (Matthew-Maich et al., 2000). Two frameworks to assist with portfolio development and assessment are presented below. Detailed, graduated guidelines for portfolio development and review are provided in Table 6.10.

Table 6.10 *A Guide to the Stages in Portfolio Development and Review/Assessment*

What to Do	How to Do It	Who Is Involved
Develop a framework and documentation for portfolio	Link the syllabus (if any) to the overall learning objectives of the learning program Differentiate between the essential and the desirable outcomes Write appropriate guidance notes for learners, supervisors, assessors, and other people involved Devise appropriate forms/checklists, etc. that will be used for review and assessment	Clinical tutor, college tutor, postgraduate dean, GP advisor, course organizer, and/or others as appropriate to the individual training program.
Establish means for supporting the learner during portfolio development	Identify educational supervisors and/or mentors Implement training for those involved in providing support	As above
Introduce a portfolio to learners	Present (rather than distribute) and explain documentation–may be appropriately done during induction Name individuals designated to support and review the portfolio	As above

continued

Table 6.10   *A Guide to the Stages in Portfolio Development and*
Review/Assessment   continued

What to Do	How to Do It	Who Is Involved
Develop individual action plan	Identify current level of learning in key areas for review	
	Identify areas for future development	
	Agree key learning objectives, linking individual learning needs and relevant syllabus	
	Write these in assessable format, with criteria for assessment if not already included in portfolio documentation	
	Agree on means for meeting needs and objectives	
	Educational supervisor and individual learner through negotiation	
Identify sources of evidence of learning appropriate to identified learning needs	Agree which objectives may be met through natural work patterns, and which will need specific training input	Education supervisor and learner
	Identify and arrange training where appropriate	
	Agree what types of evidence would be considered appropriate to demonstrate learning achievement	
Gather and document evidence of learning	Ensure that appropriate evidence of learning is gathered and its rationale for inclusion in the portfolio is established	
	Supplement with reflective accounts of learning as appropriate	
	Learner in collaboration with mentor if appropriate	
Monitor progress	Review learning objectives and progress towards their attainment	Learner with mentor and/or educational supervisor
	Ensure evidence relates to and demonstrates how learning objectives have been addressed	
	Revise learning objectives if necessary	

Table 6.10   *A Guide to the Stages in Portfolio Development and Review/Assessment   concluded*

What to Do	How to Do It	Who Is Involved
Assess/review portfolio	Select and provide rationale for evidence that demonstrates achievement of learning objectives under review	Learner with reviewer/assessor
	Ensure validity, sufficiency, authenticity of evidence, and currency of learning	Reviewer/assessor
	Agree that evidence meets defined assessment criteria	Learner with reviewer/assessor
	Plan further learning opportunities if necessary	Learner with reviewer/assessor
	Devise new learning objectives and personal learning plan	
Report results to appropriate bodies	Complete documentation	Educational supervisor/Clinical tutor
	Make recommendations for progression/additional support needed	

Challis, M. (1999). AMEE Medical Education Guide No. 11 (revised): Portfolio-based learning and assessment in medical education. *Medical Teacher, 21*(4), 370–386. Reprinted with permission.

Another portfolio assessment/development framework, "The Integrated Proficiency-Criterion Framework," integrates the National League for Nursing (1992) outcome criteria with Benner's (1984) stages of professional proficiency and is presented in Table 6.11.

The research related to portfolio development has focused on three areas of portfolio use: nursing practice (Cayne, 1995); health care education (Mitchell, 1994); and nursing education (Matthew-Maich, 1996; Oechsle, Volden, and Lambeth, 1990). The benefits of the portfolio process for the owner have been described as a spur to action and an opportunity for critical reflection and placing value on personal experiences as learning (Cayne, 1995; Matthew-Maich et al., 2000), assisting students to meet learning needs, develop self-awareness, and validating accomplishments (Oechsle et al., 1990). Other gains include personal and professional growth; developing critical thinking skills; gaining insights into existing oppressions and strategies to break free; gaining a voice and fostering a sense of community with other nurses through sharing nursing stories (Matthew-Maich et al., 2000; Sorrell, Brown, Silva, and Kohlenberg, 1997). The portfolio represents an effective, learner-centered strategy to facilitate both reflection and the tenets of PBL, resulting in multidimensional growth of the practitioner developing it.

Table 6.11   *The Integrated Proficiency-Criterion Framework*

Level of Proficiency (Outcome Criterion)	Novice	Advanced Beginner	Competent
Critical Thinking	Early development of decision-making ability with a limited view of possible options.	Has the ability to realize options but follows a systematic process for decision making.	Seeing multiple options and has the ability to differentiate possible benefits from each.
Communication Skills (written, verbal, and nonverbal)	Learning methods of communication with clients, families, and groups. Identification of effective communication patterns.	Beginning analysis of therapeutic conversation. Differentiation of therapeutic from nontherapeutic communication with clients, families, and groups	Demonstration of effective communication with clients, families, and groups. Demonstration and evaluation of teaching/learning activities.
Therapeutic Nursing Interventions	Beginning psychomotor skills acquisition. Practicing well-client psychosocial therapeutics.	Advancing psychomotor skills and psychosocial therapeutics, directed at clients, families, and groups with health deviations.	Evidence of safe psychomotor skills and individualized psychosocial therapeutics of clients, families, and groups.
Professional Development	Identification of components of professional nursing practice. Beginning followership.	Demonstration of knowledge adequate for safe nursing practice. Effective followership.	Integration of knowledge and self-evaluation. Beginning leadership.
Personal Development	Reflection of personal value system.	Clarification of personal values. Acceptance of diversity.	Identification of learning as a lifelong process. Integration of ethical values into nursing practice. Development of sensitivity to diversity.
Scholarship	Beginning understanding of principles of research-based and theory-based practice.	Beginning application of research-based and theory-based practice.	Analysis and review of nursing research, including application to nursing care.

Adapted from Benner (1984) and National League of Nursing (1992). Wenzel, L., Briggs, K., and Puryear, B. (1998). Portfolio: Authentic assessment in the age of the curriculum revolution. *The Journal of Nursing Education, 37*(5), 208–212. Reprinted with permission.

Small Groups

> . . . Groups provide real world learning by solving real life problems.
> (Carkhuff, 1996, p. 210)

Small group reflective dialogue with a skilled facilitator represents another strategy to nurture critical reflection, and PBL tutorials and clinical sessions comprise opportunities for reflective dialogue. Small groups foster reflective practice as experiences are reflected upon, shared, validated, their meaning explored, and new insights and learning gained, within a supportive culture (Graham, 1995).

Reflective dialogue that is integral to the PBL process facilitates double-loop learning as teachers and students become partners in learning, engaged in dialogue to critically examine issues (Carkhuff, 1996). He goes on to highlight the faculty's role as modeling both group and reflection skills to solve real life problems while establishing expectations of "equality, accountability, responsibility, and authority" (p. 212), and developing the following reflection skills, as outlined by Boud et al. (1985): self-awareness, description, critical analysis, synthesis, and evaluation. Andrews (1996b) emphasizes that, "reflecting with an experienced, committed supervisor will enhance the process and help to legitimize reflection as an important learning activity in the clinical setting" (p. 513).

Sharing within a small group context may foster growth, yet it may also create anxiety or feel threatening for some participants. Increased anxiety levels lead to insecure feelings and hesitancy to self-disclose, while conversely, when participants feel safe they take risks and share personal experiences and feelings (Haddock, 1997). Reflective dialogue may also surface repressed emotions caused by enhanced self-awareness and client contact. "More rigorous attempts may be required to maintain the boundary and thus the safety of the group, and to obtain supervision, in order to deal more effectively with problems arising" (Haddock, 1997, p. 381). When the reflective dialogue session is a postclinical conference or debriefing, Pierson (1998) cautions us that the facilitator must have a strong commitment to designating consistent time for this and not fall prey to the temptation of spending more time "doing" in the clinical area.

Self-Assessment/Self-Evaluations

> Reflection and self-assessment are fundamental to initiating appropriate
> self-directed learning and change. (Westberg and Jason, 1994, p. 278)

Wolff (2000) states the aim of "self-evaluation is to develop the ability to evaluate oneself in an accurate and constructive way" (p. 2). Reflection provides the information for self-evaluation and Westberg and Jason (1994) suggest that reflective learners can then gain the most from their experiences. Ultimately, skills in self-evaluation are necessary for competent performance, professional autonomy, and for lifelong learning (Arthur, 1995; Saylor, 1990; Wolff, 2000).

Assessment of processes and attitudes embodies PBL principles and is the central focus of student evaluation (Nendaz and Tekian, 1999). In PBL, self-evaluation is not only concerned with knowledge, problem-solving skills, critical thinking, communication, and group process but also with the ability to appraise one's own performance in terms of strengths and areas for improvement. Westberg and Jason (1994) attest that when students are responsible for self-assessment, they are more likely to take responsibility for their own learning and to do what is needed. Other benefits accrue in terms of reduced anxiety over grading, enhanced communication between student and faculty, improved motivation for learning and improved performance (Gordon, 1992). Woods (1994) adds that from a learning perspective, self-evaluation is a natural outcome of the PBL format and "it completes the loop in the learning cycle . . . learn more . . . learn better . . . increases one's self-image and self-confidence" (p. 8–4). Bartels (1998) suggests that by focusing on student self-evaluation "we nurture their tendencies to carry with them a developing picture of their progress" (p. 133).

Woods (1994) believes that acquiring skills in self-evaluation is the most difficult part of PBL. Students are often uncomfortable with self-evaluation if they are not prepared and reflection and self-evaluation take time (Westberg and Jason, 1994). Another potential issue is related to the faculty in a PBL program since, as Woods (1994) points out, empowering students "with this responsibility can be threatening" (p. C-5). It also demands that faculty must make the evaluation process explicit and shift from assessing content to assessing the students self-evaluation process.

Westberg and Jason (1994) suggest some specific strategies and tools that foster reflection and self-evaluation. Reflective and self-evaluation activities need to be developed and "infuse virtually all their learning." In PBL, students have repeated opportunities over the course of their program to self-evaluate their performance in both PBL tutorial groups and clinical settings. Clear goals by which the students can monitor their progress are needed, so it is important to state the outcomes in writing that students are asked to self-evaluate, along with specific criteria for evaluating those outcomes. As well, expected outcomes should evolve from curriculum goals and students' developmental abilities, so they change with each level of a PBL program (Arthur, 1995).

In her critical review of the literature, Arthur (1995) points out that there is a lack of literature on student self-evaluation in nursing programs. In examining self-evaluation in any health discipline, Arthur (1995) summarized, and Nendaz and Tekian (1999) concur, that the psychometric properties of self-evaluation measures need improvement. While Arthur (1995) endorsed self-evaluation for formative purposes, Nendaz and Tekian (1999) noted two PBL medical programs that have used self-evaluation summatively. For the most part, self-evaluation can be used for a combination of formative and summative purposes.

RESEARCHING CRITICAL REFLECTIVE OUTCOMES: THE VERDICT TO DATE

> It is the general conception of any field of inquiry that ultimately deter-
> mines the kind of knowledge the field aims to develop, as well as the man-
> ner in which that knowledge is to be organized, tested and applied.
> (Carper, 1978, p. 13)

While the origins of reflection and reflective practice are rooted in the early
work of Dewey (1933), much of the current emphasis on reflective practice
in nursing can be attributed to Mezirow (1981, 1990, 1991) and in particular
to Schön (1983, 1987, 1991) who elucidated the role of reflection in professional practice. As a means of resolving the divergence between theory and
practice and for transforming nursing education (Clarke, 1986, Gaines and
Baldwin, 1996; Harden, 1996; Watson, 1995), reflection has been advocated
as somewhat of a panacea. However, Fitzgerald (1994) states that "reflection
is not a panacea for nursing's many dilemmas—it is a way of learning more
about our work" (p. 78). The foray of nursing research into reflection and
reflective practice is in its infancy. This section will explore the nursing
research to date in the realm of reflection in nursing education.

The use of Schön's work on reflection-in-action as a theoretical base and
Mezirow's levels of reflectivity as a measurement of reflection have been used
as the focus of studies in nursing education. Richardson and Maltby (1995)
used a reflective diary, which is viewed as an effective method to promote
reflection and learning, with 30 undergraduate nursing students. The
findings indicate that the highest number of reflections occurred at the
lower levels of reflectivity. While only 6 percent of scores were found at the
higher levels, two-thirds of the students did attain conceptual and theoretical
reflectivity. The researchers also raised questions regarding students' appre-
hension of expressing feelings and felt that "assessment of their diary may
inhibit the reflective process and hinder development of the qualities and
skills required for reflection" (p. 241).

Wong et al. (1995) contributed an impressive study which offers a coding
system for measuring reflective journals to arrive at three categories: nonreflec-
tors, reflectors, and critical reflectors. The system is efficient to use and has a
high interobserver reliability (refer to Table 6.8). As we noted earlier, Wong
et al. (1995) reported that the majority of nursing students made the connection between pure and new knowledge and that 11 percent adopted a wide
multidimensional reflective perspective including transformative learning.

Several studies have explored nursing students' perceptions of the
effects of using the reflective processes. Emergent themes from a study by
Davies (1995) with first-year nursing students included reduced anxiety in
clinical practice, progression from a passive to an active learning style, assistance with solving clinical problems and understanding rationale for
practice, identification of individual learning needs, and most significantly
the emergence of client-centered care as the major focus of reflection.

Shields (1995) noted in her study, also with first-year students, that they valued reflection as a means of learning which led to behavior change, stimulated problem-solving, and increased personal and professional awareness leading to improved patient care. Second-year nursing students, when asked to examine reflection as a learning tool, responded that while it provided an opportunity to look back at a clinical situation, the purpose of reflection as a part of evaluation needed to be more clearly defined and that they needed help in developing reflective skills (Getliffe, 1996).

In a quantitative study, Lowe and Kerr (1998) used an experimental design with matched pairs of students, where one group was exposed to reflective teaching methods and the other group to the conventional teaching methods. They then measured student performance on a specially designed test covering a biological science module to determine whether student learning was affected through the introduction of a reflective learning situation compared to the conventional approach. Based on their hypothesis that a combination of personal experience and formal learning would result in "deep learning," the authors expected student nurses would score higher when taught by reflective methods. Their findings indicated no statistically significant differences between the groups. They surmised that the reflective method was as effective as following the conventional approach, in that students could be introduced to a new topic, a new teaching method and still produce a good final grade.

In summary, a growing body of literature has been presented suggesting that reflection and reflective practice is an effective learning process for professional and personal growth and may offer a catalyst for the transformation in nursing education so urgently required. However, the next section offers a different debate.

CRITIQUING REFLECTION AND REFLECTIVE PRACTICE: A FLAWED CONCEPT OR 'BEING A NURSE'

. . . [U]se of reflection as a learning strategy or tool for professional development is seriously flawed. (Mackintosh, 1998, p. 556)

. . . [R]eflection has led to behavior change, problem-solving, and personal and professional awareness as well as improved patient care. (Shields, 1995, p. 452).

As nursing education has shifted to curricula grounded in humanism and critical theory, reflection has increasingly become a significant and integral component of nursing education. In laying out the various theoretical and conceptual underpinnings of reflection, one can see that they are intuitively pleasing because they beckon us, with personal and emancipatory growth, critical and innovative thinking, a deeper understanding of nursing knowledge and practice and a way to manage the myriad of changes and demands as we start the new millennium. However, there is another side to the argument that needs to be addressed before we can continue to maintain its role in nursing education.

Much of the criticism with respect to reflection and reflective practices has been directed toward a lack of conceptual clarity, theoretical inconsistencies, missing elements, and unproven benefit to nursing and patient outcomes (Andrews, Gidman, and Humphreys, 1998; Atkins and Murphy, 1993; Foster and Greenwood, 1998; James and Clarke, 1994; Mackintosh, 1998; Smith, 1998). Another criticism is directed to the difficulty associated with how Mezirow's transformation of meaning, for example, occurs or takes place, since he presents no clear framework, set of guidelines or uniform instrumentation. Similarly, Schön is frequently cited in the nursing literature and yet he too offers little in the way of practical guidance for the development of teaching strategies (James and Clarke, 1994). Efforts to address these concerns have been presented through Burrows' (1995) Framework for Reflection on Action (Table 6.4) and Johns' (1995) Framework for Structured Reflection (Table 6.6), both of which can be utilized to guide the learner to reflect at an appropriate level.

Other issues related or connected to reflection continue to be raised. Memory and recall are linked to reflection, and Newell (1992) contends that reflection theories do not consider how these mediate the accuracy of the reflective process. On the other hand, Smith (1998) criticizes reflection models for not taking into account positive feelings and thoughts which can prompt critical reflection and suggests that these can be just as influential.

So, despite endeavors to provide theory-based approaches to reflection, concern continues to be expressed about the use of reflection within nursing. Indeed, Andrews (1996b) questions whether the process of reflection will ever be trusted by a "profession that relies upon safety and proven methods" but concludes that reflection contributes to the social elements of "being a nurse" and so is worthy of continuing exploration. Wilkinson (1999) provides a useful summary of the current status of reflection and summarizes the main concerns to keep in mind when engaged in reflective practice in Table 6.12.

So, debate and research need to continue rather than be tossed aside because "only by such means can the nature of reflection in nursing be truly understood and educational strategies evolve for the development and promotion of reflective skills" (James and Clarke, 1994, p. 89). Even as the debate continues, the learning that occurs through reflection within any curriculum, and in particular within a PBL curriculum, is apparent in the following quotes from students who participated in the studies of Matthew-Maich et al. (1997, 2000). Perhaps we can accept the contribution of reflection to the learning of these students as sufficient endorsement of its place within nursing education until further evidence suggests otherwise.

Table 6.12 *Summary of the Main Issues to Consider When Engaged in Reflective Practice*

- Complement technical rationality knowledge by using reflective practice to access tacit knowledge.
- Reflection does not occur simply by knowing about it—it depends on active strategies such as reflective writing in diaries or portfolios, and/or clinical supervision with or without the use of a model of reflection.
- Supervision by peers—one-to-one or in a group—appears to be the most effective form of clinical supervision to facilitate reflection.
- Practice-generated theory accessed through reflection can challenge espoused theory which is out of context with the diversity and complexity of real life nursing care.
- In nurse education curricula, reflection must be supplemented by nurse educators who tackle the complexities of practice with their students in real practice settings.
- Reflection can successfully occur before action, in action, or on action.
- All experience should be considered as a potential precursor to reflection, particularly habituated experiences.
- Reflective practitioners need to delineate between that which is reflection and that which is recollection.
- Reflective practice should encompass critical analysis of personal self-awareness and the social context of health and health care.
- Caution should be expressed about the ethical challenges of becoming a reflective practitioner in relation to enhancing self-evaluation and confidentiality.
- Reflection is under-researched—reflective practitioners should consider designing their own investigations or contributing to the work of others.

Wilkinson, J. (1999). Implementing reflective practice. *Nursing Standard, 13*(21), 36–40. Reprinted with permission.

SAMPLINGS OF REFLECTION: IN THE STUDENTS' WORDS

Reflecting helped me to realize that I have thoughts and feelings that can be expressed through my work; through the way I carry myself as nurse. It also helped me to build self-confidence and esteem and to be all that I want to be! The best part of writing in my journal was expressing my feelings about things I don't normally talk about everyday. In the future I will continue to express my feelings in journal style. It's like talking to someone who listens except it's only paper with personality.

Reflection helped me to realize that I can do anything I want to do; I can learn more about myself and how I have made a difference for others and myself. It has also been the writing of a journey full of experiences that I have taken a part in and that is waiting to continue to create more memories. The best part was that I got to know more about myself and the abilities that I have that I never knew existed.

Reflecting on my practice allowed me to see the positive side of things that I do in the clinical day, not just the negative. Reflecting allowed me to discover I am not as unskilled as I previously felt about myself, nursing is a part of my individuality and my personality. The best part was watching yourself become more skilled and confident; watching yourself learn and grow. Learning from experiences and finding out for yourself where your strengths and weaknesses are. You get feedback from staff and instructors, but you also get feedback from yourself. In the future I will continue to use reflective practice because nursing is a profession in which learning and growing does not stop. I will always require upgrading and additional skills to practice at the level where I feel I want to be. Taking reflective practice with me will keep me on my toes and correct inadequacies when needed. For future students I suggest concentration on implementing reflective practice throughout the nursing course. It allows you to see yourself grow and become the professional person that you thought you'd never become. In fact, some of the nurses you are amazed and awed at, may one day be you!!

Through reflection I discovered that I know and understand much more than I thought I did. The best part was looking back and realizing "I am a nurse!" This was an incredible feeling! For future students I suggest using reflection to enhance themselves not only as nurses but as people.

Writing these reflective journals has helped me develop my self-awareness skills. When I first found out that we would have to write journals every week using the LEARN format (which I remember doing in first year), I though "oh, no, not this again. It is such a waste of time." However, my experience from first year did not compare to my experience this year with the journal. I found the journal writing to be very helpful. It helped me to "talk" about my feelings and explore the reasons for my feelings. Often time I would be writing the analysis section of the journal entry and I would be typing away and pause and think to myself "is this really why I felt this way?" I really had to be introspective to understand my feelings. I also think that by exploring my feelings, I was better able to help my patient's explore and understand their feelings. I also found the journal helpful in assisting me to identify alternative solutions to a problem (i.e., what to do when the patient is silent; what to say to a patient who is making inappropriate sexual comments).

. . . If something didn't work or if I was disappointed in the consequence of something I tried to initiate, I would use this process [reflection using LEARN] to figure out what went wrong, what could I have done to try and change it, what in my behavior would work better? I think that I deal with things in a more thorough fashion, with more intention. I find that I am more methodical. More critical too. I do, I feel more critical. Before I was just sort of floating around sort of letting events rule me instead of me manipulating events for a better outcome. . . .

REFERENCES

Alsop, A. (1995). The professional portfolio—purpose, process and practice, Part 1: Portfolios and professional practice. *British Journal of Occupational Therapy, 58*(7), 299–302.

Andrews, M. (1996a). Reflection as infiltration: Learning in the experiential domain. *Journal of Advanced Nursing, 24,* 391–399.

Andrews, M. (1996b). Using reflection to develop clinical expertise. *British Journal of Nursing, 5*(8), 508–513.

Andrews, M., Gidman, J., and Humphreys, A. (1998). Reflection: Does it enhance professional nursing practice? *British Journal of Nursing, 7*(7), 413–417.

Argyris, C. and Schön, D. (1974). *Theory in Practice: Increasing Professional Effectiveness.* San Francisco: Jossey-Bass.

Arthur, H. (1995). Student self-evaluations: How useful? How valid? *International Journal of Nursing Studies, 32*(3), 271–276.

Atkins, S. and Murphy, K. (1993). Reflection: A review of the literature. *Journal of Advanced Nursing, 18,* 1188–1192.

Atkins, S. M. and Murphy, K. (1994). Reflective practice. *Nursing Standard, 8*(39), 50–56.

Baker, C. R. (1996). Reflective learning: A teaching strategy for critical thinking. *Journal of Nursing Education, 35*(1), 19–22.

Baker, C. (1991). Our stories, ourselves: Reflecting on practice. *American Journal of Nursing,* October, 66–69.

Barrow, D. (1993). The use of portfolios to assess student learning. *Journal of College Science Teaching,* Dec. 1992–Jan. 1993, 148–153.

Bartels, J. E. (1998). Developing reflective learners—Student self-assessment as learning. *Journal of Professional Nursing, 14*(3), 135.

Benner, P. (1984). *From Novice to Expert: Excellence and Power in Nursing Practice.* California: Addison-Wesley.

Bevis, E. and Murray, J. (1990). The essence of the curriculum revolution: Emancipatory teaching. *Journal of Nursing Education, 29,* 326–331.

Bolt, E. and Powell, J. (1993). *Becoming Reflective.* London: Distance Learning Centre, South Bank University.

Boud, D., Keogh, R., and Walker, D. (1985). *Reflection: Turning Experience into Learning.* London: Kogan Page.

Boyd, E. M. and Fales, A. W. (1983). Reflective learning: Key to learning from experience. *Journal of Humanistic Psychology, 23*(2), 99–117.

Brockett, R. G. and Hiemstra, R. (1991). *Self Direction in Adult Learning.* London: Routledge.

Brookfield, S. D. (1995). *Becoming a Critically Reflective Teacher.* San Francisco: Jossey-Bass.

Brown, B., Blatz, S., Crooks, D., Fawcett, M., Hyndman, J., Noesgaard, C., Parisi, L., Parsons, M., Rideout, E., and Sergeant, D. (1995). *Developing a Nursing Faculty Teaching Evaluation Process Through the Use of a Teaching Portfolio.* Hamilton, ON: McMaster University School of Nursing.

Budnick, D. and Beaver, S. (1984). A student perspective on the portfolio. *Nursing Outlook, 32,* 268–269.

Burnard, P. (1988). The journal as an assessment and evaluation tool in nurse education. *Nurse Education Today, 8,* 105–107.

Burnard, P. (1991). Using video as a reflective tool in interpersonal skills training. *Nurse Education Today, 11,* 143–146.

Burnard, P. (1995). Nurse educator's perceptions of reflection and reflective practice: A report of a descriptive study. *Journal of Advanced Nursing, 21,* 1167–1174.

Burns, S. (1994). Assessing reflective learning. In A. Palmer, S. Burns, C. Bulman (Eds.), *Reflective Practice in Nursing: The Growth of the Professional Practitioner.* Oxford: Blackwell Scientific.

Burrows, D. E. (1995). The nurse teacher's role in the promotion of reflective practice. *Nurse Education Today, 15,* 346–350.

Callister, L. C. (1993). The use of student journals in nursing education: Making meaning out of clinical experience. *Journal of Nursing Education, 32*(4), 185–186.

Cameron, B. L. and Mitchell, A. M. (1993). Reflective peer journals: Developing authentic nurses. *Journal of Advanced Nursing, 18,* 290–297.

Carkhuff, M. H. (1996). Reflective learning: Work groups as learning groups. *The Journal of Continuing Education in Nursing, 27*(5), 209–214.

Carper, B. (1978). Fundamental patterns of knowing in nursing. *Advances in Nursing Science, 1*(1), 13–23.

Cayne, J. (1995). Portfolios: A developmental influence? *Journal of Advanced Nursing, 21,* 395–405.

Clarke, B., James, C., and Kelly, J. (1996). Reflective practice: Reviewing the issues and refocusing the debate. *International Journal of Nursing Studies, 33*(2), 171–180.

Clarke, M. (1986). Action and reflection: Practice and theory in nursing. *Journal of Advanced Nursing, 11,* 3–11.

College of Nurses of Ontario. (1996). *Professional Profile: A Reflective Portfolio for Continuous Learning.* Toronto: CNO.

Cranton, P. (1992). *Working with Adult Learners.* Toronto: Wall and Emerson.

Cranton, P. (1996). *Professional Development as Transformative Learning.* San Francisco: Jossey-Bass.

Cruickshank, D. (1996). The "art" of reflection: using drawing to uncover knowledge development in student nurses. *Nurse Education Today, 16,* 127–130.

Davies, E. (1995). Reflective practice: A focus for caring. *Journal of Nursing Education, 34*(4), 167–174.

Dearmun, A. K. (1997). Using reflection to assess degree students. *Paediatric Nursing, 9*(1), 25–28.

Dewey, J. (1933). *How We Think.* Chicago: Henry Regnery.

Duke, S. and Copp, G. (1994). The personal side of reflection. In A. Palmer, S. Burns, and C. Bulman (Eds.), *Reflective Practice in Nursing: The Growth of the Professional Practitioner.* London: Blackwell Scientific Publications.

Durgahee, T. (1998). Facilitating reflection: From a sage on stage to a guide on the side. *Nurse Education Today, 18,* 158–164.

Fitzgerald, M. (1994). Theories of reflection for learning. In A. Palmer, S. Burns, and G. Bulman (Eds.), *Reflective Practice in Nursing.* Oxford: Blackwell Scientific Publications.

Foster, J. and Greenwood, J. (1998). Reflection: A challenging innovation for nurses. *Contemporary Nurse, 7*(4), 165–172.

Gaines, S. and Baldwin, D. (1996). Guiding dialogue in the transformation of teacher-student relationships. *Nursing Outlook, 44*(3), 124–128.

Getliffe, K. A. (1996). An examination of the use of reflection in the assessment of practice for undergraduate nursing students. *International Journal of Nursing Studies, 33*(4), 361–374.

Glen, S. and Hight, N. F. (1992). Portfolios: An "affective" assessment strategy? *Nurse Education Today, 12,* 416–423.

Glen, S., Clark, A., and Nicol, M. (1995). Reflecting on reflection: A personal encounter. *Nurse Education Today, 15*(1), 61–68.

Goodman, J. (1984). Reflection and Teacher Education: A Case Study and Theoretical Analysis. *Interchange, 15*(3), 9–26.

Gordon, M. J. (1992). Self-assessment programs and their implications for health professions training. *Academic Medicine, 67,* 672–679.

Graham, I. W. (1995). Reflective practice: Using the action learning group mechanism. *Nurse Education Today, 15,* 28–32.

Graham, I., Waight, S., and Scammell, J. (1998). Using structured reflection to improve nursing practice. *Nursing Times, 94*(25), 56–59.

Haddock, J. (1997). Reflection in groups: Contextual and theoretical considerations within nurse education and practice. *Nurse Education Today, 17,* 381–385.

Hancock, P. (1998). Reflective practice—using a learning journal. *Nursing Standard, 13*(17), 37–40.

Harden, J. (1996). Enlightenment, empowerment and emancipation: The case for critical pedagogy in nurse education. *Nurse Education Today, 16*(1), 32–37.

Hargreaves, J. (1997). Using patients: Exploring the ethical dimension of reflective practice in nurse education. *Journal of Advanced Nursing, 25,* 223–228.

Hawks, J. H. (1992). Empowerment in nursing education: Concept analysis and application to philosophy, learning and instruction. *Journal of Advanced Nursing, 17,* 609–618.

Heath, H. (1998). Keeping a reflective practice diary: A practical guide. *Nurse Education Today, 18,* 592–598.

Heinrich, K. T. (1992). The intimate dialogue: Journal writing by students. *Nurse Educator, 17,* 17–21.

Heinrich, K. T. (1997). Transforming imposters into heroes: Metaphors for innovative nursing education. *Nurse Educator, 22*(3), 45–50.

Heinrich, K. T. and Scherr, M. W. (1994). Peer monitoring for reflective teaching: A model for nurses who teach. *Nurse Educator, 19,* 36–41.

Hodges, H. F. (1996). Journal writing as a mode of thinking for RN-BSN students: A levelled approach to learning to listen to self and others. *Journal of Nursing Education, 35*(3), 137–141.

Holly, M. L. (1989). Reflective writing and spirit of inquiry. *Cambridge Journal of Education, 19,* 71–79.

James, C. R. and Clarke, B. A. (1992). *The Development of Reflective Practice in Nursing.* Paper presented to the Third International Nurse Education Tomorrow Participative Conference. Durham.

James, C. R. and Clarke, B. A. (1994). Reflective practice in nursing: Issues and implications for nurse education. *Nurse Education Today, 14,* 82–90.

Jarvis, P. (1992). Reflective practice and nursing. *Nurse Education Today, 12*(3), 174–181.

Jensen, G. M. and Saylor, C. (1994). Portfolios and professional development in the health professions. *Evaluation and the Health Professions, 17*(3), 344–357.

John, S. (1997). Reflective practice: Implementation in pre-registration nursing. *Assignment, 3*(1), 2–8.

Johns, C. (1994). Guided reflection. In A. Palmer, S. Burns, and G. Bulman (Eds.), *Reflective Practice in Nursing: The Growth of the Professional Practitioner.* London: Blackwell Scientific Publications.

Johns, C. (1995). Framing learning through reflection within Carper's fundamental ways of knowing in nursing. *Journal of Advanced Nursing, 22,* 226–234.

Johns, C. (1998). Opening the doors of perception. In C. Johns and D. Freshwater (Eds.), *Transforming Nursing Through Reflective Practice.* London: Blackwell Scientific Publications.

Kim, H. S. (1999). Critical reflective inquiry for knowledge development in nursing practice. *Journal of Advanced Nursing, 29*(5), 1205–1212.

Kitchener, K. S. and King, P. M. (1990). The reflective judgement model: Transforming assumptions about knowing. In J. Mezirow, *Fostering Critical Reflection in Adulthood.* San Franscisco: Jossey-Bass.

Kobert, L. J. (1995). In our own voice: Journaling as a teaching/learning technique for nurses. *Journal of Nursing Education, 34*(3), 140–142.

Landeen, J., Byrne, C., and Brown, B. (1992). Journal keeping as an education strategy in teaching psychiatric nursing. *Journal of Advanced Nursing, 17,* 347–355.

Lowe, P. B. and Kerr, C. M. (1998). Learning by reflection: The effect on educational outcomes. *Journal of Advanced Nursing, 27,* 1030–1033.

Mackintosh, C. (1998). Reflection: A flawed strategy for the nursing profession. *Nurse Education Today, 18,* 553–557.

Matthew-Maich. (1996). 'Becoming' Through Reflection and Professional Portfolios in Nursing Education. MSc (T) thesis, McMaster University, Hamilton, Ontario, Canada.

Matthew-Maich, N., Brown, B., and Royle, J. (2000). Becoming through reflection and professional portfolios: The voice of growth in nurses. *Reflective Practice* (in press).

Matthew-Maich, N., Brown, B., Royle, J., and Witmer, D. (1997). The professional profile experience: Through the voice of nurses. *College Communique, 22*(4), 12.

Mezirow, J. (1981). A critical theory of adult learning and education. *Adult Education, 32*(1), 3–24.

Mezirow, J. (1990). *Fostering Critical Reflection in Adulthood: A Guide to Transformative and Emancipatory Learning.* San Francisco: Jossey-Bass.

Mezirow, J. (1991). *Transformative Dimensions of Adult Learning.* San Francisco: Jossey-Bass.

Mitchell, M. (1994). The views of students and teachers on the use of portfolios as a learning strategy and assessment tool in midwifery education. *Nurse Education Today, 14,* 38–43.

Morgan, S. (1996). Gods, daemons, and banshees on the journey to the magic scroll: The use of myth as a framework for reflective practice in nurse education. *Nurse Education Today, 16*(2), 144–148.

Murray, P. J. (1994). Portfolios and accreditation of prior experiential learning (APEL) make credits . . . or problems? *Nurse Education Today, 14,* 232–237.

National League for Nursing. (1992). *Criteria and Guidelines for the Evaluation of Baccalaureate Nursing Programs.* (National League for Nursing No. 15-2474). New York: NLN Press.

Nendaz, M. R. and Tekian, A. (1999). Assessment in problem-based learning medical schools: A literature review. *Teaching and Learning in Medicine, 11*(4), 232–243.

Neville, A. J. (1999). The problem-based learning tutor: Teacher? Facilitator? Evaluator? *Medical Teacher, 21*(4), 393–401.

Newell, R. (1992). Anxiety, accuracy and reflection: The limits of professional development. *Journal of Advanced Nursing, 17,* 1326–1333.

Oechsle, L., Volden, C., and Lambeth, S. (1990). Portfolios and RNs: An evaluation. *Journal of Nursing Education, 29*(2), 54–59.

Paterson, B. L. (1995). Developing and maintaining reflection in clinical journals. *Nurse Education Today, 15,* 211–220.

Pierson, W. (1998). Reflection in nursing education. *Journal of Advanced Nursing, 27,* 165–170.

Reed, J. and Proctor, S. (1993). *Nurse Education: A Reflective Approach.* London: Edward Arnold.

Reid, B. (1993). "But we're doing it already!" Exploring a response to the concept of reflective practice in order to improve its facilitation. *Nurse Education Today, 13,* 305–309.

Rich, A. and Parker, D. L. (1995). Reflection and critical incident analysis: ethical and moral implications of their use within nursing and midwifery education. *Journal of Advanced Nursing, 22,* 1050–1057.

Richardson, G. and Maltby, H. (1995). Reflection-on-practice: Enhancing student learning. *Journal of Advanced Nursing, 22,* 235–242.

Ryan, M. and Carlton, K. H. (1997). Portfolio applications in a school of nursing. *Nurse Educator, 22*(1), 35–39.

Saylor, C. R. (1990). Reflection and professional education: Art, science and competency. *Nurse Educator, 15*(2), 8–11.

Scanlan, J. M. and Chernomas, W. M. (1997). Developing the reflective teacher. *Journal of Advanced Nursing, 25,* 1138–1143.

Schön, D. (1983). *The Reflective Practitioner.* San Francisco: Jossey-Bass.

Schön, D. (1987). *Educating the Reflective Practitioner.* San Francisco: Jossey-Bass.

Schön, D. (1991). *The Reflective Practitioner.* San Francisco: Jossey-Bass.

Shields, E. (1995). Reflection and learning in student nurses. *Nurse Education Today, 15*(6), 452–458.

Smith, A. (1998). Learning about reflection. *Journal of Advanced Nursing, 28*(4), 891–898.

Snowball, J., Ross, K., and Murphy, K. (1994). Illuminating dissertation supervision through reflection. *Journal of Advanced Nursing, 19*(6), 1234–1240.

Sorrell, J. M., Brown, H. N., Silva, M. C., and Kohlenberg, E. M. (1997). Use of writing portfolios for interdisciplinary assessment of critical thinking outcomes of nursing students. *Nursing Forum, 32*(4), 12–24.

Stockhausen, L. J. (1996). The clinical portfolio. *The Australian Electronic Journal of Nursing Education, 2*(2).

Strackbein, D. and Tillman, M. (1987). The joy of journals—with reservations. *Journal of Reading, 131*(1), 28–31.

Trossman, S. (1999). The professional portfolio: Documenting who you are, what you do. *The American Nurse, 31*(2), 1–3.

Tryssenaar, J. (1995). Interactive journal: An educational strategy to promote reflection. *The American Journal of Occupational Therapy, 49*(7), 695–702.

Usher, K., Francis, D., Owens, J., and Tollefson, J. (1999). Reflective writing: A strategy to foster critical inquiry in undergraduate nursing students. *Australian Journal of Advanced Nursing, 17*(1), 7–12.

Van Manen, M. (1977). Linking ways of knowing with ways of being practical. *Curriculum Inquiry, 6*(3), 205–228.

Walker, D. (1985). Writing and reflection. In D. Boud, R. Keogh, and D. Walker (Eds.), *Reflection: Turning Experience into Learning* (pp. 52–68). London: Kogan Page.

Wallace, D. (1996). Using reflective diaries to assess students. *Nursing Standard, 10*(36), 44–47.

Watson, J. (1995). Postmodernism and knowledge development in nursing. *Nursing Science Quarterly, 8*(2), 60–64.

Wellard, S. J. and Bethune, E. (1996). Reflective journal writing in nurse education: whose interests does it serve? *Journal of Advanced Nursing, 24,* 1077–1082.

Wenzel, L. S., Briggs, K. L., and Puryear, B. L. (1998). Portfolio: Authentic assessment in the age of the curriculum revolution. *The Journal of Nursing Education, 37*(5), 208–212.

Westberg, J. and Jason, H. (1994). Fostering learners' reflection and self assessment. *Family Medicine, 26*(5), 278–282.

Wilkinson, J. (1999). Implementing reflective practice. *Nursing Standard, 13*(21), 36–40.

Witmer, D. (1995). Quality assurance: Professional profile portfolio. *College Communique, 22*(1), 13–14.

Witmer, D. (1996). Quality assurance: Expectations for a learning lifestyle. *College Communique, 21*(1), 6–8.

Witmer, D. (1997). Making the choice. What reflective practice option is best for me? *College Communique, 22*(1), 15–18.

Wolff, A. (2000). *The Role of the Tutor in Problem-Based Learning: A Resource Guide for Nursing Faculty.* Vancouver, BC: Wolff Consulting Ltd.

Wong, F. K. Y., Kember, D., Chung, L. Y. F., and Yan, L. (1995). Assessing the level of student reflection from reflective journals. *Journal of Advanced Nursing, 22,* 48–57.

Woods, D. R. (1994). *Problem-Based Learning: How to Gain the Most from PBL.* Waterdown, ON: Donald R. Woods.

Developing Problems for Use in Problem-Based Learning

Michele Drummond-Young and E. Ann Mohide

The centrality of the problems encountered by students in a problem-based learning (PBL) curricula to success in meeting desired learning outcomes has been well-documented (Dolmans, Gijselaers, Schmidt, and van der Meer, 1993; Majoor, Schmidt, Snellen-Balendong, Moust, and Stalenhoef-Halling, 1990). The problem provides both the starting point for learning and the key unit for structuring relevant curriculum content (Barrows and Tamblyn, 1980; Davis and Harden, 1999; Dolmans, Snellen-Balendong, Wolhagen, and van der Vleuten, 1997). Well-constructed problems are designed to focus the students' learning, arouse their interest in the content, and provide a meaningful context within which prior learning is activated and new knowledge is gained. Whitehead (cited in Davis and Harden, 1999) describes the "rhythm of education" and identifies three stages in the educational process: romance, precision, and generalization. In the PBL Model, the romance of learning and the excitement of discovery are provided by the problem.

This chapter provides a systematic and structured approach to designing a PBL problem package, which includes not only the patient scenarios but also the patient data, supporting tutor and student guidelines, resource lists, and feedback forms. Conceptual rationale based on research and expert opinion will be presented as well as practical suggestions and concrete examples for constructing effective problem scenarios. Educators who are familiar with some of the underlying tenants of PBL but who have not written a problem themselves will be provided with evidence-based rationale and many examples to facilitate the writing process. The chapter begins with an overview of what a typical problem package might look like and then goes on to discuss what the literature has to say about content selection and problem effectiveness. Seven principles of effective problem design are identified. Their conceptual underpinnings will be discussed and adapted to nursing curricula along with examples of how to apply them when creating your own problems.

COMPONENTS OF THE PROBLEM PACKAGE

Problem packages utilized in health professional schools consist of a number of component parts. First is the problem itself, which consists of *one or more scenarios*. Each scenario should describe the real-life clinical presentation upon which the problem is built. The number of scenarios and the degree to which they are developed will vary with curricular needs and the way the problem will be utilized. If, for example, the problem is about the diagnosis, treatment, and related nursing management of a patient with breast cancer, it could be developed in five scenarios to illustrate the trajectory of breast cancer and relevant cancer care concepts. Scenario One could describe the discovery of the lump and the initial primary care visit to the nurse practitioner and physician. Scenario Two could take place post biopsy in the surgical clinic where issues related to treatment options are discussed, while Scenario Three refers to the immediate postoperative period in an acute care setting. Scenario Four might focus on discharge planning while Scenario Five takes place in an outpatient cancer center where ongoing patient monitoring and prognosis are the main learning issues. There is no norm for the number of scenarios to be included in any problem, but experience suggests that anywhere between one and five seems appropriate, depending on the complexity of the case being presented and the level of students. Cases for beginning students are less complex and have fewer scenarios while those for senior students require more scenarios due to their increasing complexity. However, students generally wish to move on to another problem after five to six weeks, which allows for exploration of no more than four or five scenarios.

The second component of the problem package, termed the *patient data,* is the description of the particular patient (or family) being presented in the problem package. Included in the patient data are: personal variables such as age, ethnicity, physical appearance, and personality traits, a relevant health history, physical assessment findings, and, where relevant, laboratory and radiology results. It is these patient details that make the situation real and the problem specific; students often speak of the patients by name and describe the situations encountered long after they have moved on to other problems.

An important component of the problem package is the *tutor guide,* which contains information to assist the tutor with implementing the problem in the tutorial setting. Schools with integrated curricula often have educators facilitating problems about which they have some knowledge but no clinical experience, therefore, supplemental material describing key concepts and significant patient issues guide the tutor to ensure essential content is explored. Additional supplemental material may include helpful hints for facilitating the students' critical inquiry. This information is particularly useful in nursing programs where PBL has been recently introduced. Some schools have developed "facilitator phrase books," containing principles for effective facilitation as well as examples of questions to stimulate discussion (Mpofu, Das, Murdoch, and Lamphear, 1997).

Next in the problem package is a *learning resource list*. This is a compilation of relevant resources such as clinical experts who could act as consultants to the students, community programs and services, and educational materials such as texts, journal articles, and audiovisual resources. This seems to be an optional addition to the problem package, since some educators using PBL believe students should find all their own resources while others adhere to the belief that pointing students to some classic resources and community experts will facilitate learning, especially for beginning students.

Finally, a feedback form is included with a problem, to encourage students and faculty to comment on the usefulness of the problem and to include any new resources that were identified by the tutorial group.

PROCESS OF PROBLEM DEVELOPMENT

The actual design of the problems for a program of study consists of several steps (Figure 7.1), which we will follow to present the process of problem development. At Step One in the initial iteration of problem development, the mission and philosophy of the educational program, the outcomes for each

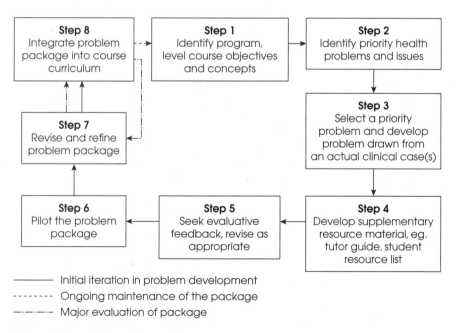

Figure 7.1 Development cycle for a PBL problem package.
© Mohide and Drummond-Young, 1996.

year, and the specific objectives for each course within the program should be reviewed. Within this context, at Step Two, the content for inclusion in course problems is selected and then, at Step Three, the specific problem is chosen for development. Each PBL problem is best developed from an actual patient situation or a compilation of several patients, since this adds to the authenticity of the problem for study. Supplementary resources are written and complied at Step Four, followed by the important activity of seeking feedback and revising the problem and its accompanying material, which is Step Five. At this point the problem is ready to be piloted within the PBL nursing course, with one or perhaps two tutorial groups (Step Six). During Step Seven, written feedback through the use of feedback forms and an interview with the tutorial group following the use of the problem provides information that can be used to refine and revise the problem as necessary. At Step Eight the problem is integrated into the course curriculum. Each problem is evaluated following its use through feedback obtained from students and a review of the currency of the information contained in it. For example, a problem concerning gastroenteritis in an 18 month old may need extensive revision if the gold standard for rehydration has changed. The problems for each course should be reviewed on a yearly basis and revisions and refinements made.

Until recently educators in PBL curricula have used intuitive guidelines as a basis from which to design problems for their curricula. Dolmans et al. (1997) made a substantial contribution to the problem design process through their review of the research on learning and cognition from which they derived the following seven principles of effective problem design, which will be referred to throughout our description of the problem development process:

- *Expected learning outcomes:* The learning outcomes expected by faculty should be embedded in the problem in a way that they are likely to be identified by learners.
- *Phase of the curriculum:* The problem should be consistent with the phase of the curriculum and stage of student learning.
- *Level of complexity:* Problems should be complex enough for learners to look broadly yet appreciate the need to work collaboratively to maximize learning.
- *Degree of integration:* Concepts from biological and behavioral sciences should be included to encourage integration of knowledge.
- *Openness of the problem:* The problem should be open-ended enough to challenge learners and sustain discussion.
- *Relevance and motivation:* The problem scenario should be relevant to practice, of sufficient interest to motivate student self-study, and should require learners to use thinking skills beyond simple knowledge and comprehension.
- *Promotion of student activity:* The problem scenario should promote active involvement in identifying and accessing resources and acquiring relevant information.

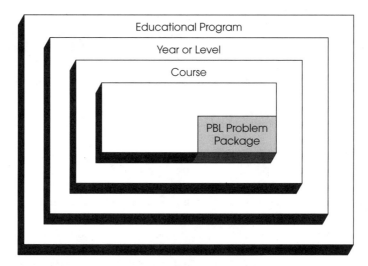

Figure 7.2 Ensuring the relationship among program components.
© E. A. Mohide and M. Drummond-Young, 1996.

What follows is a description of the process of problem development. This same process should be followed whether you are developing problems for one course within a conventional curriculum or for an entire PBL-based curriculum. We will illustrate the process of problem development with actual examples from a curriculum that uses the PBL Model for all nursing courses.

Step One: Review Expected Learning Outcomes

The first step in problem construction is a review of the relationships among the conceptual framework, the educational philosophy upon which the program is based, the expected outcomes of the educational program, the course objectives, and the level of students for whom it is intended (Figure 7.2). If these have not been clearly articulated and agreed upon by faculty, the first step is to revisit each of these issues.

Step Two: Determine the Content to Be Included

The knowledge, skills, and dispositions required to practice nursing effectively in the current and future health care context must next be determined and used as the basis for problem development. Bevis and Watson (1989) have suggested some broad guidelines for the selection of program and course content and these are:

• The legal and professional standards, governance, and guidelines (e.g., nurse practice acts, entry level competencies, and accreditation criteria).

- The demography of the community within which the school resides; the characteristics, age distribution, income level, employment trends, ethnicity, and needs of the population, and the services, agencies, and health care providers available to meet those needs.
- The purposes, philosophy, and organizational structure of the institution that sponsors the school of nursing.
- Present and projected health problems and issues and their probable management.

Barrows and Tamblyn (1980) have suggested five criteria to be used in choosing the specific problems to be developed: (1) the problems are commonly seen; (2) they represent urgent situations that require skillful, effective management; (3) they have a potentially serious outcome to which an intervention can make a significant difference; (4) they are often poorly handled; and (5) they emphasize or underline important concepts in the basic foundations of practice.

These criteria were extended by MacDonald et al. (1989) in their model for determining the priority health problems to be included in the medical school curriculum at McMaster University. Categories in their model include: (1) the prevalence and/or incidence of the problem; (2) the one-year case fatality rate [i.e., the number of individuals dying of a disease within one year of diagnosis divided by the total number of individuals with the disease during the same time period (Lilienfeld and Stolley, 1994)]; (3) the level of remaining quality of life (based often on a "best estimate" by one or more clinicians); (4) duration of deviation from health; (5) urgency of the illness condition; (6) availability and applicability of preventive measures; (7) accuracy and availability of the diagnostic process; and (8) efficacy of treatment measures. The authors developed a weighted scale, where each of the eight categories had a possible score of 0 to 2, to allow for a quantitative approach to choosing priority conditions for medical education. Although they acknowledge that the usefulness of this approach is dependent on the quality and quantity of information available, they contend that the model encourages a more holistic analysis of health care data from which to derive curriculum content.

The limitation of this approach for nursing is that it relies heavily on medical diagnostic labels and misses many of the causal factors related to the health problem being evaluated. Arthur and Baumann (1996) revised the MacDonald et al. (1989) approach, by incorporating the concept of amenability to nursing interventions, wherein "health-related issues where nursing can expect to have little impact are of lower priority than those that can benefit from the unique services provided by nurses" (p. 64). Their priority health issues formula has five components: (1) magnitude of illness, or the prevalence and/or incidence of disease; (2) the case-fatality rate which provides information about the severity of the problem; (3) lost quality of life, which the authors acknowledge is at present difficult to calculate; (4) duration of ill health, which addresses the length of time nursing interventions may be required; and (5) the concurrent burden factor, or the potential burden the problem may create within a community. The priority health issues derived from this formula are then assessed in relation to their amenability to nursing interventions, which are determined through the literature and from expert opinion and designed to achieve any or all of the following outcomes, depending on the situation:

- To decrease the magnitude of the problem
- To facilitate maximum function
- To improve quality of life
- To minimize the duration of the problem

This approach to content selection captures disease specific health problems; however since it relies on medical diagnoses, population-based health problems and issues that are of particular relevance to nursing practice and therefore important to include in a nursing curricula may be missed. Risky health behaviors such as smoking, poor nutrition, and teenage pregnancy are difficult to quantify in a formula; however, they can be ranked in terms of how well they respond to the "mission of nursing," namely, health promotion, illness prevention, and enhanced coping (Arthur and Baumann, 1996). The use of information about both amenability to nursing interventions and the common health issues and problems provides some rationale for the choice of curriculum content rather than relying only on expert opinion and faculty bias.

In summary, some method such as the Arthur and Baumann (1996) formula, is useful to identify the priority health issues for nursing practice, which might be classified as the Health Issues and Problems Theme within a curriculum. These become the focus for the problem development. All the other content themes of the curriculum, based perhaps on a careful analysis of the criteria suggested by Bevis and Watson (1989), are then embedded in one of these priority health problems. For example, content themes might be Nursing Role Theme, Communication Theme, Teaching/Learning Theme, and Concepts and Theories for Nursing Practice (all related to nursing practice), and Professional Evolution and Health Care System Theme (all derived from system issues). Through such a process core knowledge for the practice of nursing is identified and problems are developed for use of PBL tutorials. An example of the content areas for an intermediate level PBL course are included in Table 7.1.

Phase of the Curriculum

Selection of content for any course is also influenced by the phase of the curriculum (Guideline #2, Dolmans et al., 1997). The problem should be consistent with the phase of the curriculum and sequencing of the teaching/learning experiences for which it is being used. It should enable

Table 7.1 *List of content areas by curriculum theme*

Nursing Role Theme	Professional Evolution Theme
Nursing role, acute care	Collaboration and decision making on
Rehabilitation	multidisciplinary teams
Community resources	Conflict identification
Assessment	
Individual	Teaching/Learning Theme
Family	Application of education theory with
Community	patient/families
Goal setting/planning	Discharge planning
Accountability	Self-care
Advocacy	
	Health Care System Theme
	Risk factors for disease
Concepts and Theories for Nursing Practice	Morbidity/mortality
Growth and development	Introduction legal issues
Coping	Public Hospitals Act
Role theory	Occupational Health and Safety Act
Separation anxiety/bonding	
Family theory	Priority Health Issues
Self-esteem/self-image	Cancer
Pathophysiology	Cerebrovascular accident
Group theory	Ischemic health disease
	Asthma
Communication Theme	Diabetes mellitus
Use of terminology/documentation	Adolescent health issues including
Interpersonal communication	smoking and gender identity
Dyads/Families	Gastroenteritis

students to build on and activate prior knowledge (Davis and Harden, 1999; Dolmans et al., 1997). The sequencing of the learning is based on the curriculum framework and is approached in a number of ways. "Many nursing programs begin with the simple and move to the more complex in both conceptual learning and clinical practice. Some argue that health and healthy clients should be introduced first, since health in its broadest sense, is central to nursing. Others argue that students come into the program with a predetermined image of nursing as a technical profession, so their learning readiness should be captured by providing in-hospital experiences and later move to health, which is a very complex concept" (*BScN Programme Handbook*, 1999, p. 16). The sequencing of the learning which evolves from the curriculum plan serves to establish the placement of essential concepts for beginning, intermediate, and senior students in order to ensure that the core content and entry to practice competencies are learned when students are both cognitively and developmentally prepared for the content, for example, have had the foundational knowledge and life experiences or appropriate clinical exposure to build upon and make the content meaningful.

If the sequencing of the concepts in your program moves from health to illness, the emphasis for the problems at various stages of the program may appear as follows:

Beginning Level   Health as a broad concept and contexts affecting health (various settings, growth and development, economic, social and cultural determinants)

Intermediate Level   Illness/disruption in health and coping (acute/chronic/community)

Senior Level   Health as a holistic concept, promotion, illness prevention in a variety of community and institutional settings

Therefore health problems that most naturally emphasize the concepts essential to a given level should be placed accordingly. An example of a beginning level problem is given in Box 7.1. It is based in part on a number of regional priorities identified by a local health survey and relates to the overall emphasis for beginning students on broad concepts of health.

This problem is designed for students to explore content areas related to: (1) the determinants of health such as income level; (2) the normal growth and development of a school-aged child; (3) the significance of nutrition in relation to learning; and (4) the role of the public health nurse in the elementary school system. The chart data describing Jeannie indicates

---

Box 7.1   Jeannie Bradley—School-aged child

Scenario One

Jeannie is a seven-year-old grade two student at Earl Kitchener School. She lives with her parents and three-year-old sister, Gracie. At the beginning of the school year there was no apparent difference between Jeannie and her peers in terms of academic performance. However, her teacher has noticed that over the last few months Jeannie has been "falling behind" the others, particularly in language skills (reading, spelling, and writing). Jeannie appears to be overly tired and shows a lack of interest and motivation. Occasionally she has fallen asleep in class. When asked if she is getting enough sleep at night she states she goes to bed at 8:30 p.m. on school nights.

Jeannie's teacher contacts you, the public health nurse, in order to ask for some advice.

© *School of Nursing, McMaster University.*

she lives with her parents and has a younger sibling. When the students are asked what important features need to be assessed in this situation they will recognize, from their prior learning and life experience, that family life has a major influence on children and that there are a number of ways in which family life affects children. They may discuss what is important for normal family functioning and for healthy living, which should lead to the exploration of some of the determinants of health such as unemployment, poverty, and nutrition. Cues such as the child's age and grade should initiate questions, such as "What are the cognitive tasks of a normal seven-year-old?" "What might affect a seven-year-old's ability to accomplish these cognitive tasks?" As the author of a PBL problem be sure you have a clear understanding of the curricular content students have been exposed to previously through compulsory electives and non-nursing courses. For example, they may have completed courses in Introductory Psychology, and Growth and Development of the Child, and students should be making connections and application between knowledge attained in these courses and Jeannie's situation (Guideline #4, Dolmans et al., 1997).

Step Three: Select a Priority Health Issue and Develop the Problem

Once the content has been selected, there are many issues to consider in developing the actual problems for study, among them choosing the format to be used, ensuring the openness of the problem, embedding cues to specific learning outcomes, and promoting both integration of content and student activity.

Format for Problem Presentation

Problems can be presented to students in one of several formats: (1) as written scenarios, where the relevant history and clinical findings are provided in a sequential manner; (2) through a standardized patient, where people trained to simulate an actual patient in every detail are interviewed and examined by the students; (3) with videotapes, where the scenario is presented through a video-clip; and (4) using computer formats, wherein students ask questions, request additional information, and suggest actions. Other less frequently used presentations are newspaper clippings and actual patients as well as policy guidelines and research proposals for the purpose of studying issues relevant to population health (Davis and Harden, 1999; Jayawickramarajah, 1996; Pham and Blumberg, 2000).

Harden (1983) has identified the following factors to keep in mind when selecting the appropriate format to present problems to students:

- The ability to communicate the necessary information
- Ease of use
- Ease of production

This last factor is largely influenced by the resources available to produce the problem. Programs in large universities or colleges will likely have technical assistance and qualified support staff to assist. Those with standardized patient programs will have a means to train patient simulators to act out the patient roles identified in the problems. The other major influence on format choice is whether your program is offered on–site or uses a distance modality. Web pages or PC Challenges, used for both online synchronous tutorial work as well as in the live tutorial setting are making PBL accessible to a larger cohort of students (Harden, 1998; also see Chapter 14). Since the underlying principles of effective problem design are the same for all formats and since the written format is used most often, it will be used to illustrate problem development in this chapter.

Openness of the Problem

Barrows (1985) proposes that problems should be ill-defined, providing cues that leave the potential learning issues open enough to permit analysis of the clinical situation, while at the same time having "one central theme, similar to a mystery story, rather than multiple themes" (Hafler, 1991, p. 153). There are two major areas to consider in relation to ensuring the problem scenario is open enough to sustain discussion (Guideline #5, Dolmans et al., 1997). First of all, clinical information should not be pre-interpreted. Students must learn to deal with the kind of raw data they will encounter in the clinical setting. Drawing their own conclusions about the data is the first step in clinical decision making and constitutes hypothesis generation, one of the preliminary steps in the PBL process. So, instead of reporting hypertension or clinical depression, the author should include the blood pressure reading and the symptoms of affective disorder that the patient in the scenario is experiencing. This will give the student the latitude to "explore the hypothesis space." In addition to beginning the clinical decision-making process, pre-interpreting the data also pre-sets the learning issues in an explicit way and does not stimulate students to define for themselves what is relevant to learn or to generate alternate learning issues, which contravenes some of the basic tenets of PBL. Students should both define for themselves what is important to learn and be actively involved in the learning process (Barrows and Tamblyn, 1980). Second, avoid including judgments and stereotypes that cloud or prejudice the students' perception of the patient or situation in the problem scenario, except when the intent is to identify and develop a learning theme or concept. An example of this may be related to the diagnosis of AIDS and health provider attitudes.

Embedding Content for Learning

Since the mission of nursing is so broadly based and the range of possible content to include in any problem is immense, it is important to choose carefully the content for any one problem and to design it so that students are not overwhelmed by the potential learning possibilities (Guideline #1, Dolmans et al., 1997). The challenge for problem development is to engage the student in an appropriate learning direction, and the first opportunity lies in the title of the problem (Pham and Blumberg, 2000). A broad title such as the name of the individual in the problem and a general area of focus, like family violence, chronic illness, or rehabilitation, creates a mind-set from which the student will have a greater likelihood of interpreting the cues to the embedded content.

Developing tools such as a "learning concept grid" can also assist the faculty and tutorial group, by making explicit the content areas to be addressed in the problem. Concepts to be explored through the course are listed and, at the completion of each problem, the faculty member and students identify which concepts were explored and use the list as a guide in the selection of subsequent problems for study. An example of a learning concept grid for Jeanette Lalonde, Scenario One, a problem within an intermediate level course, is presented in Table 7.2. Similar concept grids can be

Table 7.2 *An example of a learning concepts grid*

Example: Paper Problem/ Problem and Scenario	Concept	Specific Issues/Problems/ Nursing Diagnoses Explored
J. Lalonde Scenario 1	Coping	Fear and anxiety related to unknown etiology of lump and anticipatory fear of possible diagnoses of cancer.
	Pathophysiology	Types of breast cancer.
		Other conditions which may cause breast lumps.
	Self-care/health promotion	Self-breast examination. How to do it? What are the benefits? What are its uses as a screening tool?
		Potential knowledge deficit related to not knowing how to do breast examination or the potential benefits of this form of self-care.
	Epidemiology	Incidence of breast cancer in this age group.
		Causes of breast cancer.
		Potential risk of breast cancer related to presenting symptom of breast lump and increasing incidence of breast cancer.
	Role of the nurse	The role of the nurse in an outpatient surgical clinic.
		Physical assessment and health teaching for a woman with a breast lump.

developed for each problem package within a course, since they are a kind of quality control, to ensure that the content for a particular course is indeed included in the problems developed for the course.

Cues to the content in the problem should be written clearly in order to avoid distracting ambiguity and so that students can recognize and process the information to be gained (Schuwirth et al., 1999). Lack of clarity about the meaning of salient details or terms of reference can inhibit the exploration and elaboration that initiate the inquiry process. Jargon should be avoided since it leads to ambiguity and preoccupies the student with a search for the unknown, moving the focus of exploration from the embedded concepts. Such short forms as COPD (chronic obstructive pulmonary disease) or SOBOE (short of breath on exertion) are often uncommon language to students with limited exposure to the clinical setting and therefore should be written in full.

The problem scenario should contain sufficient cues to guide the student and to stimulate discussion through posing critical questions and giving explanations (Dolmans et al., 1997; Davis and Harden, 1999). Box 7.2 gives an example of how the cues to the content elicit a search for explanations.

This scenario, describing the entry into the health care system of Jeanette Lalonde, is intended for Intermediate Level students, where the focus is acute illness. Breast cancer was selected because it remains the most commonly diagnosed malignancy in women. Canadian statistics demonstrate that the incidence of breast cancer is increasing by 1.5 percent per annum. As the population ages the incidence of breast cancer is expected to increase further (Logan, Aitken, and Evans, 1999). This problem is a prototype of breast cancer detection and diagnostic management which students are likely to encounter in their current clinical practicums and have perhaps encountered in their personal lives. The concepts in this scenario become shaped by the health problem and the other contextual variables. In this scenario, learning to cope with anticipatory fear of potential diagnosis of breast cancer is a central theme, and this is congruent with the learning concepts grid, where coping is one of

---

Box 7.2   Jeannette Lalonde-Acute Illness

Scenario One

Jeannette Lalonde is a 50-year-old woman who began an exercise class in October. About mid-October she noticed a lump in the upper outer quadrant of her left breast. She consulted her family physician about the lump. The family physician palpated the lump and ordered a mammogram. The mammogram indicated an abnormality. At this point Mrs. Lalonde was referred to a surgeon.

You are the nurse assigned to Mrs. Lalonde when she comes in for her first visit with the surgeon. You will be conducting the initial assessment.

© School of Nursing, McMaster University.

the concepts highlighted for study. Students should learn about coping theory and search the literature to learn how general coping concepts are applied to the patient with breast cancer. Cues to the need to learn about the epidemiology and early detection of breast cancer are presented by the patient's age and initial detection of the breast lump. Obvious learning questions related to this cue would be: "How common is breast cancer?", "In what age range is it most prevalent?", and "How sensitive and specific are diagnostic tests such as mammograms and biopsies?" Here, as with any PBL problem, students move from the specific health problem, breast cancer, to the embedded principles or concepts, for example, incidence and prevalence of breast cancer, efficacy of diagnostic tests, issues in coping with uncertainty, and then generalize this learning to other contexts in both their clinical and academic settings (Davis and Harden, 1999).

The issue of effectiveness of problems in stimulating the intended learning outcomes has been of interest to researchers as well as problem developers, and investigators have focused primarily on the congruency between student-generated learning issues and predetermined faculty objectives established for a given problem (Majoor et al., 1990; Dolmans et al., 1993; Mpofu et al., 1997).

The most extensive work in this area has been conducted by Dolmans et al. (1993) and Mpofu et al. (1997). They define effective problems as those that enable the student to identify learning issues that have a high degree of correspondence with the objectives that were pre-set by the faculty. Such problems assist students with accomplishing the intended learning outcomes for the course, by leading them to learn core content (Mierson, 1998). However, if problems are poorly constructed, students may not identify the appropriate learning issues and therefore fail to cover required content.

Dolmans et al. (1993) investigated the relationship between faculty objectives and student-generated learning issues by addressing three specific questions:

a. To what degree are faculty objectives reflected in student-generated learning issues?
b. To what extent do students miss certain objectives and are these faculty objectives classifiable?
c. Do students generate learning issues not expected by faculty? Are these relevant to course content and why do students generate these issues?

Data were collected during a six-week course offered to a cohort of 120 students in the second year of a medical school program. The course consisted of 12 problems based on 51 pre-set faculty objectives. Group facilitators were asked to record all the learning issues generated by students in their tutorials. Twelve pairs of experts were asked to judge the congruency between the faculty objectives and the student generated objectives for each problem. It was assumed that a faculty objective was identified when the two raters agreed that the learning issue corresponded with the objective. If the raters failed to agree or if both raters agreed that there was no correspondence, then an objective was assumed not to have been identified by the student.

In response to the first question, the twelve tutorial groups identified on average 64 percent of the faculty objectives. For 10 of the 12 problems the congruence between learning issues and objectives were close to the average.

Analysis for the second question revealed about 15 percent of the faculty objectives were not perceived by students as relevant to their learning. Three major categories of mismatches were identified. First, the tutors' objectives that also related to other curricular activities, such as knowledge learned in skills labs and other courses, or those perceived by students as having been covered in another context did not qualify as a learning issue. Second, the tutors' objectives spanning more than one problem, such as "the influence of the environment on health," were seen as too broadly defined and additional skill in focusing the learning question and searching the database were required. For this reason the students avoided them. Finally, psychological and social objectives were seen by medical students as having less priority than physiological objectives and therefore were often neglected.

The third question addressed mismatches consisting of learning issues identified by students that were not expected by faculty. These mismatches revealed four categories of learning issues:

1. Those related to prior knowledge deficiencies. Faculty expected this content to be known since it was covered in prior courses.
2. Those focusing on patient management and intervention rather than physiology and pathophysiology. These were concepts intended for study later in the curriculum.
3. Those where students attempted to integrate information learned in other courses. These issues were intended for a different educational experience, such as skills training and were outside of the mandate of the course.
4. Those arising from students' personal interest in and experience with the health problem or issue.

A later study by Mpofu et al. (1997), using a similar method with a cohort of entry-level medical students, supported the above findings. Most significant was their conclusion that broadly defined objectives, along with tutor and student inexperience, influenced the ability of students to cover intended course content and subsequent learning outcomes.

For the most part, students in both studies were able to identify what they needed to know. This seems to relate to the quality of the problem, as well as the facilitator and student familiarity with the stages or steps in the PBL process (Dolmans et al., 1993; Mpofu et al., 1997; Davis and Harden, 1999). Beginning students require some assistance with the inquiry stages of PBL, when they are exploring the cues to the embedded content. Unlike medical curricula, nursing curricula tend to be more biopsychosocial or holistic with a greater focus on health and the quality of life, making psychosocial issues more likely to surface while pathophysiology may be perceived as a lesser priority. Therefore, learning objectives or concepts should be clearly defined for each problem especially those that are likely to be ignored by students. Orienting the student to the focus of the course will help to minimize the possibility of missing important learning issues relevant to the problem.

Promoting Integration of Learning

An understanding of the overall educational program is also useful when deciding how to integrate learning outcomes from other courses into your problem scenario (Guideline #4, Dolmans et al., 1997). It is well-known that learning basic science concepts within the context of a health problem enhances the students' ability to integrate the information (Barrows, 1985; Norman and Schmidt, 1992). As you construct the problem keep in mind that students from traditional information-oriented educational approaches tend to compartmentalize their knowledge to specific courses (Dolmans et al., 1993). Therefore, it is important to provide some means of triggering the need to integrate knowledge from other courses. The majority of nursing programs have undergone a process of adaptation of PBL into pre-existing programs of study, resulting in a hybrid PBL curriculum, where the majority of nursing courses are taught using an integrated approach and other courses use a combination of lecture, seminar, and tutorial formats. Therefore, providing an overview of concurrent courses in the course manual, for which you are developing the problem, will make this information available to both tutors and students. This should assist with reinforcing integration of the content as an explicit expectation.

As the author of the problem scenario it would be useful to have a blueprint of both prior and concurrent courses, for example, critical appraisal of the literature, epidemiology, population health and the sciences such as physiology and pathophysiology. This will assist you with identifying what is prior learning, what is more recent learning and therefore needs to be reinforced, and what degree of cognitive sophistication should be expected of students to manage the integrated concepts. For example, if intermediate students have not yet taken a course in critical appraisal of research, we should not expect them to critically appraise a study they may have retrieved in response to a learning issue but rather expect them to respond to some pre-set questions related to the author, content level, and currency of the information in their journal article or text. (See Chapter 5 for more detail on learning information management skills.)

It is also of great benefit to the student to integrate the knowledge and experience obtained through their concurrent clinical practice which might be taking place in an acute or chronic care setting or in the community. This adds relevancy to the problem and gives the student an opportunity to spend more time reflecting on the health care delivery system than may be available

---

Box 7.3 Jeannette Lalonde–Acute Illness

Scenario Two

The surgeon performed a needle aspirate. The pathology report showed infiltrating ductile carcinoma of the breast tissue. Mrs. Lalonde discussed various treatment options and their effectiveness with the physician and the nurse. After consideration of treatment effectiveness and the implications of treatment on her ability to care for her family and perform her farm duties, she decided to have a mastectomy. Surgery was scheduled for the following week. As a nurse in the surgical clinic you will be involved in Jeanette's preparation for surgery.

© *School of Nursing, McMaster University.*

---

while in a busy practice setting where other issues take precedence. Knowledge and skills from other courses are integrated in the following example.

The learning issues within the scenario shown in Box 7.3 include: (1) the pathophysiology of adenocarcinoma; (2) treatment options available; (3) body image/self concept; (4) grief and loss; (5) family coping; and (6) patient teaching and pre- and postoperative care. Cues such as "various treatment options" and "their effectiveness" might lead the student to ask "What are the treatment options for Jeanette Lalonde?", "How effective are these options?", and "What are the risk factors involved with these options?" The next cue "implications of the treatment on her ability to function" leads the student to ask if some treatments are more debilitating than others, with longer term adverse effects. Mrs. Lalonde has chosen to have a mastectomy. This is likely to lead the intermediate student, who has had prior exposure to the concepts of self-esteem and body image, to question the impact of losing a breast and to wonder what the literature has to say about body image post mastectomy. These students also have prior knowledge of the normal function of the musculoskeletal system. This knowledge will be mobilized by the cue that our Mrs. Lalonde works on a farm, a job that requires both stamina and stresses the musculoskeletal system, and leads to questions about the amount of muscle that is removed with a mastectomy and the impact that has on her functional capacity. Other questions such as "What is adenocarcinoma?" and "What pre- and postop teaching is required for Jeanette?" are more explicit in the scenario. Thus, the cues presented in this scenario will engage the student, stimulate interest, and elicit elaboration through building on previous learning.

Level of Complexity

When writing problems for an integrated curriculum one should keep in mind that themes will be revisited at later stages in the curriculum, so that the level of complexity of the problems should increase over time (Guideline

#3, Dolmans et al., 1997). Each scenario should build on prior exposure to the concepts within the theme, adding new learning outcomes and presenting fresh learning opportunities. For example, using the theme of communication, the following learning opportunities might be presented. As an introduction to professional communication, students might study a problem that triggers learning issues such as distinguishing between social and professional communication, identifying stages of the interview, and developing the skills of focusing and following. These goals might be met using a problem about a normal, healthy woman who is perimenopausal.

The subsequent examination of the communication theme might build on prior learning by focusing on active listening skills and the technique of active inquiry. These goals might be met through a problem where a patient is seeking help with smoking cessation. In this situation the student would develop skills in interpreting affect and content. The interpretations will assist the student with hypothesizing about the strengths and barriers associated with smoking cessation.

A more advanced level of development of effective communication skills could come through the opportunity for self-awareness, more in-depth analysis, and increased sophistication with interview techniques, through an encounter where therapeutic interventions with a grieving patient are required. The student would become more self-aware by exploring his/her own feelings related to loss and grieving and how these feelings impact on the nurse-patient relationship.

In order to maintain a stimulating level of complexity, every visit to a theme should result in (Harden and Stamper, 1999, p. 141):

New knowledge or skills

More advanced application of areas covered

Increased proficiency or expertise through further practical experience

Relevance to Practice and Motivation for Self-Study

The problem scenario should be relevant to real-life clinical practice (Guideline # 6, Dolmans et al., 1997; see also Arthur and Baumann, 1996; Davis and Harden, 1999; MacDonald et al., 1989; Pham and Blumberg, 2000). Research on human memory indicates that there is better recall if the context in which the information is learned is similar to the context in which it is applied (Brown, Collins, and Duguid, 1989; Godden and Baddeley, 1975; Tulving and Thomson, 1973). The contextual information in the scenario should depict the appropriate health care services and providers available to meet the needs that result from the health issues or problems in the region where the school is located. This provides the students with the types of health problems and context that are similar to those they will be exposed to in their clinical practicum, and therefore, will enable them to more effectively recall what they have learned through the problem.

As the author of the problem, it may be helpful to consult with clinicians who work with the types of patient you are writing about, to discuss the sorts of issues such patients encounter and how they are likely to be treated. These consulting clinicians can be a valuable resource to authors who have some knowledge of the area about which they are writing but little clinical exposure, since they will be able to review the problem scenarios and patient data for internal consistency. Supporting patient data such as health history, physical examination findings, and diagnostic results may be based on one case or a number of cases. If a number of cases are used to develop your prototype problem, ensure there is congruency among the presenting symptoms, health history, and diagnostic results to avoid ambiguity about the content to be studied. For example, a sixteen-year-old female with a three-year history of Insulin Dependent Diabetes Mellitus (IDDM) who is ambivalent about giving in to peer pressure to drink alcohol, has a slightly high blood sugar and has a chronic yeast infection, presents as a congruent picture of a recently diagnosed adolescent struggling to come to terms with her diabetes.

In addition to developing data related to the health problem or issues, it is important to provide details about the patient family and social history. Personal characteristics give "life" to the individual(s) in the scenario and provide cues to elaborate on the psychosocial issues relevant to nursing care. The role of the nurse should also be clearly identified. This provides the student with a perspective from which to understand the learning outcomes and also makes explicit the unique contributions and services provided by nurses.

Promotion of Student Activity

The problem should motivate the student to self-study and should require learners to use thinking skills beyond knowledge and comprehension (Guideline # 7, Dolmans et al., 1997). In order for students to learn effectively in PBL the problem must provide (Schmidt, 1993; Charlin, Mann, and Hansen, 1998):

Active processing of information

Activation of prior learning

Meaningful context

Opportunities for elaboration and the organization of knowledge

Constructing a context similar to the student's clinical setting, using a patient population they will encounter, and providing a clear role for the nurse will enhance interest in the content to be studied since students are given both a perspective from which to view the problem and can easily relate to it. The problem should also sustain discussion about the embedded content which will engage and stimulate the student to seek further explanations. As the students attempt to identify relevant factors in order to understand the issues described in the problem they make use of pre-existing ideas, opinions, and prior knowledge. This provides them with the direction and the extent of study that needs to be undertaken in order to acquire a deeper understanding of the problem (Barrows, 1985). Through this analysis of the cues and the application and reorganization of prior knowledge, the students are able to identify what they know and what they need to learn. Current theories in the science of learning and cognition emphasize that students should be actively engaged in acquiring knowledge and should take a major role in defining the content (Schmidt, 1993; Dolmans et al., 1997).

Active involvement in identifying and accessing resources leads to independent study, which is a core component of effective PBL. Resource acquisition and application are integral to student learning outcomes and are strongly influenced by learning issues. Therefore, close attention must be paid to those factors that shape the student's selection of learning issues and resources (Blumberg, Michael, and Zeitz, 1990; Dolmans et al., 1993; van den Hurk, Wolfhagen, Dolmans, and van der Vleuten, 1999). A recent study by van den Hurk et al. (1999) contributes to our understanding of how learning issues impact on independent study. They collected interview and questionnaire data from a cohort of 69 percent of the students from years one to four in a medical program in Holland, to explore three key areas related to the impact of learning issues on various aspects of their independent study: (1) the impact of the tutorial group process on generating useful learning issues; (2) the influence of learning issues on independent study; and (3) the variables associated with the choice of resources during independent study.

First, they found that well-structured tutorial discussion, where students listen to each other, influences learning issue selection, and the tutor—whose task it is to promote both stimulating and relevant exchange of ideas—ultimately guides the discussion in the tutorial group. Tutors therefore require both content knowledge and process facilitation skills in order to succeed with this very significant role in the learning process (Schmidt et al., 1996). This once again underscores the importance of providing the PBL faculty tutors with adequate guidelines to support their role in tutorial.

Second, they found that learning issues were the predominate influence on initiating study and determining what content should be studied. Junior students tended to be more reliant on learning issues and focused solely on that content whereas experienced students were more spontaneous, expanding their focus as they came across concepts that "piqued their interest." Third, lists of recommended resources and preset objectives were the most important factors in student selection of resources for independent study, since they provided a baseline from which to work and saved the students a lot of time. These findings reinforce the usefulness of reference lists which might include key articles, clinical experts, and appropriate subject headings to assist the students with searching for the most recent journal articles in the content area. Other less traditional resources that might be included are lectures, independent learning packages, and audiovisual presentations specific to the problem under study. These are particularly useful in countries where the literature in a specific topic area may be limited. Some schools have developed a sequencing of information management skills to assist their entry-level students to become more effective and efficient with research skills, and a comprehensive discussion of strategies to nurture information management skills is presented in Chapter 5.

Active engagement with the problem. can also be facilitated through feedback to students about their learning. Concerns about whether they are learning what they need to know dominates the literature on student perceptions of PBL (Ishida, 1995; Khoiny, 1995; Rideout, 1998; Solomon and Finch, 1998). Although this should not present a problem since students emerge from PBL with lifelong learning skills, it still seems to trouble those who are making the transition from information-oriented education to PBL (Davis and Harden, 1999). Mixed methods of validating how effectively the small group has worked with problems are useful. First, a powerful mechanism for receiving feedback about content acquisition as well as group process occurs in the final step on the PBL process, when the group reflects on their learning and group process issues. Second, the learning concepts grid described earlier in the chapter can be used to provide feedback to students that they explored the relevant content embedded in the problem. Third, some problems have a set of multiple choice questions placed in the tutor or student guide which can be used at the end of a problem to provide formative feedback on the knowledge acquisition These are not used as a summative evaluation measure since this approach to content evaluation has been found to direct the learning activities to only the content that is being tested (Dolmans and Schmidt, 1994). A final suggested method of providing formative feedback and encouraging student learning is the use of either oral or written journals, which are found to promote deeper learning such as integration, assimilation, and generalization. This strategy promotes analysis and evaluation of the students' learning experience in relation to the problem and group process. It is generally considered an important aspect of turning experiences into learning by questioning and evaluating what has been learned (Boud, Keogh, and Walker, 1995; also see Chapter 6). Evaluation of the student's ability to apply concepts related to communication techniques can be accomplished by interacting with a standardized patient. This resource not only provides an opportunity for evaluation but it also adds an emotional and behavioral dimension to the cognitive learning triggered by the problem scenario. The student interview with the standardized patient should be accompanied by clear outcome objectives and parameters for feedback. Further discussion related to the standardized patient as a resource in PBL is available in Chapter 12.

Step Four: Develop Supplementary Resource Material

A point of debate in problem development concerns the degree of compre-hensiveness of the patient data included in the problem package. Should it have some missing data such as one might encounter in real practice, for example, inadequate or absent assessment information, or should it reflect "best practice." On the one hand, general opinion on this issue seems to favor inclusion of comprehensive patient data to support the problem narrative especially in problems used with beginning students. Bordage and Lemieux (1991) argue that the provision of problems reflecting best practice are important since clinicians tend to recognize patterns in new clinical situations and relate them to how they resemble or differ from the prototype. On the other hand, senior students tend to have sufficient clinical knowledge and exposure to enable them to identify gaps in the client data. Another consideration when presenting the patient data for the problem is choosing the structure to follow, such as Gordon's functional health patterns.

A variety of resource materials are an integral part of the problem package, of which the patient scenarios we have described above are only part. The availability of standardized patients to portray the patient is a useful adjunct for learning. The development of written content and process guidelines for tutors to use in encouraging learners to generate ideas, question, integrate, and reflect on the issues and concepts triggered by the scenario can be helpful. Additional means of supporting student learning and tutor comfort, especially for those who may not have content expertise in the area, include scenario specific information such as written preset problem objectives or essential concepts, a list of present and possible patient problems, and a resource list with key resources related to the clinical case. These will assist the tutor with promoting a lively discussion and focusing the group. Overall, effective questions should stimulate and challenge the student's assumptions, explanations, knowledge base, ability to identify learning issues, and self-directed learning skills.

Step Five: Seek Evaluative Feedback; Revise as Appropriate

Once the problem has been developed it should be reviewed by an objective reader who has: (1) a fairly good idea of the curriculum themes and how essential content is sequenced; (2) prior experience writing problems; and (3) familiarity with the clinical orientation of your problem. This person should give feedback on any duplication or gaps with relation to content as well as determine the level of complexity for the intended students. Any suggestions for revision should be incorporated into the problem, which is now ready for use with tutorial groups.

Step Six: Pilot the Problem Package

A next step in the problem development process is to pilot the problem package with two tutorial groups: one with an experienced PBL tutor who is familiar with the health problem and the other with a tutor who is less experienced in PBL and/or with the clinical content. This "test" problem should be piloted on a voluntary basis, and used in place of one of the regular problems offered in the designated course. Each of the tutorial groups could then provide the author with feedback on their ability to work with the new problem. The author may want to develop a feedback form that targets any areas of concern regarding the new problem. The pilot process avoids the potential of a very useful, and often labor-intensive problem, being axed from the curriculum, by catching flaws related to implementation at an early stage.

Steps Seven and Eight: Revise and Refine Problem Package and Incorporate into the Curriculum

In these final steps, any last revisions are made to the problem which is then incorporated into the curriculum. The half-life of curricula is estimated to be five years, which necessitates periodic close review of both content and process (Arthur and Baumann, 1996). Therefore, it is important that all the existing problems be reviewed in order to maintain relevancy of the content to both practice and placement in the curriculum. Any scientific advancement that would impact on how the problem is presented, change the diagnostic assessments or treatments or alter the prioritization of the health problem or issue will have an impact on its significance to the curriculum. One fairly efficient way of keeping up-to-date with this information is to enable students and tutors to respond to the problem by filling out a semi-structured feedback sheet that invites them to revise and update any changes in practice and literature or human resources.

DEVELOPING PROBLEM WRITING SKILLS: FACULTY EXPERIENCES

Although educational principles essential to the development of effective problems have been discussed in this chapter, little has been said about the educator's experience of constructing PBL problem packages. The experiences of novice authors in a baccalaureate nursing program that recently adopted PBL provide insight into the benefits and concerns for faculty and resulted in some practical suggestions to assist faculty members with problem development (Hengstberger-Sims and McMillan, 1993). Adequate faculty support such as workshops, mentoring and providing dedicated time for faculty to develop their case writing skills were described as essential to promoting the development of quality problem packages.

Mohide and Drummond-Young (1996) also explored the problem development experiences of faculty teaching in an undergraduate baccalaureate nursing program with a well-established PBL curriculum. The processes, satisfactions, and challenges associated with authoring problem packages were surveyed. Almost all participants reported that they experienced one or more sources of satisfaction, the most frequent source of which was the sense of having made a significant concrete contribution to the curriculum. However, 80 percent of the "authors" experienced problems associated with the process, including a lack of explicit and consistent guidelines for problem development, no prototype problem packages to serve as examples, and a lack of identified experienced faculty to serve as mentors or resources for those who were involved in writing up cases for the first time. The survey results also suggested the need for improved consistency in formatting problem packages. Faculty found inconsistency in ways the many component parts of problems were developed, which distracted from the delivery and flow of the problem and was both time consuming and frustrating. Faculty authors also identified the need to establish a means of maintaining quality control of the problems already developed. Faculty were concerned that some "old problems" were no longer priority issues or health problems and that since the curriculum had undergone recent revision they no longer fit where they were placed in the teaching/learning sequence.

The overall content analysis from this study resulted in the development cycle for PBL problem packages which was presented in Figure 7.1. This cycle depicts a stepwise approach to problem construction and maintenance, which could be used in conjunction with the seven educational principles discussed earlier in this chapter, in order to provide a critical path for problem construction.

CONCLUSION

Crafting skillful problem packages for PBL is an art. In this chapter the importance of selecting content and designing the problem scenarios on evidence-based rationale has been acknowledged and applied to curriculum development. Utilizing a systematic population-based approach to identifying relevant health issues or problems facilitates both the currency and representativeness of curriculum content. The problem packages should reflect health problems and issues students will be exposed to in their current and future practice as well as provide learning opportunities to develop problem-solving skills and application of knowledge. Research into learning and cognition has given us well-grounded principles from which to construct engaging problem scenarios that will effectively promote active learning to meet essential learning outcomes. Well-structured problems activate prior knowledge and stimulate students to elaborate on cues to the embedded content. They also elicit student-generated learning issues that have a high congruence with preset faculty learning objectives for the scenario.

This chapter has confirmed the crucial importance of the PBL problems to student learning and satisfaction. Authors developing problem packages require dedicated time for the task of writing, a prototype problem to refer to, and input from clinical experts in order to ensure internal congruency of the component parts of the problem package. The guidelines developed by Dolmans et al. (1997) should be used to guide the process. Great problems make great learning!

REFERENCES

Arthur, H. and Baumann, A. (1996). Nursing curriculum content: An innovative decision-making process to define priorities. *Nurse Education Today, 16(1),* 63–68.

Bachelor of Science in Nursing Programme Handbook. (1999–2000). *School of Nursing, McMaster University,* Hamilton, ON.

Barrows, H. S. (1985). *How to Design a Problem-based Curriculum for the Pre-clinical Years.* New York: Springer.

Barrows, H. S. (1988). *The Tutorial Process.* Springfield: Southern Illinois University.

Barrows, H. S. and Tamblyn, R. M. (1980). *Problem-based Learning: An Approach to Medical Education.* New York: Springer.

Bevis, E. O. and Watson, J. (1989) *Toward a Caring Curriculum: A New Pedagogy for Nursing.* New York: NLN.

Blumberg, P., Michael, J. A., and Zeitz, H. (1990). Roles or student-generated learning issues in problem-based learning. *Teaching and Learning in Medicine, 2,* 149–154.

Bordage, G. and Lemieux, M. (1991). Semantic structures and diagnostic thinking of experts and novices. *Academic Medicine, 66,* S70–S72.

Boud, D., Keogh, R., and Walker, D. (1995). *Reflection: Turning Experience Into Learning.* London: Kogan Page.

Brown, J. S., Collins, A., and Duguid, P. (1989). Situated cognition and the culture of learning. *Educational Researcher, 18,* 32–42.

Charlin, B., Mann, K., and Hansen, P. (1998). The many faces of problem-based learning: A framework for understanding and comparison. *Medical Teacher, 20,* 323–330.

Davis, M. H. and Harden, R. M. (1999). AMEE Medical Education Guide No. 15: Problem-based learning: A practical guide. *Medical Teacher, 21(2),* 130–140.

Dolmans, D. H., Gijselaers, W. H., Schmidt, H. G., and van der Meer, S. B. (1993). Problem effectiveness in a course using problem-based learning. *Academy of Medicine, 68(3),* 207–213.

Dolmans, D. H. and Schmidt, H. G. (1994). What drives the student in problem-based learning? *Medical Education, 28,* 372–380.

Dolmans, D. H., Snellen-Balendong, H., Wolhagen, I. H., and van der Vleuten, C. P. (1997). Seven principles of effective case design for a problem-based curriculum. *Medical Teacher, 19,* 185–189.

Gijselaers, W. M. (1996). Connecting problem based practices with educational theory. In L. Wilkerson and W. Gijselaers (Eds.), *Bringing Problem-based Learning to Higher Education: Theory and Practice.* San Francisco: Jossey-Bass.

Godden, D. R. and Baddeley, A. D. (1975). Context dependent memory in two natural environments: On land and underwater. *British Journal of Psychology, 66,* 325–331.

Hafler, J. P. (1991). Case writing: Case writers' perspectives. In D. Boud and G. Feletti (Eds.), *The Challenge of Problem-based Learning.* New York: St. Martin's Press.

Harden, R. M. (1983). Preparation and presentation of patient-management problems. *Medical Education, 17,* 256–276.

Harden, R. M. (1998). AMEE Guide No. 12: Multi-professional education: Part I—Effective multi-professional education: A three-dimensional perspective. *Medical Teacher, 21,* 7–14.

Harden, R. M. and Stamper, N. (1999). What is a spiral curriculum? *Medical Teacher, 21,* (2), 141–143.

Hengstberger-Sims, C. and McMillan, M. A. (1993). Problem-based learning packages: consideration for neophyte package writers. *Nurse Education Today, 13,* 73–77.

Ishida, D. N. (1995). Learning preferences among ethnically diverse nursing students exposed to a variety of collaborative learning approaches including problem-based learning. Unpublished doctoral dissertation, University of Hawaii.

Jayawickramarajah, P. T. (1996). Problems for problem-based learning: A comparative study of documents. *Medical Education, 30,* 272–282.

Khoiny, F. E. (1995). The effectiveness of problem-based learning in nurse practitioner education. Unpublished doctoral dissertation, University of Southern California.

Lilienfeld, D. E. and Stolley, P. D. (1994). *Principles of Epidemiology.* New York: Oxford University Press.

Logan, D. M., Aitken, S. E., and Evans, W. K. (1999). Breast Screening. *Journal SOGC,* July, 779–785.

MacDonald, P. J., Chong, J. P., Chongtrakul, P., Neufeld, V. R., Tugwell, P., Chambers, L. W., Pickering, R. J., and Oates, M. J. (1989). Setting educational priorities for learning the concepts of population health. *Medical Education, 23,* 429–439.

Majoor, G. D., Schmidt, H. G., Snellen-Balendong, H. A., Moust, J. H., and Stalenhoef-Halling, B. (1990). Construction of problems for problem-based learning. In Z. M. Nooman, H. G. Schmidt, and E. S. Ezzat (Eds.), *Innovation in Medical Education: An Evaluation of its Present Status.* New York: Springer.

Mierson, S. (1998). A problem-based learning course in physiology for undergraduate and graduate basic science students. *Advances in Physiology Education, 20*(1), S16.

Mohide, E. A. and Drummond-Young, M. (1996). *Developing Paper Problems for Small Group Learning in Baccalaureate Nursing Programmes: A Survey.* In Global Connection in Learning, First International Conference of the Nursing Education Research Unit, McMaster University, Hamilton, ON, June.

Mpofu, D. J., Das, M., Murdoch, J. C., and Lamphear, J. H. (1997). Effectiveness of problems used in problem-based learning. *Medical Education, 31,* 330–334.

Norman, G. R. and Schmidt, H. G. (1992). The psychological basis of problem-based learning: A review of the evidence. *Academic Medicine, 67,* 557–565.

Pham, K. and Blumberg, P. (2000). Case design to emphasize population health concepts in problem-based learning. *Education for Health, 13*(1), 77–86.

Rideout, E. (1998). The experience of learning and teaching in a non-conventional nursing curriculum. Unpublished doctoral dissertation, University of Toronto.

Schmidt, H. G. (1993). Foundations of problem-based learning: some explanatory notes. *Medical Education, 27,* 422–432.

Schmidt, H. G., Machiels-Bongaerts, M., Hermans, H., Ten Gatre, O., Venekamp, R., and Boshuizen, H. (1996). The development of diagnostic competence: a comparison between a problem-based, an integrated, and a conventional medical curriculum. *Academic Medicine, 71,* 658–664.

Solomon, P. and Finch, E (1998). A qualitative study identifying stressors associated with adapting to problem-based learning. *Teaching and Learning in Medicine, 10(2),* 58–64.

Schuwrith, L. W., Blackmore, D. E., Mom, E., van den Wildenberg, F., Stoffers, H. E., and van der Vleuten, C. P. (1999). How to write short cases for assessing problem-solving skills. *Medical Teacher, 21,*(2), 144–150.

Tulving, E. and Thomson, D. M. (1973). Encoding specificity and retrieval processes in episodic memory. *Psychological Review, 5,* 352–373.

van den Hurk, M. M., Wolfhagen, I. H., Dolmans, D. H., and van der Vleuten, C. P. (1999). Student-generated learning issues. A guide for individual study? *Education for Health, 12(2),* 213–221.

The Faculty Role in Problem-Based Learning

Angela C. Wolff and Elizabeth Rideout

> . . . *[A] good tutor maximizes tutorial opportunities by being active in a variety of ways: in planning and preparing, in listening, in encouraging critical thinking, in enriching, in offering spoken and unspoken feedback . . . and is restrained in the transmission of information. The active tutor should have a plan for each tutorial, but rarely invoke it; should have knowledge, but not unload it; should have questions, but not feel compelled to ask them. (Glick, 1991, p. 1)*

The faculty role is central to problem-based learning (PBL), and there is consensus that adoption of that role requires a profound reframing of the assumptions and fundamental beliefs about learning and teaching (see, for example, Barrows and Tamblyn, 1980; Barrows, 1988; Boud and Feletti, 1991; Creedy, Horsfall, and Hand, 1992; Kalain and Mullan, 1996; Schmidt, 1983; Stinson and Milter, 1996; Tipping, Freeman, and Rachlis, 1995; Walton and Matthews, 1989; Wilkerson and Hundert, 1991). To be effective, faculty enacting the PBL tutor role must depart from the more didactic *chalk and talk approach* that emphasizes the dissemination of information and become facilitators of learning, where the emphasis is on questioning student logic, values, and beliefs; assisting students to clarify their learning needs and select resources for self-study; and facilitating student discussion and evaluation.

While some faculty may find sharing control in the classroom and relinquishing their status as expert cause for uncertainty, those who embrace PBL approaches discover a sense of freedom and relationships that are empowering to students and rewarding to faculty. As such the adoption of PBL has profound implications for faculty and this chapter will focus on the various components of that change. It begins with an overview of the PBL faculty role, including descriptions of effective, and ineffective, faculty behaviors. An issue that has received considerable attention is the relative importance to student learning of expertise in content compared to skill in group process, and the empirical evidence related to this topic will be provided. Finally, faculty development programs are acknowledged as essential for adoption of the PBL faculty role. The features of a variety of programs that have been devised to assist faculty in the transition will conclude this chapter.

THE ROLE OF FACULTY IN THE PBL MODEL

The importance of the faculty role in the PBL Model, and strategies for successful enactment of the role, have been investigated from the perspectives of both students and faculty, and described by a number of writers. As the following section indicates, there is significant congruence among the descriptions of the faculty role.

Student Perceptions of the Importance of the Faculty Role

Students describe the faculty role as crucial to effective learning in PBL tutorials. This was made abundantly clear in a recent study by Rideout (1999), where students in a PBL program provided the following comments on the role and influence of the faculty:

> *I think the tutors are vital in moving the group and having us cover things that are important because tutors know better than [we do] what is important and what we should be getting out of this.*

> *The tutor's role was certainly that of guidance for the group.*

> *The tutor's role is to make sure we don't miss the big things and to redirect us if we get off topic.*

> *The tutor said it was her goal to help us come together and I want you to feel free to express yourself and if you get off track maybe we can help you back on, if not, if you are going in the right direction I will encourage you.*

> *The group was good because of the tutor. (She) helped us identify our own issues, if someone was standing back she would help us deal with it. She facilitated.*

Similar comments are evident in the work of Virtanen, Kosunen, Holmberg-Marttila, and Virjo (1999) in their study of medical students in Finland, who described the tutor role as facilitating the group rather than leading it, and helping to keep the group focused. Specific comments included:

> *The tutor probed in the right direction but did not lecture.*

> *The tutor does not say a lot. He can stir things up if necessary.*

von Döbeln (1996) described her experience as a student in a PBL medical program in Sweden similarly, emphasizing the importance to her learning of tutor involvement in group dynamics, and in helping the group become aware if they became embroiled in a discussion that was peripheral to the problem of current interest. She acknowledged: "A possible trap for tutors is to interfere too much and not allow students to solve problems in their own way. It is not easy being a good tutor" (p. 96).

Faculty Perceptions of the Faculty Role

Faculty in the Rideout (1999) study described their role as that of guide and advocate. In fulfilling such a role, the faculty tutor is there to challenge students to explore issues in depth, ensure students develop correct and current information, and set standards of achievement. Faculty also describe the importance of "letting students know you know what they are talking about" and "challenging students if they have incorrect information." They also acknowledge that all this must take place within a supportive environment, in an atmosphere of trust and caring facilitated by the tutor. Similar descriptions were reported by authors such as Stinson and Milter (1996), who noted the teacher observes, corrects, and encourages the performance of students, and Gijselaers (1996) who described the role as "a balance between allowing the students to discuss issues and intervening to make sure that critical issues are identified" (p. 19).

The need to adapt the role to the level of student has also been acknowledged (Rideout, 1999). Words like *coaching, cajoling, guiding* were used to describe the role in interactions with beginning students, while collaborating, relinquishing control, and becoming more of a mentor were the role expectations in the senior year of the program. These role descriptions mirror those of Barrows (1988), who spoke of the role change as moving from modeling to coaching to fading.

The words of students are perhaps most informative on this issue:

I saw the tutor as a very strong role in guiding and learning. They coached and cajoled you, especially in first year.

The tutor became more of a collaborator with the student. By fourth year the tutor totally backed off, they never told you what to do, it was more what did you do today and where do you want to go from here?

They stepped out and took on more of a mentor role. They helped me, and moved from dictator teacher to more of a mentor role.

In second year she took on leadership roles. In fourth year she was willing to relinquish control. She was a great role model.

Effective and Ineffective Faculty Behaviors

Personal and professional qualities of *helpful* faculty have been noted by several authors. Mayo, Donnelly, and Schwartz (1995) suggest that the effective or outstanding faculty tutor demonstrates the ability and patience to listen to students. Since faculty who provide direct answers can "short circuit" the entire learning process, effective tutors must possess the fortitude not to provide answers prematurely or force personal views when students fumble. Furthermore, skilled faculty tutors support the group in choosing a course of action and guiding them through the steps of the PBL process. They keep the dialogue focused, provide constructive feedback that focuses on behaviors rather than personality traits, and act as role models by illustrating their ability to apply the principles of PBL. Qualities identified by Barrows (1988) include the importance of active reflection upon their tutoring practices so that insight and improvement can occur. He asserts that tutors know they have been successful when the tutorial group can function independently or with minimal guidance, and effective faculty tutors recognize this.

Rideout (1999) found that faculty tutors were considered helpful when they: (1) demonstrated knowledge and expertise, including being up-to-date clinically; and (2) interacted with students in ways that displayed enthusiasm, interest in students and their learning, empathy and patience, support, flexibility, and attention and involvement in student learning. These behaviors were exemplified in the following quotes:

The tutors I found most helpful were those who expected more, were very organized, were on the ball, and knew exactly what you were doing.

The traits of a good tutor included being attentive to group needs, being part of the group, involved in all the decisions. We looked to her as a peer. She was involved in all that we were doing, we would listen to her.

Particular behaviors that *hindered* the learning process have been identified by writers such as DesMarchais (1991) who reported that students identified tutors who did not intervene and who seemed unconcerned with group process as unhelpful, while Kaufman and Holmes (1996) recounted tutor weaknesses in managing group process, including being too directive, letting the group get off topic, being disrespectful to students, and having no sense of humor.

Tutor qualities and behaviors that hindered learning have also been identified by Rideout (1999) as: (1) being severe and harsh in student-tutor interactions (e.g., being outspoken, abrupt, critical, and/or rigid); and (2) demonstrating a lack of sufficient engagement with students (e.g., being disorganized, wishy/washy, not punctual, too laid back, inconsistent, and subjective; and not dealing with issues of group process). The situations described below exemplify the behaviors perceived by students as negative for learning:

She is very intense, and a lot of "you don't know this or that," a lot of constructive criticism and not very much that was good. I need to be told I am doing something well also.

We were very on edge, trying to figure out what she wanted, and "if I say something, is it going to get me in trouble." You would say something and the tutor might say "no, I don't think so" and we would be very unsure. The group was stressful and the whole atmosphere was very tense.

I have been in groups where the tutor was very directive and we ended up doing something we didn't feel was important. In that kind of environment we ended up feeling frustrated and dreading the next class.

We were left to do a lot on our own and not given much incentive to get moving.

She could have been a little more active, it took us so long to get going, she could have given us a few more suggestions.

Not surprisingly, the positive and negative faculty actions described above are not dissimilar to those identified in the extensive literature that describes more or less desirable faculty behaviors in non-PBL curricula (see, for example, Cust, 1996; Reilly and Oermann, 1999; Wong and Wong, 1987).

Content Versus Process Expertise

The voices of students and faculty indicate that a broad range of behaviors and skills are required in order that effective and enjoyable learning occurs. Although they allude to the issue of the relative importance of content knowledge compared to group process expertise required for the role, they do not provide a clear answer. Is one area of expertise more important to student learning than the other, or do the best results come from a combination of subject and process expertise? For the answer to this question, we turn to the research literature.

There is some evidence to support the contention that tutors should have content expertise. Davis, Nairn, Paine, Anderson, and Oh (1992) studied student-tutor interactions during one PBL course within a curriculum that was otherwise traditional in structure and process. Twenty-one tutorials—where one-half were led by tutors with content expertise and the others led by nonexperts—were taped, and the data analyzed. The researchers found scores on end-of-course multiple choice examinations and ratings of tutors by students were greater in groups led by content experts compared to those with nonexpert tutors. A trend to a slightly higher percentage of time devoted to teacher-led activities in the expert-led groups was noted. In a similar study, Eagle, Harasym, and Mandin (1992) examined the quantity and appropriateness of the learning issues identified within groups led by content experts compared to nonexpert led groups, and they concluded that twice as many learning issues were identified by groups led by content experts. The tutorials were not taped, so the differences in behaviors of the two types of tutors were not available for examination.

The influence on learning of process expertise was the subject of a study by Silver and Wilkerson (1991), who compared four tutorial groups where two tutors had content expertise and two did not. The groups were taped and tutor comments analyzed for the amounts of time taken up by comments of students and tutors and the patterns of exchanges during tutorials. Expert tutors were more likely to take a directive role in the tutorials, speaking more often and for longer periods, and providing more direct answers. The investigators concluded that the use of expert tutors resulted in more teacher-directed discussion, which is at odds with the educational philosophy and benefits of student-directed interaction on learning outcomes.

Altogether these studies suggest that both process and content expertise are required by tutors but, prior to the work of Schmidt, van der Arend, Moust, Kox, and Boon (1993) and Schmidt and Moust (1993), the best mix of the two areas of proficiency was unclear. Schmidt et al. (1993) explored the effects of content and process expertise on students' achievement scores, self-study time, and student ratings of tutor behaviors. Using data collected from 336 tutorial groups within seven different PBL programs, they concluded that students guided by content experts spent more time on self-directed study and achieved somewhat better scores on end-of-unit achievement tests than students guided by nonexpert tutors. It is noteworthy that there was also a positive although somewhat lesser effect on student achievement scores when tutors had process expertise only. Furthermore, content and process expertise were correlated, leading Schmidt and his colleagues to conclude that subject-matter knowledge and process-facilitation skills "are intimately intertwined in the behaviors of effective tutors and that both contribute to the learning of students" (p. 790).

Further evidence comes from a second study conducted by Schmidt and Moust (1995) using 524 tutorial groups representing a variety of health sciences programs. These authors analyzed correlations among tutor behaviors and students' self-study time, reported interest in subject material, and level of achievement. The researchers concluded that students learned best when the tutor combined content expertise with personal qualities that created an atmosphere for learning, namely, a commitment to students' learning and an ability to express oneself in a language understood by students. Not surprisingly they concluded that students' learning is enhanced by tutors who demonstrate strength in both content and process. Overall the study findings and the related literature point to the fundamental importance of the faculty tutor as an influential factor in effective learning outcomes and a sense of achievement for students. To date, much of the literature has focused on the overall perceptions and attitudes of medical educators and students. Nevertheless, the findings support the conclusion that expertise in both content and process are required for optimal learning for students and satisfaction for tutors.

Specific Strategies for PBL Faculty

Each stage of the PBL process presents special challenges for faculty and students. Although some or all of the actions described below are equally relevant in non-PBL situations, it is only within the PBL Model that they are all required on a regular basis to assist students to attain and apply new knowledge. All of the PBL sessions focus to a greater or lesser extent on helping students develop the skills and dispositions of group process, self-directed learning, critical thinking, critical reflection, and information management—what Barrows (1988) refers to as *metacognition,* and particular faculty strategies related to these outcomes are discussed in more detail in the chapters in Section Two. Some general approaches that faculty should use to facilitate the PBL process follow.

Getting Started: The First PBL Session

One of the first issues that faculty will confront is how to begin the first PBL session of a course with a new group. Drawing on previous experiences of initiating groups will certainly be useful, since many of the activities should be the same. Introductions are an important starting point, and there are many ice breakers that can make this time both engaging and effective (see, for example, Westberg and Jason, 1996). It is during this initial activity that the climate begins to be established. An attitude of acceptance and openness encourages everyone to participate and lets group members discover each others' particular interests, areas of expertise, and hopes and fears about the course. If students have completed other PBL courses, it is useful to inquire about their likes, and dislikes, about their previous experience, and their expectations for this new course. By expressing interest in each student and asking questions, faculty model the desired behaviors of students. Once the group members have introduced themselves, some discussion of process issues is useful. This activity results in what some faculty call "ground rules" or "group norms." This introductory session is also a time for the faculty member to share group and course expectations. Expectations regarding attendance, promptness, completion of group tasks, and ongoing group evaluation are some of the common topics that should be debated and decisions taken.

In addition to setting the emotional climate, the first session also provides an opportunity to begin to establish the educational climate. Clarifying that it is acceptable, indeed encouraged, to say "I don't know" is important, and that saying "But I will find out" is even better! Challenging the opinions and information that students bring to the group is another important norm that can be discussed in the first session. Certainly it is important to make it clear that students are expected to take increasing responsibility, as the course progresses, for monitoring the task and maintenance activities within the group.

Helpful Hints for Facilitating PBL Groups

The first steps for a group confronted with a PBL problem are the analysis of the problem and identification of learning issues. The emphasis here is on stimulating inquiry and critical thinking through the use of thought-provoking open-ended questions such as:

- Are there other possibilities you may not have thought of?
- What is the evidence to support that idea?
- Would you explain that a bit more?
- What do you mean?

- I'm not sure I'm clear just what you plan to explore further, it seems a bit broad to me.
- Let's stop and review what we know now about the issue.

Once learning issues have been identified and clarified, students discuss and finalize the kinds of resources they will search out. This may include using the resource lists that are often available, but it will always include some debate about the merits of alternate resources and identification of new options. The faculty member assists this process by challenging the choices if they are unclear, suggesting alternatives, assisting students to consider resources other than textbooks and journal articles, and generally ensuring that students leave with a clear direction. For example, a student may say he or she will look at the community resources relevant to a particular problem. Here the faculty member should question the student to ensure that she or he is specific about just what community agencies might be approached, for what purpose, and the plan for contacting the resource. This level of intervention on the part of the tutor should decrease as the students gain experience with the PBL process, and, in fact, students would take offense if the faculty member did not become less active in their questioning over time.

Once the students have completed their information search, they return for the next step of the process, where they share and critique the new information. During this time, the faculty tutor focuses on ensuring that the discussion is at a level of rigor, depth, and breadth appropriate for the stage of the group. The tutor again challenges the students by asking for fuller explanations, for clarification of points made, and for links with other new and prior knowledge. All group members are encouraged to participate and again the tutor models the expected behaviors and becomes less active in the questioning and linking activities as the students become more skilled.

At this session the faculty tutor also asks students to describe the resources they used during the period of self-directed study and the process used to access the resources (e.g., computer searches, internet, interviews with resource people, and visits to community settings). As Barrows (1988) comments, students often express frustration that resources were not available or did not contain the quality or quantity of information expected. Finding the right resource is difficult, but the process is assisted by a thorough orientation, practice, and feedback. These strategies are described in detail by Bayley, Bhatnagar, and Ellis in Chapter 5. Students are also expected to critique the resources they bring to the session. The tutor aids this process by again asking such challenging questions as (Barrows, 1988, p. 38):

- What was the date of publication of that book?
- Who were the authors of that article and are they authorities in the field?
- How do you know the information is reliable?

During this stage of sharing new learning, it is often a temptation for each student to deliver a "minilecture" on the topic they chose to pursue during self-study. Here again the faculty must be prepared to intervene, to prevent the outcome that Barrows (1988) describes as: "the power of their new learning will be lost if they just sit there and, in essence, lecture to each other about what they have learned in their study" (p. 39). Instead students should be encouraged to debate the consistencies and inconsistencies in the information being presented, compare it with their prior knowledge of the subject, and begin to apply it to the patient problem. Again the faculty member's role is to challenge, ask for fuller explanations, help students make connections and summarize key issues. Some useful questions include:

- Do we have the entire explanation now?
- Do we have all the facts we need to move on?
- How does this information support or not support our original hypothesis?
- How will this information help us to manage the patient situation?

The final stage of the PBL process is the evaluation of the learning that has taken place, what Barrows (1988) refers to as the "debriefing or the conscious integration of what has occurred" (p. 40). Again the faculty tutor plays a key role, by encouraging students to review what they have learned from the exploration of the problem. Some suggested questions include:

- What have we learned from this problem?
- How might this new information be used in your clinical practice?
- In what way has working through this problem helped with understanding (how nutrition affects diabetes, for example)?

Discussion like this helps to make the learning explicit and thus more likely to be retained for later use.

Attending to Group Process

Concurrently with interventions to assist students to develop their critical thinking, self-direction, and information management, faculty must also be attending to the group process issues that arise and helping students to become collaborative learners. There are many important issues confronted by most groups that will require interventions by the faculty tutor and these are discussed in depth by Benson, Noesgaard, and Drummond-Young in Chapter 4. As well, readers are referred to the wealth of literature on the topic of group process that provides useful guidance to the new and seasoned PBL tutor (see, for example, Barrows, 1988; Brookfield and Preskill, 1999; Corey and Corey, 1997; Sampson and Marthas, 1990; Tiberius, 1990; Westberg and Jason, 1996; Woods, 1994; Wolff, 2000).

COMPONENTS OF FACULTY DEVELOPMENT PROGRAMS

For many, adopting the faculty tutor role as described earlier is merely an application of their current role in a non-PBL curriculum. For others, the change requires a considerable shift in philosophy and beliefs about being a teacher, as well as changes in behavior. Faculty members have reported decreased levels of self-confidence and feeling of uncertainty about when and how to intervene in a tutorial group (Bernstein, Tipping, Becovitz, and Skinner, 1995; Creedy and Hand, 1994). To ease the role transition and maximize their role, it is essential that faculty receive orientation and ongoing support (Moust, deGrave, and Gijselaers, 1999; Stern, 1998). We will now consider the essential ingredients in an effective faculty development program, and describe the various programs that have been offered. While the list of issues to be considered in faculty development is long, the predominant challenges faced by faculty are: (1) reframing the theoretical basis of education, (2) developing an understanding of PBL, (3) acquiring and maintaining the qualities of effective tutors, and (4) developing leadership for the future (Irby, 1996).

Reframing the Theoretical Basis of Education

The first step toward adopting the PBL approach is a redefinition of the word *teacher*. Whether consciously or not, most faculty members teach "in ways that suggest we equate telling with learning and that we view teachers as the ultimate sources of knowledge" (Wilkerson and Hundert, 1991, p. 16). With the PBL Model, faculty first need to redefine their relationship to the content to be learned and the students to be taught. Barrows and Pickell (1991) suggest that faculty need to make themselves vulnerable and admit they do not know all the answers. Reframing views of the educational process also requires faculty to develop increased levels of professional and personal awareness of self in relation to others (Creedy and Hand, 1994; Wilkerson and Hundert, 1991). Such an awareness can be achieved through reflection on one's current teaching ideologies, approaches, and practices. This fresh image of faculty as facilitators of learning is a major pedagogical shift for those new to PBL approaches. Before faculty members can move on to where they need to go, they need to have awareness of who they are as faculty and what beliefs they hold. Such reflection indirectly shapes one's future action (Olson and Singer, 1994; Schön, 1987) and has been found to promote the development of competence (Wolff, 1998).

As faculty are rethinking assumptions about teaching and learning, they should also be introduced to the PBL Model and to the theoretical underpinnings of the model. The goal here is to assist faculty to question their old "ways of knowing" and become aware of PBL as an alternative approach to education. Both the theoretical basis for PBL and the research regarding

PBL provide rationale. So this first step in the faculty development process serves to explain why a new model of education is needed and provides rationale for one model that is both congruent with current educational theory and effective in practice.

Experiencing the process of PBL is a persuasive approach to increasing acceptance of the model. As Irby (1996) notes: "Reading and talking about PBL are not as powerful as experiencing the method. When they (faculty) experience the power of learning in this mode at an emotional level, their assumptions about teaching and learning will be challenged" (p. 74). Participating in a PBL session should be an essential first step in any faculty development program.

Acquiring Effective PBL Skills

Next faculty must achieve competence as skilled facilitators of the PBL process, which includes the complex and sometimes conflicting roles of consultant, learner, mediator, challenger, negotiator, director, evaluator, and listener. As Irby (1996) indicates, these are indirect forms of instruction that facilitate conversation, dialogue, and debate rather than the transmission of information, and identifying and practicing these roles is an essential feature of becoming an effective faculty tutor. Irby (1996) goes on to say that: "Faculty development programs (to help faculty acquire PBL skills) should be skill based with clearly articulated guidelines and rationale" (p. 75). Practicing the faculty tutor role in a small group, videotaping the practice sessions and obtaining feedback based on rationale are powerful strategies for learning new skills. It is useful to incorporate examples and exercises that highlight situations that faculty new to PBL often describe as difficult to deal with, such as giving up control, not delivering a lecture if the topic is close to the faculty member's heart, providing feedback on student performance and confronting group conflicts. Participation in such highly interactive sessions can be stressful, so it is essential that a safe environment be provided for faculty members as they take risks and practice these new skills.

Maintaining and Building on PBL Skills

This third component of a faculty development program for PBL has several aims. First, it is important to review and critique the experience of teaching in the PBL approach. Wilkerson and Maxwell (1988) suggest regular meetings of faculty teaching in a particular course. Such meetings provide the opportunity for faculty members to learn from and work with one another, dealing with both the content and process of tutoring. These meetings offer the benefits of ongoing collegial support and dialogue, and promote personal reflection.

Second, a focus on developing advanced conceptual knowledge about PBL and advanced teaching skills should be incorporated. Reviewing relevant literature and determining alternate strategies for dealing with new or recurring difficult situations in tutorials would be useful at this stage. As Irby (1996) states: "This is less skill oriented and more a process of reflection on experience and reconceptualization of ideas" (p. 75). A seminar format is appropriate here, where faculty share common problems and successes, experts can be called upon to provide their insights, and other mediums such as the series of videotapes for tutor training prepared by Maastricht University can be used to stimulate discussion.

Developing Effective Leadership Skills

The final component of a faculty development program should focus on the future, through inclusion of knowledge and skills in leadership and educational research for those faculty who have an aptitude and interest in leadership positions. Irby (1996) suggests activities such as workshops and fellowships aimed at leading groups, developing courses and curriculum, evaluating programs, and conducting research.

FACULTY DEVELOPMENT PROGRAMS

The aim of all faculty development programs should be to instill a positive attitude toward the PBL approach, promote confidence in the ability to serve as faculty tutors, and result in a change in focus from a teacher-centered to a student-centered educational philosophy (Kaufman, 1995). Below are five representative programs that embody these desired outcomes and incorporate all or most of the components discussed above.

Program 1

Benor and Mahler (1989), who developed their program for the medical faculty at Ben Gurion University, believe that programs for new PBL tutors should be continuous, multiphasic, interdisciplinary, appropriate in the provision of feedback and support, and considerate of individual variability of both needs and capabilities. To incorporate these beliefs, their program includes four phases. The *first phase* of the process features a two-day orientation workshop aimed at the attitudinal domain, and attendance is a prerequisite for academic promotion. Teacher philosophy, educational approaches, and identification of individual faculty needs are topics for discussion in small group sessions. The *second phase* consists of a three-day workshop introducing faculty to educational language, concepts, and basic instructional methods of PBL. The focus is on the cognitive and attitudinal domains necessary for the acquisition of generic knowledge to foster self-acceptance as faculty. This workshop is structured in small group modules with a larger plenary discussion and short lecture summary.

The *third phase* builds on the knowledge of education and the clarification of values attained through the Phase One and Two workshops, and focuses on the development of general faculty tutor skills, including high-level questioning, self-learning about the problem-based approach, writing test items, being a preceptor of students, and other topics based on specific tutor need. Each of five workshops ranges from three to four days in length and concentrates on a different aspect of the PBL Model.

The *fourth phase* targets a small group of faculty who have completed the previous phases, with the purpose of developing selected individuals for educational leadership. Faculty members attending these sessions are expected to further develop their own instructional abilities and acquire the detailed educational knowledge required to educate other faculty and to conduct research.

Benor and Mahler (1989) incorporated an evaluation component in their program, which included pre- and post-test questions that evaluated the cognitive components and the degree of satisfaction with the workshops. Faculty facilitating PBL groups were also evaluated by students on completion of the course through live or videotaped observations of their tutorials. Repeated observations of 60 faculty for two years revealed a significant change in faculty performance, in particular, an increased interaction among students within groups. While many components of this faculty development program are incorporated in programs implemented elsewhere, three unique features about this program are: the gradual acquisition of facilitation skills, from general to specific; the acknowledgment of individual differences among faculty members; and the emphasis on motivation and encouragement of faculty member involvement.

Program 2

The faculty development program of the University of Sherbrooke medical school, described by Grand'Maison and Des Marchais (1991), has three overall components. First, a two-day preparatory workshop focuses on the application of educational principles (e.g., student-centered learning, student motivation, and community-oriented education) to medical education. This workshop is obligatory for all medical faculty preparing to adopt the PBL tutor role. The format includes individual and group work, discussions, and a plenary session.

Next are workshops designed to prepare faculty specifically for their roles in PBL education. All new faculty members tutoring in the PBL program are required to attend a comprehensive one-day PBL introductory workshop, where participants learn about the theoretical foundations of PBL and student-centered learning, acquire beginning tutor skills, and construct PBL scenarios. Following this, new tutors must participate in a comprehensive three-day tutor training program, where the aim is to assimilate the PBL methodology and provide a safe environment for faculty to engage in the tutor role. In preparation for this, participants are asked to observe six hours of tutorials and identify their specific learning needs. Then, during the workshop, they concentrate on mastery of the particular tutoring skills they have identified. This latter program has also been modified and offered as a one-day refresher course to experienced tutors.

The Sherbrooke approach also includes an optional program for faculty members interested in assuming leadership and training roles in medical education. The program has three components: participants complete 17 self-instructional packages which cover basic concepts and major themes in medical education; they participate in 100 hours or more of training which focuses on developing a student-centered philosophy and facilitating the learning process; and finally they join in a half-day meeting every three weeks to discuss the module assignments.

A strength of this program is its emphasis on developing a base of knowledge about medical education in general, followed by the gradual acquisition of tutoring skills and the reinforcement of the newly developed skills. Although no systematic evaluation of the program was reported, Grand'Maison and Des Marchais (1991) concluded that high faculty member participation in the series of four faculty development programs resulted in a more student-centered educational philosophy and greater interest in medial education. These changes had a significant impact on implementation of the PBL curriculum.

Program 3

The McMaster University Program for Faculty Development is multidisciplinary and consists of three foundational workshops regarding PBL. Each workshop is interactional and lasts two days (Branda and Sciarra, 1995). The first workshop orients new faculty members to issues and skills involved in PBL. The first day participants enact the learner role by working through hypothetical interdisciplinary health scenarios within a tutorial guided by an expert facilitator. On the second day sessions are held on topics such as the use of resources (standardized patients, anatomy modules) and the development of PBL problems.

The second workshop emphasizes the role of the faculty tutor in small group learning. Beginning competence in the PBL process is developed though actual experience with a small group of students, who are volunteers from the various health sciences programs of nursing, medicine, physiotherapy, and occupational therapy. Feedback to faculty engaging in the PBL tutor role is provided by the workshop facilitator, peers, and students, with the latter found by participants to be most valuable (Branda and Sciarra, 1995).

A third workshop, described by Branda and Sciarra (1995) but no longer offered on a regular basis, focused on the principles of student evaluation and the development of evaluation measures. This workshop resulted in a publication available for purchase that summarizes the content of that workshop entitled "Evaluation Methods: A Resources Handbook" (see www.fhs.mcmaster.ca/ped).

A one-year leadership development program is also offered which prepares faculty to assume leadership roles in education. Participants take part in a variety of activities: they may implement a small research project, take a credit course in educational theory, attend a series of classes, or define any other activity that assists them to develop the necessary skills for effective leadership and management. Four two-day retreats are held over the 12-month period, to encourage discussion of the progress on individual projects. Each participant is also assigned a faculty mentor whose role is to provide support and guidance (Branda and Sciarra, 1995).

What is absent from the McMaster Faculty Development program is any planned follow-up or additional training and support for new faculty. Once they have completed the two introductory workshops (unless they are chosen to take the Leadership Development Program), they are left to receive any additional guidance and support from within their own department, with no formal provision to ensure that this occurs.

A strength of these faculty development workshops is the actual experience of participating in, and facilitating, tutorials and therefore encountering the range of common PBL issues. The only program evaluation data documented by Branda and Sciarra (1995) came from their observations of changes in faculty behavior that occurred during the introductory workshops.

Program 4

Creedy and Hand (1994) describe their approach for preparing nursing faculty to teach in their Bachelor of Science in Nursing Program at Griffith University, Australia, in which participants attend a seven-month professional development program which involves in-service sessions, planning sessions, and teaching observations. To facilitate adoption of PBL teaching practices, participants are encouraged to speak with colleagues, reflect on their actions, and provide support to one another. An interpretative case study method was used to examine changes over the course of the program in participants' thinking about teaching in general and the PBL method in particular. The data collection methods included personal reflective journals, classroom observations, groups discussions, and four semistructured interviews conducted before, during, upon completion of, and three months after completion of the program. These data were not used to evaluate the faculty development program per se, but were used as a basis for developing future faculty development programs, namely, strategies that foster reflection; opportunities to exchange information and share resources; and the development of peer support networks (Table 8.1). Their overall conclusion is that effective faculty development programs should provide a sense of control and power to the faculty learning process.

Table 8.1   *Factors Influencing Faculty to Change Their Teaching Style*

Factor	Description
Developmental nature of the conceptual change	Effective use of the new pedagogy takes place over time, similar to a developmental process. Educators moved from not knowing about the innovation to application of the innovation.
Influence of stress on conceptual change	Personal factors may influence a teachers willingness to adopt a new teaching and learning pedagogy. Stress can be inversely related to change, and lower levels of self-confidence, tolerance, and inability to cope interfere with adoption of the innovation. Faculty could not change until they were comfortable to do so.
Use of reflection is integral to the change process	To support the change process, it is necessary for the educational institution to provide a climate that is supportive of reflection (e.g., allowing and encouraging time for group team meetings). Faculty should be encouraged to reflect on both a personal and professional level.

Source: Adapted from Creedy and Hand, 1994.

Program 5

A quite different model of faculty development was devised for use in the medical school at Harvard University and has been used subsequently at the University of California Los Angeles (UCLA) (Wetzel, 1996; Wilkerson and Hundert, 1991; Wilkerson, 1996; Wilkerson and Irby, 1998). Their model begins with a precourse workshop of two hours (contrasted with the two-day introductory workshops used on other programs) where participants experience a PBL tutorial. Following that orientation, the program is "course-driven" meaning the general skills training is accomplished within the particular course in which the faculty member is teaching (Irby, 1996). Faculty members meet individually with an educational consultant from within the faculty development program, to preview the PBL problems and expected content to be discussed in the course. Weekly tutor meetings are held throughout the course, to discuss any issues and problems the tutors might be having, and to preview the case/problem for the coming week. Observation and feedback are other components of the program, wherein the consultant observes tutorials and gives feedback on a regular basis throughout the course. At the end of each course, faculty meet to discuss common issues, approaches, and revisions. A one-day workshop is held each year to discuss the tutorial process and any problematic issues that may have arisen in their groups. Thus the Harvard/UCLA program is more individualized and continuous than the other programs described and could be said to be more congruent with the learner-centered, self-directed philosophy of the PBL Model.

The evaluation of the effectiveness of the program focused on the satisfaction of tutors with the PBL faculty role. The majority described positive outcomes of the PBL process, but suggested that an incentive program for teaching should be established concurrently in any school moving to the teaching-intensive PBL Model (Nayer, 1995).

GENERAL CONCLUSIONS ABOUT FACULTY DEVELOPMENT PROGRAMS

First, successful adoption of the PBL Model depends largely on the acceptance of the institution and participation by all those who teach (Wilkerson and Maxwell, 1988). Successful programs should be designed with faculty involvement and those responsible for instituting the PBL method should encourage an alteration of the organizational environment to ensure specific individuals are allocated to the faculty development task. This includes the appointment of an effective leader, as well as the designation of consultant experts who have read the literature and who can determine faculty members' needs (Holmes and Kaufman, 1994; Wilkerson and Maxwell, 1988).

Second, faculty development programs for PBL must be experiential, so faculty "walk the talk" of participating in PBL, and thereby learn and practice the principles of PBL (Barrows and Pickell, 1991). Programs that expect faculty to develop their own learning objectives and engage in the learning program are congruent with PBL. As such, faculty should be expected to develop any specific and personal learning goals and seek out the necessary resources. Group sessions should allow faculty to role play their approach to various representative issues confronted in PBL sessions. The group facilitator acts as a coach, observing and giving feedback.

Third, written materials should be developed to enhance participants' knowledge base. One such resource is an orientation guide developed for faculty adopting the PBL Model (Wolff, 2000). This orientation guide, entitled *The Role of the Tutor: A Resource Guide for Nursing Faculty* is a user-friendly, concise, thorough resource that provides a background on PBL and focuses on particular strategies faculty can use in specific situations. It is a useful complement to the interactive workshops that should be the centerpiece of any PBL faculty development program.

Fourth, a process should be instituted for ensuring collegial support is offered to all PBL faculty. Personal contacts and social support play major roles in influencing individuals to adopt an innovation. Such support can take a variety of approaches, including regular faculty tutor meetings held at the beginning, during, and at the end of a course and observations of tutorials and feedback by peers.

Fifth, developing a method of rewards and recognition for teaching will reinforce faculty commitment to a new approach to education. Incorporating methods of faculty evaluation, acknowledging excellence in teaching through faculty and university awards for teaching, and including contributions to education as an expectation for tenure and promotion are some of the methods used to encourage and reward PBL teaching and continual learning.

Finally, the outcomes of the faculty development program should be evaluated. Although the aforementioned programs included some degree of evaluation, it was often limited. When devising a new program, it is recommended that a method of evaluation be built into the program. The desired outcomes should be made clear and specific and a model of program evaluation selected. Economic evaluations have been underrepresented in the literature on PBL. Therefore, an approach to cost analysis should be considered an integral component of outcome research. Studies should be conducted that use rigorous and appropriate methods of design and analysis.

CONCLUSION

Success of any curriculum that incorporates the PBL Model is dependent on a cadre of faculty who have a commitment to the method, the self-awareness and intellectual sensitivity to adopt and maintain the role, the ability to facilitate group learning, and sufficient expertise in the subject being explored by students to ensure rigor in learning. Faculty development is therefore crucial to prepare faculty for this new role. The most comprehensive faculty development programs featured in this chapter extend over a substantial period of time thereby allowing for the learning and change process to occur. These programs incorporate all domains of learning while featuring experiential learning. Typically, these programs also provide ongoing support to new problem-based learning tutors.

Overall, successful programs foster unconditional acceptance among faculty, offer support, acknowledge the feelings conjured by the change process, and utilize the influence of key educational leaders. Over a significant period of time, the focus of such programs should promote professional, instructional, organizational, and leadership development. Finally, all programs for faculty development should include formal and rigorous evaluation of their outcomes and cost effectiveness.

REFERENCES

Barrows, H. S. (1988). *The Tutorial Process*. Springfield, IL: Southern Illinois University School of Medicine.

Barrows, H. S. and Tamblyn, R. M. (1980). *Problem-Based Learning: An Approach to Medical Education*. New York: Springer.

Barrows, H. S. and Pickell, G. C. (1991). *Developing Clinical Problem-Solving Skills: A Guide to More Effective Diagnosis and Treatment.* New York: W. W. Norton.

Bernstein, P., Tipping, J., Bercovitz, K., and Skinner, H. A. (1995). Shifting students and faculty to a PBL curriculum: Attitudes changed and lessons learned. *Academic Medicine, 70*(3), 245–247.

Benor, D. E. and Mahler, S. (1989). Training medical faculty: Rationale and outcomes. In H. G. Schmidt, M. Lipkin, M. W. de Vries, and J. M. Greep (Eds.), *New Directions for Medical Education: Problem-Based Learning and Community-Orientated Medical Education* (pp. 248–259). New York: Springer-Verlag.

Boud, D. and Feletti, G. (1991). *The Challenge of Problem-Based Learning.* New York: St. Martin's Press.

Branda, L. A., and Sciarra, A. F. (1995). Faculty development in problem-based learning. *Annals of Community-Oriented Education, 8,* 195–208.

Brookfield, S. and Preskill, S. (1999). *Discussion as a Way of Teaching: Tools and Techniques for Democratic Classrooms.* San Francisco: Jossey-Bass.

Corey, M. S. and Corey, G. (1997). *Groups: Process and Practice.* Pacific Grove, CA: Brooks/Cole.

Creedy, D., Horsfall, J., and Hand, B. (1992). Problem-based learning in nursing education: An Australian view. *Journal of Advanced Nursing, 17*(6), 727–733.

Creedy, D., and Hand, B. (1994). The implementation of problem-based learning: Changing pedagogy in nurse education. *Journal of Advanced Nursing, 20*(4), 696–702.

Cust, J. (1996). A relational view of learning: Implications for nurse educators. *Nurse Education Today, 16,* 256–266.

Davis, W. K., Nairn, R., Paine, M. E., Anderson, R. M., and Oh, M. S. (1992). Effects of expert and non-expert facilitators on the small-group process and on student performance. *Academic Medicine, 67*(7), 470–474.

DesMarchais, J. E. (1991). From traditional to problem-based curriculum: How the switch was made at Sherbrooke, Canada. *Lancet, 338,* 234–237.

Eagle, C. J., Harasym, P. H., and Mandin, H. (1992). Effects of tutors with case expertise on problem-based learning issues. *Academic Medicine, 67*(7), 465–469.

Gijselaers, W. M. (1996). Connecting problem-based practices with educational theory. In L. Wilkerson and W. M. Gijselaers, (Eds.), *Bringing Problem-Based Learning to Higher Education: Theory and Practice.* San Francisco: Jossey-Bass.

Glick, T. (1991). The role of the tutor and learning agenda in the problem-based tutorials. Harvard Medical School, Office of Educational Development: *Tutoring Excellence, 1,* 1–2.

Grand'Maison, P. and Des Marchais, J. E. (1991). Preparing faculty to teach in a problem-based learning curriculum: The Sherbrooke experience. *Canadian Medical Association Journal, 144*(5), 557–564.

Holmes, D. B. and Kaufman, D. M. (1994). Tutoring in problem-based learning: A teacher development process. *Medical Education, 28,* 275–283.

Irby, D. M. (1996). Models of faculty development for problem-based learning. *Advances in Health Sciences, 1,* 69–81.

Kalain, H. A. and Mullen, P. B. (1996). Exploratory factor analysis of students' ratings of a problem-based learning curriculum. *Academic Medicine, 71*(4), 390–392.

Kaufman, D. (1995). Preparing faculty as tutors in problem-based learning. In W. A. Wright (Ed.), *Teaching Improvement Practices: Successful Strategies for Higher Education* (pp. 101–126). Bolton, MA: Anker.

Kaufman, D. M. and Holmes, D. B. (1996). Tutoring in problem-based learning: Perceptions of teachers and students. *Medical Education, 30,* 371–377.

Mayo, W. P., Donnelly, M. B., and Schwartz, R. W. (1995). Characteristics of the ideal problem-based learning tutor in clinical medicine. *Evaluation and the Health Professions, 18*(2), 124–136.

Moust, J. H. C., de Grave, W. S., and Gijselaers, W. H. (1999). The tutor role: A neglected variable in the implementation of problem-based learning. In Z. M. Nooman, H. G. Schmidt, and E. S. Ezzat (Eds.), *Innovations in Medical Education: An Evaluation of Its Present Status.* New York: Springer.

Nayer, M. (1995). Faculty development for problem-based learning. *Teaching and Learning in Medicine, 7*(3), 138–148.

Olsen, J. R. and Singer, M. (1994). Examining faculty beliefs, reflective change, and the teaching of reading. *Reading Research and Instruction, 34*(2), 97–110.

Reilly, D. E. and Oermann, M. H. (1999). *Clinical Teaching in Nursing Education.* Sudbury MA: Jones & Bartlett.

Rideout, E. (1999). Doing it: The roles, influences and behaviors of tutors. In J. Conway, and A. Williams, (Eds.), *Themes and Variations in PBL.* Callaghan, Australia: PROBLARC.

Sampson, E. E. and Marthas, M. (1990). *Group Process for the Health Professions.* Albany, NY: Delmar.

Schmidt, H. (1983). Problem-based learning: Rationale and description. *Medical Education, 17,* 11–16.

Schmidt, H. G., van der Arend, A., Moust, J. H., Kox, I., and Boon, L. (1993). Influence of tutors' subject-matter expertise on student effort and achievement in problem-based learning. *Academic Medicine, 68*(10), 784–791.

Schmidt, H. G. and Moust, J. H. C. (1995). What makes a tutor effective? A structural-equations modelling approach to learning in problem-based curricula. *Academic Medicine, 70*(8), 708–714.

Schön, D. A. (1987). *Educating the Reflective Practitioner.* San Francisco: Jossey-Bass.

Silver, M. and Wilkerson, L. (1991). Effects of tutors with subject expertise on the problem-based tutorial process. *Academic Medicine, 66*(5), 298–300.

Stern, P. (1998). Skills for teaching: A problem-based learning faculty development workshop. *American Journal of Occupational Therapy, 52*(3), 230–233.

Stinson, J. E. and Milter, R. G. (1996). Problem-based learning in business education. in L. Wilkerson, and W. H. Gijselaers, (Eds.), *Bringing Problem-based Learning to Higher Education: Theory and Practice*. San Francisco: Jossey-Bass.

Tiberius, R. G. (1990). *Small Group teaching: A troubleshooting Guide*. Toronto, ON: OISE Press.

Tipping, J., Freeman, R. F., and Rachlis, A. R. (1995). Using faculty and students perceptions of group dynamics to develop recommendations for PBL training. *Academic Medicine, 70*(11), 1050–1052.

Virtanen, P. J., Kosunen, E. A., Holmberg-Marttila, D. M. H., and Virjo, I. O. (1999). What happens in PBL tutorial sessions? Analysis of medical students' written documents. *Medical Teacher, 21*(3), 270–276.

von Döbeln, G. (1996). Four years of problem-based learning: A student's perspective. *Postgraduate Medicine, 72*, 95–98.

Walton, H. J. and Matthews, M. B. (1989). Essentials of problem-based learning. *Medical Education, 23*, 542–558.

Westberg, J. and Jason, H. (1996). *Fostering Learning in Small Groups: A Practical Guide*. New York: Springer.

Wetzel, M. S. (1996). Developing the role of tutor/facilitator. *Post graduate Medical Journal*, 474–477.

Wilkerson, L. (1996). Faculty development in the New Pathway. In J. Carver and J. Adelstein (Eds.), *New Pathways to Medical Education*. Cambridge: Harvard University Press.

Wilkerson, L. and Maxwell, J. A. (1988). A qualitative study of initial faculty tutors in a problem-based curriculum. *Journal of Medical Education, 63*(12), 892–899.

Wilkerson, L. and Hundert, E. M. (1991). Becoming a problem-based tutor: Increasing self-awareness through faculty development. In D. Boud and G. Feletti (Eds.), *The Challenge of Problem-based Learning* (pp. 159–171). London: Kogan Page.

Wilkerson, L. and Irby, D. M. (1998). Strategies for improving teaching practices: A comprehensive approach to faculty development. *Academic Medicine, 73*(4), 387–396.

Wolff, A. C., (1998). *The Process of Maturing as a Competent Clinical Teacher*. Unpublished master's thesis, University of British Columbia.

Wolff, A. C. (2000). *The Role of the Problem-based Tutor: A Resource Guide for Nursing Faculty*. Unpublished manuscript.

Woods, D. (1994). *Problem-Based Learning: How to Get the Most from PBL*. Waterdown, ON: Woods.

Wong, J. and Wong, S. (1987). Towards effective clinical teaching in nursing. *Journal of Advanced Nursing, 12*(4), 505–513.

Evaluating Student Learning

Elizabeth Rideout

E valuation of student learning has long been a controversial matter in education generally, and it is a particularly thorny issue among those who adopt problem-based learning (PBL). Swanson, Case, and van der Vleuten (1991) begin their description of strategies for student evaluation in PBL curricula by stating that "assessment can drive student learning in antithetical directions and there is little agreement among PBL advocates on methodologies for assessment" (p. 260). Although the literature reveals no imperatives in the choice of evaluation strategies, there seems to be consensus that any evaluation system adopted in a PBL curriculum must assess not only the accumulation of knowledge but also reflect the development of particular skills and abilities, including critical analysis and application of knowledge, self-awareness, self-directed learning, and teamwork. There also seems to be agreement on several guidelines to consider when choosing a process of student evaluation, which are derived from the writings of educators in general as well as those with a particular focus on PBL, including Frederiksen (1984), Neville (1995), Norman (1994), Norman, Wakefield, and Shannon (1995), and van der Vleuten and Verwijnen (1990).

EVALUATION GUIDELINES

Guideline 1

Evaluation methods *influence both student and teacher behaviors*. Expressions like "evaluation drives learning" and "teaching to the test" reflect this guideline. Forms of evaluation that test students on facts, for instance, will undermine the adoption of new learning approaches and reinforce the memorizing of out-of-context information. Similarly, the use of methods that do not influence overall outcome in a course of study can be dismissed by students as not worthy of their time or commitment.

Guideline 2

Evaluation methods must be *congruent with the educational philosophy* under-lying the curriculum, which, in the case of PBL, is learner-centered and focused on process as well as content. Methods of evaluating content mastery must reflect—and encourage—the problem-based, self-directed approach to learning, and incorporate process outcomes as well. Therefore methods must be used that determine accomplishment in all these areas.

Guideline 3

Since it is unlikely that any one form of evaluation can appraise all the required domains of learning, an effective system will probably require two or more methods of evaluation—the *multiple methods guideline.*

Guideline 4

Any system must include both *formative and summative evaluation,* to ensure that information is provided about ongoing progress as well as end-of-course achievement. Students should have the opportunity to maximize their learning through regular feedback and self-evaluation as they progress through a course of study.

Guideline 5

Students should be informed at the beginning of each course about the specific evaluation activities to be used. Guidelines should be explicit and criteria for evaluation must be available to the students. This guideline can be summarized as the *no surprises* rule.

Guideline 6

Since the PBL Model emphasizes active learning on the part of students, the evaluation system chosen should reflect this guideline. *Active student involve-ment* can be demonstrated in a number of ways such as: (1) offering students the choice of methods of evaluation for all or part of a course; (2) using "active methods" that assess behaviors, such as communication skills or physical assessment; and (3) having students give feedback about the methods used during and at the end of each course within a curriculum.

Guideline 7

Standards of *reliability, validity,* and *acceptability* should be considered in the critique of any evaluation strategy. When these are satisfactory, there is a greater sense that an assessment measure is fair, rigorous, and relevant to the desired learning outcomes.

STRATEGIES FOR EVALUATION

"There is tremendous latitude for choice in the design of an evaluation system; the challenge is to ensure that the choice ultimately rests on a careful and unbiased assessment of the relative importance of each (outcome) goal" (Norman, 1994, p. 6). In the following pages, the various evaluation methods that are used currently in PBL programs are described, with the exception of student self-evaluation (a cornerstone of PBL) which is discussed elsewhere in this book. The strengths and limitations of the various methods are presented, and examples are provided. They are described in alphabetical order, since they all have a place, but none should be considered a necessary part of a PBL assessment system (Nendaz and Tekian, 1999). Instead, the desired outcomes for each course within a program, and the nursing program overall, should direct the selection, in conjunction with the guidelines described above.

Clinical Reasoning Exercise

The clinical reasoning exercise is an oral or written examination consisting of multiple questions (scenarios) administered within a 30–60 minute period, with only a brief assessment for each case (Neville, Cunnington, and Norman, 1996). Students are presented with scenarios that represent the course content and which target the particular aspect of the decision-making process being emphasized. For example, if the emphasis in the course is the generation of possible hypotheses to explain a patient situation, the scenario will present a patient who has a particular set of concerns and the student will be asked to develop the most likely diagnosis and suggest reasonable hypotheses. The evaluator is provided with a list of the sample answers, a firm time line is set (usually three to five minutes per scenario), and students are rated on a seven-point scale, with anchors of unsatisfactory, borderline, good, or excellent. Both written and oral formats of the test have been used. The written form achieved slightly higher interrater reliability, was more efficient of faculty time but was less acceptable to students, who preferred the oral format. There was a high correlation between the oral and written formats. The number of scenarios comprising the examination can range from 10 to 20, depending on the course outcomes and content. There are no reports of the use of this strategy in nursing programs, although the student outcomes being tested, the congruency with the PBL Model, the ease of administration, and the level of reliability and validity associated with it suggest it would be useful and appropriate in nursing education.

Essays

Written assignments or essays are used frequently in PBL programs, generally related to issues selected by students in relation to overall curriculum objectives. With their emphasis on self-selection of topic, self-directed information searching, and presentation of data in a clear and focused manner, written assignments are viewed as a relevant evaluation method within the PBL approach (Palmer and Rideout, 1995). However, issues of reliability and validity of written essays have been raised repeatedly (Neufeld, 1985; Nichols and Miller, 1984; Day et al., 1990). Some authors believe they have no place in summative student evaluation (Norman, 1991) while others believe faculty have the experience and objectivity to grade written work in a conscientious manner (Stenhouse, 1975). There is also some evidence that careful orientation of faculty to the purpose of the assignment, and the use of clear and discrete criteria for grading, can increase reliability of essays (Nichols and Miller, 1984). In most curricula, students are expected to develop good writing skills and to be able to review, critique, and make conclusions about a body of literature related to a specific issue of interest. As long as this is the case, essays will continue to be used as an evaluation measure. However, because of the questions of reliability, they should be only one evaluation measure in any course of study.

An example of an essay used for evaluation of junior students in a Population Health course in a PBL curriculum is presented in Figure 9.1. Performance on this essay represents 35 percent of the final grade in the course.

Modified Essay Questions

An evaluation method associated with the PBL approach is the Modified Essay Question (MEQ) (also called Problem Analysis Questions by DesMarchais, Dumais, Jean, and Vu [1993]). The MEQ is a serial, structured examination presenting one or more clinical cases in a booklet format (Feletti, 1980). Each MEQ consists of a brief scenario reflecting a clinical situation and one or more questions pertaining to it, with additional information provided on subsequent pages, and more questions posed. The questions generally address data collection, analysis, and management of the presenting situation. An example of an MEQ appropriate for a senior level nursing student is presented in Figure 9.2. This MEQ consists of three parts; it would be printed on three consecutive pages, with instruction to the student not to go back and work on previous pages.

MEQs are intended to examine the ability to explore and manage patient problems and to assess relevant knowledge. Sample answers are developed and the criteria for evaluation are stated and provided to students in advance (Figure 9.3).

Acceptable levels of interrater reliability and validity have been reported for MEQ exams, although the intercase reliability is reported to be problem-

Due: To be handed in the week of _____.

Length: Between 2500 and 3000 words

Style: Typewritten and double spaced, APA

Process:

1. During the first few weeks of the course, identify an unresolved health issue that you become aware of from any source (e.g., a newspaper article). The task is to follow and collect evidence that pertains to this issue over the succeeding weeks.

2. Begin the paper by: (a) defining the health issue, and (b) identifying its place and priority within the health care system.

3. Discuss the implications of this health issue, with reference to the structure of the health care system and the forces which influence (a) the health status of populations and/or (b) the development of health policy.

4. Summarize your stand on the issue and discuss the long-range effects of your position. Provide rationale for each identified long-range effect on the health of populations.

5. The paper should demonstrate the student's ability to integrate the concepts learned in the course. There should be a *logical, problem-solving approach to the issue, with sound rationale and evidence for statements made.* Critical analysis must be apparent.

Note: The topic should be discussed with your tutor. Developing an outline would be helpful.

A **health issue** can be broadly defined. Examples include: Should the government look after us from "cradle to grave" even if we are leading unhealthy lifestyles? What is the role of the nurse in Primary Health Care? Is the management of industrial waste a concern for the health professions? What are the health implications of abortion on demand/pro-life stands? How will we care for the growing elderly population? How will nurse practitioners fit into the health care system? How will the reduction in the numbers of acute care beds affect the health of the population? What are the implications of needle exchanges/drug cafes for health status?

Figure 9.1 Example of Essay Assignment
© School of Nursing, McMaster University.

atic, therefore requiring tests that include several problems or cases. Some authors suggest that a minimum of five cases are required (Knox, 1989; Stratford and Smeda, 1995). Despite concerns about the number of cases needed to achieve acceptable levels of reliability and validity, the use of MEQ's in PBL programs continues to be reported (Foldevi and Svedin, 1996; Neville, 1995; Hammar, Forsberg, and Loftas, 1995).

Scenario 1, Part 1

Cassie is a 10-year-old girl who has been receiving treatment for Acute Lymphoblastic Leukemia. She was admitted last night to the pediatric ward with neutropenia and a temperature of 39.5 degrees. Today as you begin your shift you find she is lying in bed—pale, anxious, restless, and occasionally crying. Cassie tells you she is having a lot of pain.

1. Suggest a number of explanations (hypotheses) for Cassie's appearance and behavior and give your rationale.
2. What subjective and objective data would you collect to assess Cassie's pain? Provide rationale for your suggested data collection.

Scenario 1, Part 2

Cassie's parents are obviously upset and want you to relieve the pain as soon as possible. They have never seen their daughter so ill and upset and they are very distressed. Cassie continues to complain of severe abdominal pain.

3. Given these additional data, what are your explanations now concerning Cassie. What additional data would you collect? Why?
4. Outline your nursing interventions to deal with Cassie's pain and give reasons for them. Outline how you would know if your management of Cassie's pain has been effective.

Scenario 1, Part 3

How do you think you did on this scenario? Identify any gaps in your knowledge/understanding of this situation. Identify action you would take (if any) to improve your performance on this scenario.

Figure 9.2 Modified Essay Question (MEQ)

Instructions: For each of the evaluation items, please read both statements I and II and then circle the most appropriate number on the rating scale below.

1. Hypothesis generation

Unable to suggest any initial explanations; didn't seem to know where to start	Accurate and appropriate initial description of most likely explanation (mechanism); also suggests reasonable alternative explanations.

| 1 | 2 | 3 | 4 | 5 | 6 | 7 |

Figure 9.3 Modified Essay Question (MEQ) Criteria for Evaluation

2. Data gathering and interpretation

Unsystematic approach to asking for information; no idea of important items; inaccurate rationale for clinical data collection.

Suggests clinical information to be collected; selects >80% of key data items; provides accurate rationale for data collection.

1   2   3   4   5   6   7

3. Interim problem formulation

Inaccurate and imprecise statement of main problem(s); suggestions, alternate explanations absent or weak. Does not incorporate new information.

Accurate and precise outline of main problem(s) with credible explanation and reasonable proposals for alternate mechanisms. Incorporates new information.

1   2   3   4   5   6   7

4. Supplementary data gathering

No ideas about additional data; rationale inadequate or incorrect.

Suggests additional clinical information; provides accurate rationale; additional data are related to main problem.

1   2   3   4   5   6   7

5. Management plan

Unable to identify any appropriate plan for nursing care; proposed options are irrelevant and off target.

Proposes a realistic plan for nursing care; able to prioritize appropriately.

1   2   3   4   5   6   7

6. Knowledge (current)

Demonstrates poor knowledge base relative to the scenario. Unwilling or unable to think through unfamiliar concepts.

Demonstrates outstanding knowledge of concepts; able to apply these to explanations of underlying mechanisms in the case.

1   2   3   4   5   6   7

7. Self-assessment ability

Unwilling or unable to assess own performance; any statements were imprecise or vague; unclear about own strengths and weakness.

Clear and systematic assessment of own performance, with appropriate balance of strong and weak points; good ideas for further improvement and how to achieve this.

1   2   3   4   5   6   7

continued

8. Overall assessment

Major Errors/ Omissions	Some errors/ omissions	Some Minor Difficulties	Adequate	Good	Very Good	Excellent
1	2	3	4	5	6	7

Comments:

Summary:

Figure 9.3   Modified Essay Question (MEQ) Criteria for Evaluation   *concluded*

Multiple Choice Questions

Evaluation strategies in traditional health professional programs have relied primarily on examinations using Multiple Choice Questions (MCQs) aimed at the measurement of changes in knowledge. The reliance on MCQs has been viewed as contrary to the PBL Model for two reasons: (1) students are believed to study for the test rather than for their own learning; and (2) MCQ examinations do not assess the more process-oriented PBL outcomes (Norman, 1991; Swanson et al., 1991; West, Umland, and Lucero, 1985). Also, unless all students study the same problems in the same order and focus on the same learning issues, MCQs would be complex to prepare since several versions of the exam would be needed in order to assess the wide variety of possible learning outcomes. Despite these limitations, there are certainly PBL programs that use MCQs, but only as one of several components of an evaluation plan (Neville, 1995). As the evaluation guidelines outlined earlier suggest, students should be evaluated on all the intended outcomes of a course or program. If factual knowledge is an intended outcome and faculty believe MCQs are the most effective evaluation method, then MCQs should certainly be included. However, of key importance is the inclusion of other methods to assess other intended outcomes such as clinical decision making and self-directed learning.

Table 9.1   *Example of an OSCE station to assess physical assessment skills in a beginning level student.*

Mr. Jones has come to the clinic for a general health assessment. Please complete a physical assessment of his respiratory system. Please describe aloud what you are doing and describe your findings.

The Objective Structured Clinical Examination

The Objective Structured Clinical Examination (OSCE) was developed in response to criticisms of the direct observation method of evaluating clinical practice in general, and clinical skills in particular, primarily because of its potential for testing a wide range of knowledge and skills during one examination period (Harden, Stevenson, Downie, and Wilson, 1975; McKnight et al., 1995). In an OSCE, students rotate around a series (up to 20) of timed stations (lasting anywhere from 5 to 25 minutes) where they may be asked to take a patient history, perform some part of a physical examination, teach/counsel/advise a patient, perform a skill, or interpret and/or document findings. An example of an OSCE scenario for use with beginning level nursing students in a health assessment course is presented in Table 9.1.

A standardized form with specific criteria for scoring is prepared in advance. An example of the criteria is presented in Figure 9.4.

A plethora of studies have investigated the reliability and validity of the OSCE (for example, Cunnington, Neville, and Norman, 1997; Roberts and Brown, 1990; Roberts and Norman, 1990; Stratford et al., 1990) and the overall conclusion is that high interrater reliability is generally achieved while intercase reliability is poor, indicating that competence is situation or case specific. This low correlation among stations requires an increasing number of testing stations for a stable estimate of performance to be achieved (Salvatori and Brown, 1995). Content and construct validity have been demonstrated although criterion validity is weak.

There are obvious advantages to using the OSCE as a method of evaluating clinical competence including: the ability to test a wide range of skills in a relatively short period of time; low preparation time since a bank of stations, once developed, can be used on numerous occasions (Stevens and Brown, 1989); and flexibility in the format, allowing for choice of stations and range of competencies to be tested. The inclusion of the OSCE as one component of the medical licensing processes in Canada is evidence of its acceptance as an evaluation method (Reznick et al., 1993). The disadvantages include the large number of stations (a minimum of 10 is suggested) that are required to get a reliable estimate of overall competence and the associated costs and logistics of organizing a large scale OCSE for large numbers of students (Nayer, 1993).

Assessment Skill	Circle One	Observer's Comments
A. Inspect		
1. General appearance		
• Color	Yes (1) No (2)	_____
• Posture	Yes (1) No (2)	_____
• Comfortable/apprehensive	Yes (1) No (2)	_____
• Use of accessory muscles	Yes (1) No (2)	_____
2. Chest wall configuration		
• AP chest diameter	Yes (1) No (2)	_____
• Symmetry of chest movements	Yes (1) No (2)	_____
3. Assessment of respirations		
• Rate	Yes (1) No (2)	_____
• Rhythm	Yes (1) No (2)	_____
• Depth	Yes (1) No (2)	_____
B. Palpate		
1. Chest wall expansion during inspection		
• Symmetry of expansion	Yes (1) No (2)	_____
C. Percuss		
1. Percuss posterior chest		
• Compare sides	Yes (1) No (2)	_____
• Avoid percussing over bone	Yes (1) No (2)	_____
D. Auscultate		
1. Instruct patient to take slow, deep breaths in and out of mouth during auscultation	Yes (1) No (2)	_____
2. Auscultate posterior chest		
• Compare sides	Yes (1) No (2)	_____
• Avoid auscultating over bone	Yes (1) No (2)	_____
3. Auscultate anterior chest		
• Compare sides	Yes (1) No (2)	_____
• Avoid auscultating over bone	Yes (1) No (2)	_____
4. Describe breath sounds		
• Quality of breath sounds	Yes (1) No (2)	_____
• Quantity of breath sounds	Yes (1) No (2)	_____
• R/O adventitions sounds	Yes (1) No (2)	_____

Figure 9.4   Criteria for evaluation of OSCE station

Assessment Skill	Circle One	Observer's Comments
E. Analysis		
1. Describe findings		
• General impression of respiratory status	Yes (1) No (2)	_____
• Detailed explanation of findings	Yes (1) No (2)	_____
• Accuracy of descriptions	Yes (1) No (2)	_____

Portfolios

Student-centered learning is, by definition, an individualized approach to education. Within the guidelines of the curriculum framework, objectives, and goals, students are encouraged to identify their own ways of learning—the emphasis is on "learning how to learn" as well as gaining awareness, knowledge, and skills needed for professional practice. The PBL Model purports to facilitate the development of self-evaluation skills which are essential for reflective practice (Schön, 1987). Because student-centered learning also emphasizes student autonomy in selecting learning opportunities and demonstrating competencies in a variety of ways, the evidences of learning selected by each student will of necessity also be unique and individualized. While students have the opportunity to demonstrate learning in tutorials and through required course assignments, they also need to have the vehicle through which they can demonstrate and reflect upon their individual learning. Journal keeping and personal learning portfolios are strategies that provide students the freedom to explore the personal meaning of their educational experiences and demonstrate their increased self-awareness and skills in self-evaluation. The student has the responsibility to select those pieces of work that best reflect learning. If used as a summative evaluation measure, a portfolio can also give students the opportunity and vehicle through which to respond to (reflect upon) feedback provided through prior formative evaluation, and demonstrate how they have incorporated that feedback into subsequent learning.

While portfolios do provide an individualized evaluation format for students, there is concern regarding the appropriateness of assigning a grade to the personal reflective component of student submissions, since the presence of an external "evaluation" may intimidate students and limit the very self-disclosure the strategy purports to encourage. As with any evaluation strategy, it is essential that portfolios be introduced with careful consideration of the learning outcomes they are appropriate to measure, and if components of them are to be graded, the criteria must be clearly developed. Portfolios are labor intensive for students and faculty alike, and therefore should be used judiciously.

Progress Testing

Most of the methods of student evaluation described in this chapter, although congruent with the philosophy and process of PBL, have varying levels of reliability and validity and have been reported to leave students unsure, indeed anxious, about whether they have learned what they need to know in order to function as competent health professionals (Blake et al., 1994; van der Vleuten and Verwijen, 1990). However, there continues to be reluctance to reintroduce traditional MCQ examinations into PBL curricula because of the reasons noted in the section on MCQs, namely, the steering effect on student activity and an emphasis on knowledge acquisition and de-emphasis on the other learning outcomes valued in PBL. A response to this dilemma is Progress Testing, which was developed concurrently at the University of Missouri—Kansas City School of Medicine and The University of Maastricht, The Netherlands, and subsequently introduced into the medical program of McMaster University (Arnold and Willoughby, 1990; Blake et al., 1996; Boshizen, van der Vleuten, Schmidt, and Machiels-Bongaerts, 1997; van der Vleuten and Verwijnen, 1990). Whether called the Quarterly Profile Exam (as at the University of Missouri) or the Personal Progress Index (PPI) (McMaster University), the test consists of an examination given to all students at regular intervals throughout a program consisting of up to 300 multiple choice questions that together form a sample from the entire cognitive domain of the discipline. Performance on the examination is used for formative evaluation only, with the results going to students and an advisor not involved in the summative evaluation of the student. The results are used to provide feedback to students about their developing knowledge base (which has been shown to grow exponentially over the years in the programs) and to identify students who are not performing at the expected level, so that remedial activity can be made available. Students have reported that Progress Testing is valuable, fair, and does not cause them to change their study habits and preparation for tutorials (Blake et al., 1996).

Self-Selected PBL Evaluation Strategies

As students progress in a program using the PBL approach, it is useful to provide them with increasing choice of the methods by which they will be evaluated. Although the faculty will want to continue to specify the methods for the largest portion of summative student assessment, it is also in the spirit of PBL to have students select the methods for a component of their assessment. With this rationale, one approach that has been used in nursing is the

Table 9.2   *Sample plan for selected PBL evaluation strategies*

1. Invented Dialogue

I have chosen this since I really want to explore how I would react to a patient who is sad and tearful having been given bad news. Since I might not get the chance to try this out with a standardized patient, I will use this technique to try out an approach and get some feedback from the tutor. Being with someone who has just received bad news worries me. Doing this learning strategy will help me decide how I might handle such a situation.

Due date: Week of October 16

Percent of grade: 10%

2. Critical Incident Reflection

I will choose two incidents from PBL that I will describe and analyze, using the LEARN approach. I will use one group process issue and one content issue. I really want to become more assertive in expressing my viewpoint so I will be alert for a situation where I wished I had been more assertive (or where I was assertive and I want to think about where I was). I also want to be more critical of what others present in the group so I will look for that too.

Due Date: Week of November 2

Percent of Grade: 20%

incorporation of Selected PBL Strategies that comprises a percentage of their final grade. Students select from a variety of options and prepare a plan which includes their rationale for choice of methods. A sample plan is presented in Table 9.2.

In this example the student chose two options, "invented dialogue" and "critical incident reflection." In the former, a dialogue, or "carefully structured conversation" is developed (Angelo and Cross, 1993, p. 203), which is related to the issues being explored in PBL. The student then analyses the dialogue using communication theory. Evaluation is based on the analysis, using preset criteria. In the critical incident reflection, students choose particular events from PBL sessions to analyze. Although such reflection and analysis is an ongoing expectation within PBL, by including it as a PBL strategy students also receive a portion of their grade for a thoughtful critique of an incident.

Another option for inclusion as a PBL strategy is "directed paraphrasing" (Angelo and Cross, 1993), where students select one or two journal articles relevant to the problem they are studying in their PBL course. The guidelines for this strategy ask the student to summarize and restate the information in a clear and concise manner; demonstrate critical analysis of the material (including comparing and contrasting the findings); and describe application of knowledge to the problem. Guidelines and criteria for evaluation are provided to the student.

In another alternative, entitled "Unleash Your Creativity," students choose their own individual strategy and develop the criteria against which they will be evaluated. For example, a student may elect to demonstrate the application of educational principles in patient education, by developing a picture book to teach children about medication use, using both text and pictures. Evaluation criteria would relate to the rationale for the book, based on literature about growth and development, and teaching/learning principles. Students might also choose to incorporate feedback from children who used the book.

The strategies described above are clearly not unique to PBL, but what makes their use particularly congruent with the PBL Model is the degree of control given to students to select not only the specific strategies they will use, but how the grading will be allocated. The concerns with these strategies are similar to those associated with essays, in particular the level of subjectivity afforded the evaluator and the possibility of a lack of consistency among evaluators.

Triple Jump

The triple jump, a method of evaluating the application of knowledge to clinical situations in a controlled setting outside the clinical environment, has been used in medical, nursing, and science programs (Allen, Duch, and Groh, 1996; Callin and Ciliska, 1983; Smith, 1993; Feletti and Ryan, 1994). In this oral evaluation method, students meet one-to-one with faculty and are presented with a problem scenario. Students are asked to generate hypotheses/hunches about the possible issues and their likely connections. They then collect data from the faculty member about the situation. Based on the additional data students then narrow or refine their hypotheses and identify learning issues. This part of the process is usually 45 minutes in length.

Students are then given time, from 2 (the usual) to 24 (uncommon but reported) hours, to conduct research. This generally involves consulting written resources but students may also choose to contact resource people. The exam ends with the student returning to do an oral report to the faculty member of the research findings and their application to the presenting problem. They also conduct a self-evaluation, commenting on what they did well, and not so well, on the exercise. This final part of the triple jump is scheduled for 30 minutes.

Although the three-step process described above is used most commonly, the triple jump can also be used as a double jump. For example, with beginning students the focus may be on patient assessment and identification of major patient issues. In this case, students would be evaluated on their ability to determine the most likely patient issues and to collect the relevant data (Step One). After a period of self-study, they would finalize their list of patient issues and define nursing interventions for one issue (Step Two). This information could then be presented to the faculty member in writing rather than orally, which is the usual method for Step Three. This modification to the triple jump has two possible advantages. First, for students who become anxious in an oral exam, it means they have done one part of the examination orally and the second part in written format. Second, it saves faculty time since she or he grades the written material which takes less time than meeting with the student for 30 minutes. Another format for the triple jump involves providing the scenario and patient data to the student, who begin with the self-study part of the jump, where they review the patient data, identify the patients strengths and problems, and determine appropriate nursing interventions for the patient. Thus, the usual Steps One and Two are combined and are done independently by the students. The students then present orally, to the faculty tutor, the appropriate nursing interventions, supported with evidence that they have collected during the exercise. Again the triple jump has become a double jump.

A double jump scenario that might be used with intermediate level students is presented in Table 9.3.

Faculty are provided with several information sources, all designed to increase the likelihood of objectivity and consistency in the administration of the examination. First, they have a list of *instructions for the students,* from which they read directly, to ensure that each learner receives the same information. There is space on this form to make notes as students go through the exercise (Figure 9.5).

Table 9.3 *Example of Double Jump Scenario*

**Practice Problem,
Problem XV**

Presenting Situation:

Mr. Gord Jakes, a 31-year-old executive, comes to his general practitioner's office with low back pain. He is active in sports and has had episodes of back pain over the past two years. Lately, these episodes have become more bothersome. You are the nurse in the office who first interviews Mr. Jakes.

Please read aloud the following instructions to the student.

Part A—Assessment and Problem Identification

Please read aloud the presenting situation on the problem card.

Now, before we get further into the problem, let's stop for a minute. Based on the opening statement only, share with me your ideas about client problems and issues and their most likely explanations (hypotheses).

Figure 9.5   Instructions for students for double jump   *continued*

Now, let's proceed with the problem. As you ask me for information from the history and physical examination, I will give you the data.

Tutor Notes:

Is there any other data you would like from the chart?

You have much more information about the client and problem now. I would like you to begin to summarize the patient's problems now.

Tutor Notes:

From this initial problem list, which are the *most important* patient issues? Give your reasons for the ranking you have chosen.

Tutor Notes:

Part B—Self-Assessment and Plan for Meeting Learning Needs and Preparation for

Step II

At this point in the problem, can you identify important gaps in your knowledge/understanding of relevant information that you want to pursue in Step II? State your plan of action for Step II.

Tutor Notes:

You now have two (2) hours to revise your problem list, rank the revised problems, and prepare a plan of care for one of this client's major problems.

You should take the problem scenario and the chart data with you for the Step II part of the exercise.

During Step II, Part A you are asked to complete in writing a revised, problem list, incorporating any new information relevant to the client situation, rank the client problems in priority, giving scientific rationale to support the problems selected and the ranking. In addition you will select one of the client's major problems with which to plan care and develop a plan of care.

In Part B of Step II, you will evaluate the exercise; both your use and management of resources and your performance during this exercise.

Tutor Notes: Following the completion of Step II, the student will return their written work to the tutor. The Problem Scenario Card and Scenario Chart Data should also be returned.

THE END!

Figure 9.5   Instructions for students for double jump, *concluded*

Second, a *list of criteria* is provided to faculty for use in grading the performance of students. These are made available to students before the exercise, to ensure they are well-informed about the expectations. A sample of the criteria found in assessing a double jump is presented in Table 9.4.

Table 9.4   *Criteria for Evaluation of the Double Jump*

	Statement I	Statement II
1. Hypothesis generation	Unable to generate relevant issues in the client situation. Major gaps in the hypotheses that are generated.	Identifies relevant issues in the client situation. Generates accurate and appropriate initial hypotheses related to the main features of the client situation. Includes physical, psychological, and social concepts.
	1 2 3 4 5 6 7	
2. Data gathering	Unsystematic data collection. Data gathered is insufficient and is not relevant to the client situation.	Systematic collection of data. Data is sufficient and is relevant to the client situation.
	1 2 3 4 5 6 7	
3. Data gathering— rationale	Is not able to state rationale for seeking specific data.	Able to state rationale for seeking specific data.
	1 2 3 4 5 6 7	
4. Data gathering— clinical reasoning	Does not recognize knowledge gaps. Unable to think through unfamiliar concepts.	Demonstrates clinical reasoning in data collection by generating further relevant questions based on data obtained.
	1 2 3 4 5 6 7	
5. Interim problem formulation— individualized	Inaccurate or imprecise statement of main client problem(s). Problems identified are not supported by data; data is insufficient or is not relevant to the problems.	Accurate and precise outline of main client problem(s). Problems are supported by relevant data.
	1 2 3 4 5 6 7	
6. Interim problem formulation—holistic	Problem list is limited to one domain of the client situation.	Problem list includes psychological, physical, social, cultural, and spiritual context of the client situation.
	1 2 3 4 5 6 7	
Total Score: _____ = _____ %		Letter Grade: _____
Divided By: 198		

© School of Nursing, McMaster University.

Table 9.5   *Tutor Guide to Expected Responses to Gord Jakes Double Jump*

- Chronic pain, related to (R/T) disc degeneration, stress at work and home as evidenced by (AEB) patient's statements of pain × 2 years, guarded posture, tense appearance.
- Knowledge deficit of effective pain relief measures AEB patient having unrelieved pain.
- Alteration in ADL R/T pain limiting his movements AEB difficulty dressing, getting in and out of bed, driving.
- Individual coping impaired R/T usual coping styles not effective for dealing with pain AEB statements of frustration, concern about being a failure.
- Altered family interactions R/T pain interfering with functioning AEB missed family outings, moving out of shared bedroom.
- Anxiety R/T role performance at work AEB palpitations and neck twitches when doing presentations, onset of pain coincides with work starting.
- Sleep-Pattern Disturbance R/T pain waking him at night AEB interrupted sleep.
- Powerlessness R/T inability to manage pain symptoms on his own AEB statements of irritability, frustration, and lack of control.
- Interruption in sexual relationship R/T pain on intercourse AEB patients' statements.
- Alteration in nutrition greater than body requirements R/T inactivity and "junk food" consumption AEB 10 kg. overweight.

Finally, a list of *expected responses* is developed for each scenario and given to the faculty member, again to assist with consistency in grading and fairness to students. The evaluation of the student should not be limited to the "expected responses," since some students identify relevant well-supported issues that are not noted on the "expected responses." The possible responses to the Gordon Jakes scenario are presented in Table 9.5.

The strengths of this evaluation method include the reinforcement of the decision-making process that is central to PBL, and the emphasis on process as well as content evaluation. The method is also very flexible, as demonstrated above with the modification of the triple jump to a double jump. Acceptable levels of interrater reliability have been reported; however, consistently low levels of intercase reliability have been described, indicating that students may do well on scenarios related to their areas of interest or strength and less well on scenarios in areas to which they have not been previously exposed (i.e., asked to complete a triple jump situation related to the childbearing cycle without having encountered either theory or practice related to this area). Norman (1994) concludes that an exam consisting of many questions (approximately 10–20) would be required to achieve satisfactory intercase reliability, and this becomes unrealistic when there is considerable faculty time required to conduct each triple jump exercise.

Because of this concern with reliability and because the method is especially congruent with the PBL Model, the triple jump exercise remains a popular evaluation strategy although it is often used for formative evaluation only. However, in a recent pilot study conducted at McMaster University School of Nursing (Ploeg, Rideout, Black, and Tompkins, 1999), there was strong support from students for continued use of this method in summative evaluation. This study will continue with plans to assess the reliability and validity of the exercise in different levels of student in the BScN program. There seems to be little doubt that the triple jump is a useful method; the question is whether it should be used for formative evaluation only, or for summative evaluation also.

Tutorial Performance

PBL emphasizes not only the acquisition of knowledge and its application in decision making and clinical practice but also the ability to be a self-directed learner and to demonstrate personal characteristics including the ability to work effectively in groups. How best to evaluate these characteristics has been the subject of much discussion, although the general conclusion is that they can only be evaluated in context by rating performance in the PBL tutorial groups (Barrows and Tamblyn, 1980; DesMarchais and Vu, 1996; Hay, 1995; Neufeld and Sibley, 1989). In considering who should rate performance, the consensus is that students and their peers should contribute to the formative and summative evaluations, with the final and summative evaluation resting with the tutor (DesMarchais and Vu, 1996; Hay, 1995).

There have been few published descriptions of how such an evaluation should be completed, or on what criteria performance should be evaluated. One example comes from the integrated medical program at the University of Sherbrooke, where the competencies expected in small group tutorials are evaluated by the PBL faculty tutor using a 44-item rating form completed at the end of each session (DesMarchais and Vu, 1996; Hebert and Bravo, 1996). Student reasoning skills on problems, communication, and small group interaction, and autonomy and self-directed learning are all evaluated. Evidence of validity of the form is based on two findings: The form is considered relevant and useful by tutors and it has been effective in identifying students in need of improvement. The internal reliability of the form was 0.98, and good correlations were noted between the rating form score and global evaluations conducted by tutors. The authors conclude that evaluating tutorial performance is an integral part of a PBL evaluation process, and the form developed at Sherbrooke is a reliable and valid instrument for evaluating students' skills and attitudes during tutorials.

Hay and Schmuck (1994) report the development of a 10-item form used in the Occupational Therapy program at McMaster University, which assesses group skills, learning skills, knowledge, and critical thinking. Tutors were able to identify very weak areas of performance and to rank-order students, although all were ranked above the B-level. It seems that, although rating forms are helpful in stating the behaviors to be evaluated within small groups, their use in differentiating levels of student performance is questionable and their ability to predict performance, as judged by other evaluation measures, is unproven (Hay, 1995; Norman, Wakefield, and Shannon, 1995). A third tutorial evaluation measure comes from the Dental School at the University of Indiana and is available in print or Web-based (Chaves, Chaves, and Lantz, 1998).

More recently a faculty group at McMaster University School of Nursing has developed a 30-item measure of Tutorial Performance, which assesses tutorial behaviors in three areas: critical thinking, group process, and self-directed learning. Psychometric testing of the measure indicates internal consistency reliability for each of the three subscales at 0.8 or above, and testing for interrater reliability testing and concurrent validity are underway currently. Qualitative feedback from students and faculty has been positive, and the intent is to use the measure for tutorial performance evaluation in all courses within the BScN program.

CONCLUSION

Evaluation of student learning, an issue of discussion and debate in the educational literature generally, has received particular attention within PBL due to concerns about balancing the evaluation of content and process in a manner that does not divert student attention away from the tutorial group activities and individual student learning. The consensus is that the first step in developing the evaluation process must be identification of the learning outcomes to be achieved and there is agreement that these include knowledge, clinical decision making, clinical performance, self-directed learning, and group skills. Evaluation measures should then be selected to assess this range of outcomes. It is generally concluded that developing an evaluation system that is congruent with the purpose and philosophy of PBL, attains acceptable levels of reliability and validity, and has no negative steering effect is an ongoing challenge (Barrows and Tamblyn, 1980; Nendaz and Tekian, 1999; Neufeld and Sibley, 1989; van der Vleuten and Verwijnen, 1990).

REFERENCES

Arnold, L. and Willoughby, T. L. (1990). The quarterly profile test. *Academic Medicine, 65,* 515–516.

Allen, D. E., Duch, B. J., and Groh, S. E. (1996). The power of problem-based learning in teaching introductory science courses. In L. Wilkerson and W. M. Gijselaers (Eds.), *Bringing Problem-Based Learning to Higher Education: Theory and Practice.* San Francisco: Jossey-Bass.

Angelo, T. A., Cross, K. P. (1993). *Classroom Assessment Techniques: A Handbook for College Teachers.* Jossey-Bass, San Francisco.

Barrows, H. S. and Tamblyn, R. M. (1980). *Problem-based Learning: An Approach to Medical Education.* New York: Springer.

Blake, J., Johnson, A., Mueller, C. B., Norman, G., Keane, D., Cunnington, J., Coates, G., and Rosenfeld, J. (1994). Progress report of the Personal Progress Index. *Pedagogue, 5*(2), 1–6.

Blake, J. M., Norman, G. R., Keane, D. R., Mueller, C. B., Cunnington, J., and Didyk, N. (1996). Introducing progress testing in McMaster University's problem-based medical curriculum: Psychometric properties and effect on learning. *Academic Medicine, 71(9),* 1002–1007.

Boshizen, H. P., van der Vleuten, C. P., Schmidt, H. G., and Machiels-Bongaerts, M. (1997). Measuring knowledge and clinical reasoning skills in a problem-based curriculum. *Medical Education, 31,* 115–121.

Callin, M. and Ciliska, D. (1983). Revitalizing problem-solving with triple jump. *Canadian Nurse, 79,* 41–43.

Chaves, J. F., Chaves, J. A., and Lantz, M. S. (1998). The PBL-Evaluator: A web-based tool for assessment in tutorials. *Journal of Dental Education, 62,* 671–674.

Cunnington, J. P. W., Neville, A. J., Norman, G. R. (1999). The Risks of Thoroughness: Reliability and Validity of Global Ratings. *Advances in Health Sciences Education.* 1997. Vol. I, 227–233.

Day, S. C., Norcini, J. J., Diserens, D., Cebul, R. D., Schwartz, J. S., Beck, L. H., Webster, G. D., Schnabel, T. G., and Elstein, A. (1990). The validity of an essay test of clinical judgement. *Academic Medicine, 65,* S30–40.

DesMarchais, J. E. and Vu, N. V. (1996). Developing and evaluating the student assessment system in the preclinical problem-based curriculum at Sherbrooke. *Academic Medicine, 71*(3), 274–283.

DesMarchais, J. E., Dumais, B., Jean, P., and Vu, N. V. (1993). An attempt at measuring student ability to analyze problems in the Sherbrooke problem-based curriculum: A preliminary study. In P. A. J. Bouhuijs, H. G. Schmidt, and H. J. M. Van Berkel (Eds.), *Problem-Based Learning as an Educational Strategy.* Maastricht, Netherlands: Network Publishers.

Feletti, G. I. (1980). Reliability and validity on modified essay questions. *Journal of Medical Education, 55,* 933–941.

Foldevi, M. and Svedin, C. G. (1996). The Linkoping curriculum: The phase examination in general practice. *Medical Education, 30,* 326–332.

Frederiksen, N. (1984). The real test bias: Influences of testing on teaching and learning. *American Psychologist, 39*(3), 193–202.

Hammar, M. L., Forsberg, P. M., and Loftas, P. I. (1995). An innovative examination ending the medical curriculum. *Medical Education, 29,* 452–457.

Harden, R. M., Stevenson, M., Downie, W. W., and Wilson, G. M. (1975). Assessment of clinical competence using objective structured clinical examination. *British Medical Journal, Feb. 22,* 105–112.

Hay, J. and Schmuck, M. (1994). *An investigation of student self-evaluations of problem-based tutorials.* Unpublished manuscript, McMaster University, Hamilton, ON.

Hay, J. (1995). Tutorial Performance. In *Evaluation Methods: A Resource Handbook.* Hamilton, ON: Programme for Educational Development, McMaster University.

Hebert, R. and Bravo, G. (1996). Development and validation of an evaluation instrument for medical students in tutorials. *Academic Medicine, 71 (5),* 488–494.

Knox, J. D. E. (1989). What is . . . a modified essay question? *Medical Teacher, 11,* 51–57.

McKnight, J., Rideout, E., Brown, B., Ciliska, D., Patton, D., Rankin, J., and Woodward, C. (1987). The Objective Structured Clinical Examination (OSCE): An alternate approach to assessing student clinical performance. *Journal of Nursing Education, 26(1),* 39–42.

Nayer, M. (1993). An overview of the objective structured clinical examination. *Physiotherapy Canada, 45,* 171–178.

Nendaz, M. R. and Tekian, A. (1999). Assessment in problem-based learning medical schools: A literature review. *Teaching and Learning in Medicine, 11*(4), 232–243.

Neufeld, V. (1985). Education for capability: An example of a curriculum change from medical education. *Journal for Education and Training Technology, 21(4),* 262–267.

Neufeld, V. and Sibley, J. C. (1989). Evaluation of health sciences education programs: Program and (student) assessment at McMaster University. In H. Schmidt, M. Lipkin, M. W. deVries, and J. M. Greep (Eds.), *New Directions for Medical Education: Problem-based and Community Oriented Medical Education.* New York: Springer-Verlag.

Neville, A. (1995). Student evaluation in problem-based learning. *Pedagogue, 5(3),* 1–7.

Neville, A. J., and Norman, G. R. (1996). Development of clinical reasoning exercises in a problem-based curriculum. *Academic Medicine, 70(1),* S105–S107.

Nichols, E. G. and Miller, G. K. (1984). Interreader agreement on comprehensive essay examinations. *Journal of Nursing Education, 23(2),* 64–69.

Norman, G. R. (1991). What should be assessed? In D. Boud and G. Feletti (Eds.), *The Challenge of Problem-Based Learning.* New York: St. Martin's Press.

Norman, G. (1994). Why evaluate? *Pedagogue, 5(1),* 1–6.

Norman, G., Wakefield, J., and Shannon, S. (1995). Overview. In *Evaluation Methods: A Resource Handbook.* Hamilton, ON: Programme for Educational Development, McMaster University.

Palmer, D. and Rideout, E. (1995). Essays. In *Evaluation Methods: A Resource Handbook.* Hamilton, ON: Programme for Educational Development, McMaster University.

Ploeg, J., Rideout, E., Black, M., and Tompkins, C. (1999). An exploration of the triple Jump as an Evaluation Method in Nursing Education. Unpublished report. McMaster University: Hamilton, ON.

Reznick, R. K., Baumber, J. S., Cohen, R., Rothman, A., Blackmore, D., and Berard, M. (1993). Guidelines for estimating the real cost of an objective structured clinical examination. *Academic Medicine, 68,* 513–517.

Roberts, J. and Brown, B. (1990). Testing the OSCE: A reliable measure of clinical nursing skills. *Canadian Journal of Nursing Research, 22,* 51–59.

Roberts, J. and Norman, G. R. (1990). Reliability and learning from the OSCE. In W. Bender, R. J. Hiemstra, A. J. J. A. Scherpbeir, and R. P. Zwierstra (Eds.), *Teaching and Assessing Clinical Competence.* Groningen, ND: Stichting TICTAC.

Salvatori, P. and Brown, B. (1995). Objective Structured Clinical Examination. In *Evaluation Methods: A Resource Handbook.* Hamilton, ON: Programme for Educational Development, McMaster University.

Schön, D. A. (1987). *Educating the Reflective Practitioner.* San Francisco: Jossey-Bass.

Smith, R. M. (1993). The triple-jump examination as an assessment tool in the problem-based medical curriculum at the University of Hawaii. *Academic Medicine, 68(5),* 365–372.

Stenhouse, L. (1975). *An Introduction to Curriculum Research and Development.* London: Heinemann.

Stevens, B. and Brown, B. (1989). *A User's Manual for Evaluation of Clinical Nursing Skills.* Hamilton, ON: McMaster University.

Stratford, P. W., Thompson, M. A., Sanford, J., Saarinen, H., Dilworth, P., Solomon, P., Nixon, P., Fraser-MacDougall, V., and Pierce-Fenn, H. (1990). Effect of station examination item sampling on generalizability of student performance. *Physical Therapy, 1,* 31–36.

Stratford, P. and Smeda, J. (1995). Modified essay questions. In *Evaluation Methods: A Resource Handbook.* Hamilton, ON: Programme for Educational Development, McMaster University.

Swanson, D. B., Case, S. M., and van der Vleuten, C. P. M. (1991). Strategies for student assessment. In D. Boud and G. Feletti (Eds.), *The Challenge of Problem-Based Learning.* New York: St. Martin's Press.

van der Vleuten, C. and Verwijnen, M. (1990). A system for student assessment. In C. van der Vleuten and W. Wijen (Eds.), *Problem-based Learning: Perspectives from the Maastricht Experience.* Amsterdam: Thesis Publishers.

West, D. A., Umland, B. E., and Lucero, S. M. (1985). Evaluating student performance. In A. Kaufman (Ed.), *Implementing Problem-based Medical Education.* New York: Springer.

Developing Clinical Opportunities and Resources for Problem-Based Learning

Joan A. Royle, Wendy Sword, Margaret Black, Barbara Brown, and Tracy Carr

C linical courses in nursing education provide the student with the opportunity to experience the dynamic interactions with clients, families, and health professionals that are essential to the practice of nursing. The practice setting provides students with the opportunity to apply decision-making skills to patient situations as events are unfolding. The knowledge and skills in self-directed learning and decision making that are acquired in problem-based tutorials are applied to actual clinical situations. In the practice setting, students have the opportunity to assess patients, formulate hypotheses, develop plans of care, implement nursing interventions, and evaluate patient outcomes while working collaboratively with health professionals. The challenge for nurse educators is to be creative and innovative in assisting students to apply the knowledge and skills they learn in their formal education to the delivery of patient care.

This chapter addresses the process of teacher-learner interaction in the practice setting and the development of the clinical learning environment to support student learning. It begins with discussion on the relevance of clinical experiences and strategies to support problem-based learning (PBL) in the clinical setting. This is followed by discussion on roles and responsibilities, and relationships between the student and the faculty tutor in the practice setting. The later section provides strategies to create better organizations and structures to support a self-directed curriculum including service/academic faculty appointments, support processes, the role of clinical preceptors, and access to evidence-based information.

THE RELEVANCE OF CLINICAL EXPERIENCES
Integration of Theory and Practice

Clinical experiences are integral to a nurse's education. Although theoretical knowledge essential to nursing practice can be learned in a classroom setting, students also need the opportunity to apply learning to actual clinical situations. Practicum courses expose students to a variety of clinical situations requiring nursing judgment. The relevance of theoretical knowledge becomes apparent to students when they are confronted with real-life issues requiring thoughtful and purposeful problem solving. Students are expected to use their knowledge and skills in a specific practice area, thereby developing their ability to integrate theory with nursing practice.

In practice situations, students become engaged in decision making about client care and use theory to give meaning to the situation, to identify problems requiring nursing intervention, and to select and evaluate interventions (Kim, 1993). Theory application in the context of a clinical experience broadens understanding of how conceptual knowledge guides nursing practice.

Enhancement of Problem-Solving and Critical Thinking Skills

While PBL in classroom settings relies on patient problems specially designed to develop nursing knowledge, critical thinking and self-directed learning, practicum experiences provide actual client situations that stimulate student learning. The nature of students' work in clinical practice settings is problem-based in that they provide care for real clients with existing or potential health problems (Reilly and Oermann, 1999). Students are required to conceptualize, apply, analyze, synthesize, and/or evaluate information and plan appropriate action (Alexander and Giguere, 1996). Because encounters with clients are often ambiguous and present variations from "normal" responses as well as unanticipated complexities, students also are challenged to be innovative (Pesut and Herman, 1999; Reilly and Oermann, 1999).

The real world presents complexities that are difficult to simulate in the classroom. Clinical experiences enable students to communicate with clients, practice skills, and integrate the social, cultural, economic, and political environments of both the client and the practice setting (Johnson, 1994). Students may need to rethink their assumptions about clients' values and beliefs and explore alternative perspectives and explanations. Challenges that nurses face in the work-world may help students to think more critically about how health care policy and funding decisions impact on nursing practice.

Promotion of Self-Directed Learning

Students often discover gaps in their knowledge as they prepare for a particular clinical experience, and they must research for appropriate resources. As students interact with clients and apply the nursing process, they see further limitations in their knowledge and clinical skill set. New issues and questions arise that highlight the need for further learning.

When students enter new clinical environments, they need to acquire knowledge and skills appropriate to the client population and practice setting. For instance, when students who have worked in acute care institutions are first exposed to community health, they have to reframe their nursing practice. Community health nurses do not provide illness care to individuals but are concerned with health promotion and preventive care at the individual, group, and community levels. Students must develop an understanding of concepts such as population health, primary health care, and social determinants of health, and the role of nurses in empowerment and political advocacy (Reutter, 2000).

Professional Socialization

Reilly and Oermann (1999) state that, "professional education must provide for a practice component where the student learns to think and act like the professional in the specific discipline" (p. 1). During clinical experiences, students are expected to take on the role of a professional nurse and learn to think as a professional nurse. Their clinical activities include the totality of nursing practice. Their nursing assessments lead to the identification of nursing diagnoses and interventions. Participation in team conferences fosters understanding of the nursing perspective within a health care team. Professional socialization is enhanced by students' awareness that their roles and responsibilities are regulated by standards of practice.

Practicums expose students to clinical role models. A study of undergraduate nursing students found that students perceived staff nurses as "creative, trusted carers, sensitive to constantly changing practice and professional contexts" as well as facilitators of client self-care and health team functioning (Davies, 1993, p. 633). Clinical experiences provide opportunities for students to learn about what nurses do in diverse practice environments.

STRATEGIES TO SUPPORT PROBLEM-BASED AND SELF-DIRECTED LEARNING IN CLINICAL COURSES

Learning Plans

The use of individual learning plans in clinical courses is consistent with a self-directed approach to learning. A learning plan is an agreement between the student and the faculty tutor delineating what the student will learn, how and within what time frame this will be accomplished, the evidence required to show that the objective has been accomplished, and how the evidence will be evaluated. Although learning plans are developed at the beginning of the course to give structure to learning and direction for clinical activities, they should be flexible so that students can take advantage of unanticipated learning opportunities. Students may choose to renegotiate learning plan objectives with their faculty tutors as new learning situations arise.

Learning plans allow students to map their own learning within the parameters of course objectives and take into account their learning needs, learning style, and the nature of the practice setting. For example, an obstetric unit provides a unique opportunity to learn about the nursing care of the postpartum mother and her newborn infant. A student might develop a learning plan objective that focuses on the development of knowledge and skill related to newborn assessment.

When creating a learning plan for a clinical course, a student should develop objectives and evidences to demonstrate the application of knowledge to practice. Objectives should be related to the three domains of learning: cognitive, psychomotor, and affective (Watson, 1991). Learning plan objectives may become increasingly complex as students progress through their nursing programs. Bloom (1956) provides a sequence of learning that can assist students in identifying appropriate educational objectives. Beginner students, for example, may focus on identifying and examining particular concepts or theories (e.g., teaching and learning theories), and apply this knowledge to specific situations. More senior students might synthesize various teaching and learning theories into a meaningful whole and apply them to client situations and evaluate client outcomes.

Student-Selected Clinical Assignments

In traditional nursing education curricula, faculty tutors often select students' clinical assignments. However, student-selected clinical assignments are more in keeping with a self-directed student-centered approach to learning (Rideout, 1994). Self-selection gives students control over their learning activities and addresses personal learning needs. During a clinical practicum, students select clients with health care needs relevant to their learning. Students can be delegated, on a rotating basis, to visit the clinical setting to choose assignments for the whole group. The final selection of clients for students would be done in consultation with unit staff to ensure their appropriateness to the students' level of knowledge and skill.

In community agencies, experiences can also be student-directed with students working one-on-one with agency preceptors. Students communicate their learning objectives, needs, and interests to their preceptors and, subsequently, negotiate assignments. Client selection might include an individual, family, or community, that is, "a group, population, or cluster of people with at least one common characteristic (such as geographic location, occupation, ethnicity, or housing condition)" (Anderson and McFarlane, 1996, p. 261). Given the varied possibilities for client-selection, it is important that students focus their learning on their personal objectives.

Documentation of Clinical Learning Activities

Problem-based and self-directed learning can be supported in practicum courses through the documentation of clinical learning activities. Clinical worksheets (see Figure 10.1) are particularly beneficial for beginning

---

Part A—Patient Care Planning

Date: _____ Student: _____

Patient Initials: _____ Room: _____ Age: _____ Language/Culture: _____

Diagnosis: _____ Surgery (Procedure/Date Performed): _____

History (health history/ADL/current concern):

Physical Assessment Data:

Relevant Laboratory/Diagnostic Data:

Nursing Care Issues/Treatments/Medications:

Patient Needs/Nursing Diagnosis: Rationale:

Part B—Clinical Reflection

Student Comments	Tutor Comments
Reflections relating to: Nursing Practice Role	
Reflections relating to: Communication	
Reflections relating to: Health Care System	
Reflections relating to: Self-Directed Learning and Self Evaluation	

Figure 10.1   Patient Care Planning Worksheet/Clinical Reflection Log

students who are developing their ability to organize their learning and reflect on their clinical experiences. Clinical worksheets can be structured so that students can document data collected, generate a problem list, suggest nursing interventions, and identify knowledge gaps prior to the clinical experience. They also provide a means for students to summarize and communicate their activities on the clinical unit. Providing documentation of client

data, problems/needs, goals, interventions, and evaluation of the effectiveness of nursing actions enhances problem solving. To give direction for
future learning, students may reflect on the care provided, clinical competencies and knowledge attained, and areas for improvement.

Senior students generally are expected to take a more critical and analyt-
ical approach to clinical learning. They could be asked to critically examine
the research literature in relation to a patient issue encountered commonly
in their clinical setting and consider the applicability of their findings to
patient care (see Figure 10.2). This would involve reviewing the way the issue
is managed currently and the factors involved in the implementation of
change. Such learning activities require students to address systematically a
clinical problem and seek new information to enhance their understanding
and clinical practice.

Concept Mapping

Concept mapping is a form of structured analysis in which concepts and
propositions are linked hierarchically in a diagrammatic form (All and
Havens, 1997; Irvine, 1995; Wilkes, Cooper, Lewin, and Batts, 1999). It is a
creative process that helps students organize their thoughts and think critically about the relationships among newly acquired data as well as about how
new information relates to previously acquired information (Elberson and
Williams, 1996). Concept maps represent an individual's personal construction of meaning specific to an area of knowledge or client situation (All and
Havens, 1997; Irvine, 1995). Concept mapping can be used prior to a clinical
experience to learn more about the nursing care for a patient with a specific
health problem, to organize data, or develop nursing diagnoses and a plan of
care for a client (All and Haven, 1997). Concept maps also can be used to
provide a summary of what has been learned (All and Haven, 1997).

Research on concept mapping suggests that the process fosters meaningful learning through better integration of the subject matter. Other
benefits of concept mapping include greater knowledge retention, enhanced
motivation for learning, and better problem solving (Irvine, 1995). Concept
maps have been found to assist students to become more independent
learners and to understand the link between science and nursing practice
(Wilkes et al., 1999).

Reflective Writing

Reflective writing is another strategy used to develop problem-solving and
critical thinking skills. Learning and understanding are maximized through
the process of documenting thought processes (Usher, Francis, and Owens,
1999). In reflecting on situations encountered in the practicum, students
learn to synthesize theory and practice, apply relevant research to experiences, and identify questions for further study (Brown & Sorrell, 1993).

Criteria	Comments

1. Selection of the Clinical Problem
- Is the problem common to nursing practice in this setting?
- Does the problem have important health benefits, potential risks and costs?
- Is there potential for change?

2. Clinical Expertise
- How is the problem currently being managed in this clinical setting?
- What policies/guidelines are currently used?

3. Clinical Research Evidence
- Were the key research articles found that are relevant to the clinical problem?
- Was the literature critically appraised?
- Is a change in practice warranted based on the research evidence?
- What are the expected outcomes from a change in practice?

4. Patient/Client/Family Preferences
- Does the patient/family have adequate information to participate in the decision?
- Have the patient/family's preferences been determined?
- Are the expected outcomes congruent with the patient's preferences?

5. Resources
- Do nurses in the setting currently have the expertise to implement the proposed intervention/practice?
- What other factors in the clinical setting influence implementation of the proposed intervention/practice?
- Is the proposed intervention/practice feasible in this clinical setting?

6. Evaluations
- Is the proposed intervention based on consideration of patient preferences, clinical expertise, research evidence and resources?
- How will the intervention be evaluated?

Date: _____ Student Signature: _____ Tutor Signature: _____

Figure 10.2 Clinical Learning Activity: Evidence-Based Nursing

Adapted from Evidenced-Based Care Resource Group. (1994). Evidence-Based Care: Setting Priorities: How important is this problem? *Canadian Medical Association Journal, 150*(8), 1249–1254.

See also, DiCenso, A., Cullum, N., and Ciliska, D. (1998). Implementing evidence-based nursing: Some misconceptions. *Evidence-based Nursing. I*(2), 38–40.

© McMaster University, School of Nursing.

Reflective writing also fosters the development of understanding and enables students to know "in a new and more intimate way" (Usher et al., 1999, p. 8). Reflection is a purposeful inter-subjective process that facilitates the interpretation of experience into meaning and, ultimately, increased self-awareness, sensitivity and change in conceptual perspective (Baker, 1996; Pierson, 1998). Strategies to facilitate reflective writing and critical thinking include the use of critical incidents, journals, and portfolios. For in-depth discussion on these strategies, the reader is referred to Chapter 6 on fostering critical reflection.

Group Clinical Debriefing

Clinical debriefing provides an opportunity for students to share clinical experiences. Students often encounter situations that raise questions about patient care, ethics, legal responsibilities, and professional practice. Discussion of issues that prompt critical reflection fosters mutual learning. In essence, clinical debriefing sessions mimic small group PBL. As students share perceptions, hypothesize possible explanations, debate solutions to problems, and suggest answers, they apply their own previously acquired knowledge and gain new insights. Students also identify learning needs and seek additional information. It is helpful for students to summarize their learning and reflect on how it may be applied in the future. Group clinical debriefing can enhance knowledge retention and transfer of learning.

Self-Evaluation

Self-evaluation provides a stimulus for lifelong learning and professional development (Arthur, 1995). The notion of self-evaluation is integral to self-directed learning and easily transferable to clinical courses. Because self-evaluation is useful for formative purposes (Arthur, 1995), evaluation of one's clinical performance should be initiated at the start of a practicum. Many of the strategies discussed in this chapter, such as reflection and concept mapping, include elements of self-assessment. Although self-evaluation is ongoing, it is more formalized at midterm and end-of-term when students document their learning and identify strengths and areas for improvement or development. At the end of a clinical course, self-evaluation has both formative and summative components. Students both identify future learning needs and evaluate their achievement of course objectives.

"Self-evaluation should be accompanied by teacher-student discussions in which the evaluation is shared and decisions are made about future learning" (Reilly and Oermann, 1999, p. 410). It is important for students to get feedback from faculty tutors, both ongoing and at specified evaluation times. Students learn through collaborative assessment, by gaining new insights into their behavior, and being exposed to new ways of thinking. It becomes a means to foster professional growth and development as well as an assessment of past performance.

ROLE OF FACULTY IN THE CLINICAL SETTING

In clinical settings, students learn to cope with change and deal with the complexities and time pressures of the real world. They can take advantage of learning situations that are rare in the controlled classroom environment. However, the successful integration of this learning is highly dependent on the skill and ability of the faculty tutor. Characteristics of effective faculty in the clinical setting may be grouped into five areas (adapted from Reilly and Oermann, 1999): knowledge and clinical competence; teaching skills; relationships with students; relationships with clinical staff; and personal characteristics.

Knowledge and Clinical Competence

Successful faculty in the clinical setting are those who enjoy nursing, are good role models, demonstrate strong clinical skills and judgment, assume responsibility for their own actions, and have a breadth of knowledge in nursing (Knox and Mogan, 1987). Their job is to externalize the largely tacit or internal knowledge and thought processes underlying practice (Taylor and Care, 1999) and facilitate the acquisition of depth and breadth in subject knowledge (Creedy, Horsfall, and Hand, 1992).

Teaching Skills

The required skills include the ability to diagnose learning needs, set goals, supervise students, and evaluate learning. The faculty tutor is not just an authority figure, but rather is an expert colearner, who teaches by discovery. Frost (1996) describes the role as that of a facilitator who shares power, control, and responsibility for learning experiences. The student negotiates learning plans, goals, and activities with the faculty tutor. Shared decision making encourages students to take responsibility for their own progress, an objective of self-directed learning. Important skills include communicating clearly, promoting independence, and correcting mistakes without demeaning the student. Risk taking and errors are viewed as useful to the student learning process.

The faculty role is not to provide information but to help students to develop their own information seeking strategies to find answers (Bevis and Watson, 1989) and build on concepts being developed. Students will tend to assume that there is a single answer to a problem, so the faculty role is to help them to deal with the reality of the clinical setting and to recognize that problems can be solved in many ways (Reilly and Oermann, 1999). Critical thinking is promoted by challenging the way students think, assisting students to resolve dilemmas, and creating a responsive environment (Conger and Mezza, 1996). Raising questions that require the student to read, observe, analyze, and reflect is essential to the faculty role (Bevis and Watson, 1989).

Students become aware through research, discussion, and experience that their current beliefs may not adequately explain phenomena. They identify anomalies and become more open to more complex levels of understanding. Faculty members encourage students to experiment with learning while protecting students and patients from harmful outcomes (Chambers, 1999).

Relationships with Students

Students value faculty who are able to interact with them in a group and one-to-one. They also value faculty who establish mutual respect and rapport and are approachable, provide support and encouragement, and listen attentively (Reilly and Oermann, 1999). The faculty member fosters positive interchanges among students, clinicians, patients, and their families. Students do not respond uniformly to teaching and learning experiences. It is important to recognize that variability may be due to differences in aptitude and motivation or to perceived fear of unwanted consequences. Successful faculty help students become more open to finding meaning and relevance in the learning encounter (Reilly and Oermann, 1999).

Relationships with Clinical Staff

Faculty who work in close collaboration with experienced practitioners are in a strong position to help the student apply theory to practice. They can update their clinical knowledge and ensure that classroom information is current and credible. However, as Ioannides (1999) points out, reflection on practice in the clinical setting is most meaningful. The student's memory is fresh and clinical staff can clarify any issue immediately. The student can reflect on past experience and new learning opportunities (Frost, 1996). Clinical practice has been called "situated learning" (Chambers, 1999; Lave, 1991) because students learn by being part of a team in the practice environment but are protected by their student status. Students confront problems as they occur, assimilate knowledge to solve the problem, and evaluate the outcomes.

Personal Characteristics

Successful faculty are those with a genuine enthusiasm that comes from enjoying nursing and being highly competent. Genuineness implies a willingness to admit mistakes and an ability to convey empathetic understanding. The clinical situation is inherently unpredictable and students find this very stressful. Their learning takes place in a public situation that makes them feel vulnerable, so they need a teacher whom they can trust. Other valued characteristics of faculty are integrity, perseverance, and courage (Gaberson and Oermann, 1999). Being truthful and fair in dealing with students, striving to do well and improve as a faculty member, courage to try new approaches, or risk taking unpopular stances are important characteristics.

CHALLENGES FOR CLINICAL TEACHING IN PROBLEM-BASED LEARNING

Although a self-directed problem-based approach has many benefits, there are several challenges to teaching in the practice setting. Self-directed learning does not mean that students can independently identify learning opportunities from the outset. Rather, students in the beginning years of a self-directed learning program are exposed to the clinical setting within a guided structure and clear objectives for the behaviors to be achieved. The program planners select practice settings and specify overall course objectives. However, students assess their own needs and select their own individual learning objectives within course expectations. As students progress through the program and gain experience, they have more latitude to select their practice setting, and to select their own clinical learning experiences. However, with the student's choice comes the responsibility to ensure the choice can be supported with relevant, meaningful learning objectives. The faculty tutor, student, and preceptor/clinician all can contribute to the review of these choices. This interdependent collaboration is vital to develop an appropriate clinical experience.

In the beginning of the program, the student may find adopting a self-directed problem-based approach to learning difficult. Therefore, having the same faculty tutor for both classroom and clinical courses may help to support the transfer of theory, skills, and knowledge between classroom and the practice setting. Once the student has become a more independent learner, consistent faculty becomes less important. However, it is important to maintain consistency in curricular concepts arising from the problems studied and the kinds of client/patient issues found across settings (Karuhije, 1997). Curriculum planners can ensure that key concepts are emphasized in concurrent classroom and clinical courses (e.g., change theory, family assessment, caring).

Working within a rapidly changing clinical environment and mastering technical skills are challenges students face in the clinical setting. The faculty member must encourage the student to consider not just the "knowing how" but also the "knowing that" (Chambers, 1999). By having the student identify personal learning goals and focus on patient-centered care, such as integrating pharmacology with medication administration, the student begins to assimilate the "knowing how" (skills) with the "knowing that" (theoretical knowledge). Another challenge is to identify new practice settings that help prepare students for the variety of care environments and support the self-directed philosophy. The settings across the program also need to reflect the appropriate level of challenges and complexity for beginning, intermediate, and senior students.

International placements provide senior students with creative environments and the opportunity to obtain a more global perspective on the role of the nurse, on health as it is experienced in other cultures, and on different health care systems. Students having international clinical experiences witness, in a meaningful way, the impact determinants of health such as women's issues and literacy have on the lives of people in different cultures.

Clinical evaluation methods can be challenging and difficult to develop. Having clearly stated expected clinical behaviors that are shared with all evaluators is important. Student learning goals and evidences are derived from these behaviors. But how these are assessed and how the evidence is interpreted can vary across settings and evaluators. Although faculty tutors in clinical settings use observations most frequently as a basis for evaluating performance (Karuhije, 1997), other methods can be used, such as journaling, client documentation, care maps, care plans, conferences, presentations, and teaching plans. These evidences incorporate theory and an empirical base. A reflective student examines the outcome of his/her care, and the relationship between what was anticipated as a result of applying theory with that of previous experience.

THE CLINICAL ENVIRONMENT

Organizational and Structural Strategies

The adoption of a problem-based self-directed model for education has both teaching and administrative implications. The organizational and structural factors fall into three categories: faculty resources, support processes, and the development of the clinical settings.

Faculty Resources

According to Benner (1984) and Benner and Wrubel (1989) there is a need to "champion bringing expert clinical nurses into the mainstream of nursing education" (Bevis and Watson, 1989, p. 135). To this end, Bevis and Watson (1989) support new alliances for the benefit of nursing. They endorse the concept of tripartite alliances which consist of teacher, clinician, and student as colearners together. This leads the expert clinician to a full participation in the education of nursing students. Moreover, a valuing and an alliance with the expert clinician will produce a graduate "committed to caring practices, those committed to relationships comprised of caring communities of nurses, with a sense of membership in and among, and with mankind" (Bevis and Watson, 1989, p. 136). Thus, the curriculum implications are intimate working relationships for students in clinical settings with clinical experts. Partnership with expert clinicians can in turn influence the development of the curriculum.

Clinical Faculty Appointments

In keeping with this concept, nursing programs need to develop a cadre of clinical faculty to tutor in the nursing program. Selected clinical staff, with a minimum of a Masters degree, may be given academic appointments within a School of Nursing in return for contributions to the education programs. Clinical faculty are expected to fulfill defined preparatory criteria such as supervising students in the clinical setting with a clinical faculty member and cotutoring in a problem-based tutorial for one semester in order to attain their clinical faculty appointment. They are then expected to meet negotiated obligations such as contributing 39 hours per year to the School of Nursing. Appointments should fit within the guidelines of the academic setting and, therefore, are usually for a three year period and are renewable. Such appointments usually start at the rank of clinical lecturer or assistant professor but incumbents have the potential for promotion. Although they continue to receive their salary from their clinical employer, they receive other rewards from the academic setting such as library and parking privileges, invitations to faculty development and program activities, opportunities for collaboration with experienced faculty researchers on clinical research projects, and awards for teaching excellence.

Clinical faculty may be located in a variety of institutions and community agencies covering a fairly broad circumference surrounding the School of Nursing. Some may choose to tutor in various problem-based tutorials, research, or community development courses. They also make valuable contributions as members of School of Nursing committees, including curriculum development, scholarly activities, research, and faculty development, and as participants in the student admission process.

However, the major contribution of clinical faculty is in the role of faculty tutor to students in their own clinical settings, where they guide the learning of the student and provide consultation with the preceptor, who in turn generally provides the direct supervision to students in their daily practice. Clinical faculty are expected to know the academic and clinical standards expected of the particular level. They guide and direct students' learning and the evaluation process throughout a clinical course as discussed earlier in this chapter under "roles of faculty in the clinical setting." Ultimately, they assume responsibility for determining if the expected clinical behaviors for the course have been met and assigning the final grades for all course assignments. Course planners or other full-time faculty should be accessible to assist in the identification and formulation of a plan of action for students experiencing difficulties. The clinical faculty member may also be a resource in the prevention and/or resolution of education/service conflicts that may arise in the clinical setting. Clinical faculty provide a valuable resource to nursing programs at a time when faculty numbers are decreasing. These appointments are an established way of fulfilling the need to see expert clinical nurses as part of nursing education described by Benner (1984) and Benner and Wrubel (1989).

Clinical Preceptors

Clinical practice for nursing students today is viewed as an educational experience that is an integral component of the curriculum. We have moved from the apprenticeship model where nursing students worked with experienced nurses and provided service in exchange for their training. Although faculty have assumed responsibility for the practice component of a student's learning, economic constraints, a shortage of nurse educators, and difficulties keeping current with changes in care delivery, result in the need for efficient and effective use of clinical resources to enhance student learning. Downsizing and health care restructuring have changed the care delivery environment and created new barriers for practitioners to fulfill their teaching functions. Most nurses are products of traditional nursing education programs. Creative strategies are needed to prepare clinical preceptors for their important contributions to student learning in a problem-based curriculum.

The literature on clinical preceptors is mostly descriptive of collaborative projects between service and academia or focuses on the selection and preparation of preceptors. Most preceptor models involve a triadic relationship among the learner, the tutor, and the preceptor (Kirkpatrick, Byrne, Martin, and Roth, 1991; Melander and Roberts, 1994; Patton and Cook, 1994; Patton and Dowd, 1994). There is agreement in the literature that nurses value the preceptor role and accept their responsibilities to help students develop their knowledge and clinical skills. Commitment to the role is associated with perceptions of benefits and rewards and the support received from employers and the educational program (Dilbert and Goldenberg, 1995). There are many benefits to collaboration between service and academia in clinical education. Unfortunately, minimal attention is given to the selection and preparation of preceptors to facilitate the transfer of PBL skills to practice. The cognitive apprenticeship model of preceptorship (Paterson, 1997; Taylor and Care, 1999), which involves a strong collaboration among students, practitioners, and faculty tutors, is consistent with a problem-based self-directed curriculum. Students participate with expert practitioners to learn the knowledge, physical skills, procedures, covert thinking, and decision-making processes, values, and culture in their field of study (Taylor and Care, 1999). There is a commitment by the faculty to prepare and structure the experience and to prepare the clinician or preceptor to assume a supportive role.

Important themes identified as basic to the student/faculty/preceptor relationships are: trust, clearly defined expectations, support systems, honest communication, mutual respect and acceptance, encouragement, mutual sharing of self, and experience (Hsich and Knowles, 1990). It is important that faculty value collaboration with clinical staff and that clinicians understand the mission and philosophy of problem-based learning. Clinical preceptors require orientation to the "how to's" of their role, as well as the theoretical aspects (Royle, Sammon, Montemuro, Blythe, and Morrison, 1998). Focus groups with clinical preceptors, conducted by Royle et al. (1998), identified the need to clarify the competencies expected of students at the completion of the placement, how students are to be evaluated, and how to deal with challenging students. Experienced preceptors requested advanced workshops to improve their skills and learn to resolve complex learner issues. The educational preparation of clinical preceptors may include formal workshops, orientation sessions, and the use of audio visual and print learning resources. A key component in the development of staff nurses for their role as contributors to student learning is the ongoing learning that takes place during regular interactions with faculty.

Support Processes

Effective implementation of a problem-based self-directed curriculum requires the development of administrative processes that are aligned with the educational philosophy. Consider, for example, the process of assigning students to clinical settings. As students progress through the curriculum, they are expected to become increasingly self-directed. The process used for assignment of clinical settings, therefore, must allow for a proportional increase in student input. The opportunity to influence the decision-making process encourages students to reflect on past experiences and examine future goals to arrive at an accurate assessment of their current learning needs. They are then able to identify the clinical setting(s) that will enable them to address those learning needs. Thus, each student's input into the assignment process in the senior years may be comprised of a list of desired settings with corresponding rationale and learning objectives for each choice. Figure 10.3 provides an example of an online clinical placement form completed by a senior student.

Clinical Information Resources

When pursuing alignment of educational philosophy and administrative processes, secondary issues related to infrastructure may arise. Continuing on with our example, the decision to allow for student input implies a commitment to ensuring access to the information required to make informed decisions. Relevant information may include a profile of each clinical setting that describes the learning opportunities available, prerequisite competencies and experiences, the organizational and/or personnel resources on-site and any additional data deemed important. The accuracy of

Name: _____ Leslie Jacobs _____

Email: _____ jacobs@school of nursing _____

Phone: [Current] _____

[Summer] _____

September 2000 _____

Previous Experience

Level 2: [T1] Pediatrics 3M
University Hospital

[T2] G1 Surgery General
Hospital

Level 3: [T1] Maternity University
Hospital

[T2] Neurosurgery General
Hospital

Other: Summer job—nursing home
working as a health care aide _____

Your *completed* Placement Preference Profile will be used to assist the BScN Program in the process of allocating available clinical placement resources. **The Profile has three components:** (1) Identification of preferred clinical foci for Level 4, (2) Objectives for each focus of interest, and (3) Personal statement (optional). Please take this opportunity to influence the decision making regarding your Level 4 placements.

Identification of Preferred Clinical Foci: _____

Please list top 3 foci of interest for Term 1. You may also identify specific settings of interest (prioritize if >1):

1. Women's Health Clinic   University Hospital
2. Fertility Clinic   University Hospital
3. Child and Family Centre   Out Patient Clinics

Please list top 3 foci of interest for Term 2. You may also identify specific settings of interest (prioritize if >1):

1. Labor & Delivery   General Hospital
2. Maternity & Post Partum   University Hospital
3. Psychiatry—In Patient   Psychiatric Hospital

Please note that choices for Term 1 may be considered for Term 2 in order to achieve optimal matching. Placement settings that are not included on SPIS (www.fhs.mcmaster.ca/nursing/placements) must be discussed with the Placement Coordinator and the Course Planner *prior to* submission of your application. All placements are subject to the availability of the placement setting and faculty resources.

Figure 10.3 Level 4 Clinical Placement Preference Profile
© McMaster University, School of Nursing.

the information is critical and, in the context of a rapidly changing health care environment, a mechanism for ensuring the descriptions are current is essential. Two key infrastructure issues emerge from this discussion. First, the educational program must establish an extensive, collaborative network of health care organizations that share the goal of achieving congruence between a student's learning objectives and what a given clinical setting can offer. Such congruence pays dividends as students are more likely to invest in a clinical experience that meets their identified learning needs, and the clinical setting will derive most benefit and satisfaction from students who are interested in the practice area.

The second issue revolves around the need for a centralized source of information, a point of convergence in the network that facilitates interaction among the health care organizations, the educational program, and the students. Although the solutions proposed for this infrastructure challenge will vary depending on the unique characteristics and needs of the network's stakeholders, one practical tool that has been used effectively is a database that interfaces with the Internet. The database is the point of convergence, receiving input from the educational program and health care organizations and retrieving the information when requested by students. The Internet-interface removes many of the access barriers as there is no need for a special software package, and users can interact with the database from any location that has Internet access.

Development of Clinical Settings

A clinical climate conducive to student learning in a problem-based curriculum is one that values learning and learners, fosters a sense of inquiry and mutual dialogue, demonstrates caring relationships for all participants (clients, families, professional and nonprofessional staff, and learners), establishes standards and realistic expectations while simultaneously providing freedom to question and test new ideas. While hospitals have been the traditional setting for clinical practice, the community including home care, clinics, schools, and residential and nursing homes, is increasingly being used as most patients/clients are receiving nursing services in their homes and other community facilities. International and outpost settings are increasingly being developed and used for student learning. To develop clinical environments that promote the achievement of learning goals and objectives, the faculty and staff of the nursing programs need to develop collaborative relationships with their service colleagues and implement programs and strategies to enhance the clinical learning environments.

Access to Evidence-Based Information Resources

Self-directed students in a problem-based curriculum quickly learn to use library and other information resources to acquire the knowledge necessary to identify and resolve the health care scenarios they encounter in tutorials. To transfer these skills to clinical practice requires that the student have access to library, Internet, and other evidence-based resources. These resources are available online in most teaching hospitals but are generally lacking in community and long-term care settings.

Professional competencies for nurses include skills in evidence-based practice which are vital for patient care and for learning. Information seeking and critical appraisal of the research literature are essential skills for both students and clinicians to answer imminent clinical questions and to plan for the long-term management of common clinical concerns. Clinicians require training in both literature searching and in critical appraisal of research evidence. Senior students and faculty tutors with these skills are able to collaborate with clinical preceptors and other members of the health care team to acquire relevant evidence-based information resources to address clinical questions. Both formal and informal preparation of staff in evidence-based practice benefits the education program by having clinicians who can serve as mentors to students and by creating clinical environments that reflect the values of the program and professional standards of practice. Electronic links between clinical settings and a health sciences library can provide students, faculty tutors, and clinicians with the information resources that they need for clinical decision making.

CONCLUSION

This chapter has explored the relationship of clinical practice to PBL, provided strategies to promote problem-based clinical learning, discussed the interaction among faculty tutors and students, and policy making to create effective environments for PBL. Prerequisites to problem-based clinical learning include problem-oriented course objectives, skilled faculty, and clinical environments that are open to problem-based learners and value the professional development of employees.

REFERENCES

Alexander, M. K. and Giguere, B. (1996). Critical thinking in clinical learning: A holistic perspective. *Holistic Nursing Practice, 10*(3), 15–22.

All, A. C. and Havens, R. L. (1997). Cognitive/concept mapping: A teaching strategy for nursing. *Journal of Advanced Nursing, 25*(6), 1210–1219.

Anderson, E. T. and McFarlane, J. M. (1996). *Community as Partner: Theory and Practice in Nursing* (2nd ed.). Philadelphia: Lippincott.

Arthur, H. (1995). Student self evaluations: How useful? How valid? *International Journal of Nursing Studies, 32*(3), 271–276.

Baker, C. R. (1996). Reflective learning: A teaching strategy for critical thinking. *Journal of Nursing Education, 35*(1), 19–22.

Benner, P. (1984). *From Novice to Expert: Excellence and Power in Clinical Nursing Practice.* Menlo Park, CA: Addison-Wesley.

Benner, P. and Wrubel, J. (1989). *The Primacy of Caring, Stress and Coping in Health and Illness.* Menlo Park, CA: Addison-Wesley.

Bevis, E. O. and Watson, J. (1989). *Toward a Caring Curriculum: A New Pedagogy for Nursing.* New York: National League for Nursing.

Bloom, B. S. (1956). *Taxonomy of Educational Objective: Cognitive Domain.* New York: McKay.

Brown, H. N. and Sorrell, J. M. (1993). Use of clinical journals to enhance critical thinking. *Nurse Educator, 18*(5), 16–19.

Chambers, N. (1999). Close encounters: The use of critical reflective analysis as an evaluation tool in teaching and learning. *Journal of Advanced Nursing, 29*(4), 950–957.

Conger, M. M. and Mezza, I. (1996). Fostering critical thinking in nursing students in the clinical setting. *Nurse Educator, 21*(3), 11–15.

Creedy, D., Horsfall, J., and Hand, B. (1992). Problem-based learning in nurse education: An Australian view. *Journal of Advanced Nursing, 17*(6), 727–733.

Davies, E. (1993). Clinical role modelling: Uncovering hidden knowledge. *Journal of Advanced Nursing, 18*(4), 627–636.

Dilbert, C. and Goldenberg, D. (1995). Preceptors' perceptions of benefits, rewards, supports and commitment to the preceptor role. *Journal of Advanced Nursing, 21*(6), 1144–1151.

Elberson, K. L. and Williams, S. A. (1996). Innovative strategies for promoting clinical scholarship: A holistic approach. *Holistic Nursing Practice, 10*(3), 33–40.

Frost, M. (1996). An analysis of the scope and value of problem based learning in the education of health care professionals. *Journal of Advanced Nursing, 24*(5), 1047–1053.

Gaberson, K. B. and Oermann, M. H. (1999). *Clinical Teaching Strategies in Nursing.* New York: Springer Publication.

Hsich, N. L. and Knowles, D. W. (1990). Instructor facilitation of the preceptor relationship in nursing. *Journal of Nursing Education, 29*(6), 73–80.

Ioannides, A. P. (1999). The nurse teacher's clinical role now and in the future. *Nurse Education Today, 19*(3), 207–214.

Irvine, L. M. C. (1995). Can concept mapping be used to promote meaningful learning in nurse education? *Journal of Advanced Nursing, 21*(6), 1175–1179.

Johnson, J. L. (1994). A dialectical examination of nursing art. *Advances in Nursing Science, 17*(1), 1–14.

Karuhije, H. F. (1997). Classroom and clinical teaching in nursing: Delineating differences. *Nursing Forum, 32*(2), 5–12.

Kim, H. S. (1993). Putting theory into practice: Problems and prospects. *Journal of Advanced Nursing, 18*(10), 1632–1639.

Kirkpatrick, H., Byrne, C., Martin, M. L., and Roth, M. L. (1991). A collaborative model for the clinical education of baccalaureate nursing students. *Journal of Advanced Nursing, 16*(1), 101–107.

Knox, J. E. and Mogan, J. (1987). Characteristics of "best" and "worst" clinical teachers as perceived by university nursing faculty and students. *Journal of Advanced Nursing, 12*(3), 331–337.

Lave, J. (1991). *Situated Learning.* Cambridge: Cambridge University Press.

Melander, S. and Roberts, C. (1994). Clinical teaching associate model: Creating effective BSN student/faculty/staff nurse triads. *Journal of Nursing Education, 33*(9), 422–425.

Paterson, B. L. (1997). The negotiated order of clinical teaching. *Journal of Nursing Education, 36*(5), 197–205.

Patton, J. and Cook, L. R. (1994). Creative alliances between nursing service and education in times of economic constraint. *Nursing Connections, 7*(3), 29–37.

Patton, J. G. and Dowd, T. (1994). A collaborative model for the evaluation of clinical preceptorships. *Nursing Connections, 7*(1), 45–54.

Pesut, D. J. and Herman, J. (1999). *Clinical Reasoning: The Art and Science of Critical and Creative Thinking.* Albany, NY: Delmar Publishers.

Pierson, W. (1998). Reflection and nursing education. *Journal of Advanced Nursing, 27*(1), 165–170.

Reilly, D. E. and Oermann, M. H. (1999). *Clinical Teaching in Nursing Education.* (2nd ed.). Sudbury, MA: Jones and Bartlett.

Reutter, L. I. (2000). Socioeconomic determinants of health. In M. J. Stewart (Ed.), *Community Nursing: Promoting Canadians' Health.* Toronto, ON: W. B. Saunders.

Rideout, E. M. (1994). "Letting go": Rationale and strategies for student-centred approaches to clinical teaching. *Nurse Education Today, 14*(2), 146–151.

Royle, J. A., Sammon, S., Montemuro, M., Blythe, J., and Morrison, F. (1998). Preparing clinical educators: Interdisciplinary collaboration. *Gerontology & Geriatrics Education, 19*(2), 31–45.

Taylor, K. L. and Care, W. D. (1999). Nursing education as cognitive apprenticeship. A framework for clinical education. *Nurse Educator, 24*(4), 31–36.

Usher, K., Francis, D., and Owens, J. (1999). Reflective writing: A strategy to foster critical inquiry in undergraduate nursing students. *Australian Journal of Advanced Nursing, 17*(1), 7–12.

Watson, S. J. (1991). An analysis of the concept of experience. *Journal of Advanced Nursing, 14*(16), 1117–1121.

Wilkes, L., Cooper, K., Lewin, J., and Batts, J. (1999). Concept mapping: Promoting science learning in BN learners in Australia. *The Journal of Continuing Education in Nursing, 30*(1), 37–44.

Developing Learning and Library Resources

Janice Bignell, Hallie Groves, and Liz Bayley

Students in a problem-based, small-group, self-directed curriculum re-quire a wide range of learning resources. Some students prefer to learn on their own from textbooks while others may search the literature for the latest journal article in a specific subject area. Some learn best using au-diovisual materials, including audio cassettes and video cassettes. Increasingly, students may sit in front of a computer for hours working through a clinical simulation, pitting their knowledge against the computer program and evalu-ating themselves by a self-test at the end. Students who are technologically in-clined can search the World Wide Web and follow-up on other resources cited or consult online texts. Others may prefer a hands-on approach, a demonstra-tion, or a consultation with an "expert." However, most students will use a com-bination of these resources.

The Problem-Based Learning (PBL) Model, with its emphasis on self-directed learning, requires that this full range of resources be available for effective and efficient learning to occur. This chapter will present an overview of the various categories of resources and will describe in some detail four particularly essential assets to a PBL curriculum: an anatomy labo-ratory, a clinical skills laboratory (CSL), a library, and a computer laboratory.

CATEGORIES OF LEARNING RESOURCES

Four categories of resources were identified as essential when PBL was first introduced (Barrows and Tamblyn, 1980) and these continue to be relevant today, even though the media used to deliver them have evolved significantly (see Figure 11.1):

1. Problems, which form the basis of the curriculum
2. Reference Resources, recommended by content experts and around which most of the study takes place
3. Information Resources, which provide general information about the course or program
4. Evaluation Resources, which are used in student evaluation

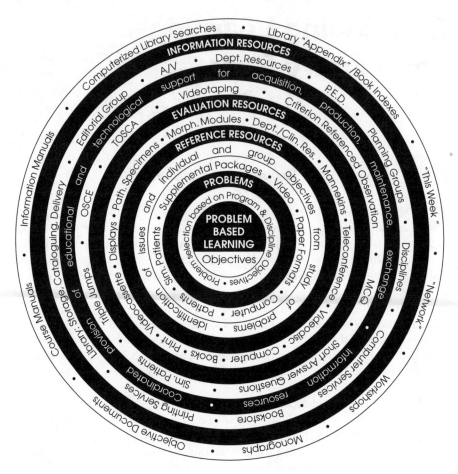

Figure 11.1   Resources for Problem-Based Learning

Problems

Problems, also called cases at various educational institutions, form the basis of the curriculum around which learning takes place in a PBL environment. Problem packages have several components. A patient problem, which may consist of several scenarios, is developed to incorporate certain learning objectives, either from a real scenario or one created to fit curriculum objectives. The setting may be hospital-based or community-based and the patient's presentation is described with minimal information given so that students can determine their specific learning issues. Chart data or nursing assessment data such as a health history and physical examination, laboratory results, and prescribed treatments are included in problem packages to provide the tutor and students with the patient details.

A tutor guide is usually provided to help elucidate the theoretical basis for the management of care and to clarify the learning objectives. A resource list of recommended references is developed by the problem author or content expert, which includes the most current and relevant editions of textbooks, journal articles, videos, Computer Assisted Instruction (CAI) packages, morphological modules, and Web pages. All of these resources should be screened and recommended by faculty. The resource list may also include resource people, for example, faculty members and clinical staff who are experts in a particular field and who can give first-hand information and experiences to the students. Although resource lists greatly increase resource usage and increase the ease of use for students, there is some controversy about whether references should be provided in a self-directed learning environment (Fitzgerald, Flemming, and Bayley, 1999).

Problem packages also include a feedback form, which elicits comments from both faculty and students about the way the problem is written, and any new and useful reference materials that students have identified. Each tutorial group is asked to complete a feedback form at the end of each problem. These comments are most helpful to faculty in their annual review of the course materials, although care needs to taken in any decision to revise or rewrite the problem based on these comments, since half the class will enjoy tackling the problem and half will not! Detailed information on the development of each of these components of problem packages can be found in Chapter 7.

Reference Resources

This category of resources represents the most extensive learning resource material available for students in their studies. These resources can take many forms.

Print

Print resources, both textbooks and journals, are housed in the library and accessible through the library catalogue. As mentioned, it is most useful and beneficial for the students' study time if these resources have been reviewed by faculty prior to being listed. Librarians may assist in updating resource lists and textbooks which become available, advise on newer publications in various subject areas, and request any new purchases. Copies of the journal articles can be made and put on reserve.

The bookstore or the printing services department prepare printed course materials which can be provided to or purchased by students. These resources contain copies of articles for students for which copyright clearance and permission has been obtained. The institutional bookstore is obviously another excellent resource for students when they wish to purchase their own copy of textbooks or CD-ROMs.

Tutorial groups may also be given copies of guidelines or protocols for management that have been developed by health professional organizations or by individual institutions and recommended for use in the various clinical settings. Hospital request forms or patient document data forms may also be available in conjunction with certain patient problems. These enable students to understand the information that must be elicited and noted in a management plan. Brochures from community agencies regarding support groups can also be included to inform students of the patient education resources that are available.

Non-Print Audiovisual Resources

Videotapes and computer applications comprise the usual choice of audiovisual resources, with laser disks being of some limited use. Slide atlases are sometimes useful, but many of these can now be found on the Web or on CD-ROM and are better utilized in these formats. A myriad of companies distribute video resources at varying educational levels. Many broadcast-quality tapes are released from television networks but these are often aimed at the general public and are not useful for university students. At times, faculty will see a program on television that might be useful in their courses; however, they need to be reminded that copying these at home, for use in the classroom, contravenes copyright laws. These programs often become available for purchase once public performance rights have been obtained.

Many video productions focus on the psychosocial aspects of a particular disease, for example, Parkinson's Disease or cancer. These are useful for students to understand the problems that patients may encounter and how they affect the family or the community at large. These issues are better dealt with in video format than in text format.

Computer Assisted Instruction (CAI) Packages

It may be assumed that in the twenty-first century the major thrust in resource development and/or acquisition will be towards computer assisted learning and interactive web-based materials (Saranto and Tallberg, 1998). While this may be true in more traditional programs it is not always the case in self-directed schools. Self-study time is limited and students want to find material in the most expedient way, so spending one to two hours working through a computer simulation package may not be the most efficient way to learn about a particular topic. If the package is interactive and the learners respond to questions and make decisions, then it will likely be used more often than one which is simply text on a computer screen. Our experience has shown that, in a collection of two hundred or so computer or CD-ROM packages, about 25 percent will be used extensively. The economic reality of this needs to be taken into careful consideration, when limited budgets are available.

The assessment of computer-based resources by faculty members can be problematic. Some faculty members have been slower to adopt computer packages as learning resources than to recommend videos. This may result from a lack of knowledge and familiarity with the media (Howard, 1990). Depending on their own learning preferences, some will like the format and some will not. Some expect the package to be all encompassing and cover the whole subject area adequately. However, very few texts accomplish this and yet they are recommended. Students now learn very differently from the way faculty learned and so having some students review the resources prior to purchase can also assist in the review process. However, the decision to purchase rests upon the faculty evaluation and budgetary considerations. Faculty may feel that existing packages are limited in the way they can teach interpretation of data, critical thinking, and decision making. However, the prospect of producing in-house materials that meet these specific needs is daunting to already overtaxed teaching staff (Houston, 1993; Saba, 1988). Very few computer-designed simulations, even those that are well-designed, will substitute for actual clinical experience, although they are useful as a pretest or for review (Rizzolo, 1990).

Acquisition of Multimedia Resources

A major issue for consideration at any institution is whether to develop resources in-house or to acquire them from outside sources. The number and variety of resources available for purchase is enormous. However, many of these were produced for a more traditional program and are not suitable for self-directed learning. Talking-head, lecture style videos do nothing to motivate learners who are used to an interactive tutorial group, since students find them boring and of limited value. Therefore, it is incumbent upon the person(s) acquiring the resources to review the material carefully prior to purchase, not only for accurate content and the technical merit of the production, but also for how interactive it is. An additional consideration in the purchase of CAI depends a great deal on the capabilities of the institutions and the library or other departments and the hardware systems available (Tallberg, 1995).

An evaluation form can be developed for this purpose, to provide information for the staff responsible for the purchase and cataloguing of new multimedia resources. In some institutions, staff in a learning resource center have this role, aided by various faculty members who are responsible for the learning objectives and content of the course or program. Where a Faculty of Health Sciences is in place, resources may be needed in similar content areas for several programs. Therefore, a coordinated acquisitions process assists all programs to find suitable resources and avoids unnecessary duplication. However, this may lead to an unbalanced collection and there may be large gaps in the overall collection. Coordinated review and evaluation help to broaden the scope of the collection while effectively allocating the limited budgets which many schools have for purchasing resources.

It is convenient and very helpful if a cadre of resource people from a variety of disciplines can be enlisted to help with the review of resources. An assessment of an external resource may be delayed for some weeks while someone is found who has the content, educational expertise, and time to assist in the process. Some institutions have tried the "A/V Showcase" concept several times a year, where a larger number of resources are brought in for review at one particular time, usually for a week.

With these factors in mind, and the fact that technology is continually changing and updating at a rapid pace, it is incumbent upon the purchaser to acquire the most useful, interactive resources and then to encourage faculty to recommend them to students. This may be done via course outlines, resource pages, electronic messaging systems, and Web pages. Feedback forms are essential at the completion of a course to evaluate the usefulness of the resources.

Development of Multimedia Resources

Video production is often less expensive and usually less time-consuming than computer productions, and making either of these in-house ensures that the resource will meet the specific needs of the users. It may be necessary to do this if other appropriate resources cannot be found. There may also be more interest from the students if the resource is authored by someone they are familiar with or from their own institution.

The reality is that some resources may take months or even more than one year to complete and by this time the need may have passed or the focus changed. Unless technical staff are readily available to assist in the production based on educational content, then the process is hampered even more. Development of resources may rely heavily on the coordinated efforts of several departments.

Audiovisual or media services may be involved in the technical aspects as well as the computer services unit, based on the needs and educational content from a particular program. Sometimes the cost of production and the investment of faculty time makes it prohibitive and purchasing becomes the only option.

Discipline-Specific Resources

These resources include morphological resources in anatomy, pathology, histology, radiology, and digital imaging which will be described later in this chapter. Some clinical departments maintain their own slide or specimen collection and the students should be made aware of these. As well, faculty need to be aware of what is available and encourage their students to utilize the areas that maintain the resources. These resources should also be listed on the resource lists that are given to students. Often faculty members from these areas will present scheduled sessions around a specific discipline.

Community Resources

Community agencies are a valuable source of information that students may find helpful to visit and attend some of the sessions they provide for patient education and advocacy. National or provincial organizations provide brochures and other useful literature which may accompany the problem as "supplemental" material.

People Resources

People resources are usually faculty and clinical or community-based staff who are content experts and experienced in the issues around which the problems have been developed. They may provide input into the problem while it is being written, as well as fielding questions from the students during the term.

Standardized patients form a major resource to provide students with a realistic approach to problem solving and to enhance their communication skills. Unfortunately, low budgets often prohibit their extensive use, but many programs realize that their value as an educational tool outweighs their cost.

Community-based people are excellent resources when students need to find out about support groups and patient education. Usually these contacts are very pleased to be able to share their knowledge with students. As these people are volunteering their time, a letter of thanks for assisting students is also well-received and fosters community involvment in the students' learning.

In many schools an electronic server has been established for student/faculty communications and various resource people in a variety of disciplines can respond to questions the students might have. Alternatively, these faculty could enhance student learning and understanding of various concepts by posting a "question of the week." This type of system may be beneficial and can stimulate discussion among the students themselves. By sharing knowledge they develop and enhance self-directed learning skills.

Other resource people may be required to provide scheduled sessions for students, for example, on physiological aspects of the clinical scenarios in the problem. Critical thinking and appraisal skills may be another lecture-style topic. While these sessions are mainly didactic, it is preferable they use interactive, interesting, and challenging methods of presentation in order to gain a good audience especially when attendance is not mandatory.

Information Resources

Information resources include course outlines or manuals where overall learning objectives are listed, class schedules are outlined, evaluation methods are described, and where additional resource sessions or resources are noted. It is useful if students receive information regarding events of particular interest that are being held throughout their institution, including visiting lecturers or guest speakers from government departments.

Evaluation Resources

Evaluation in a self-directed program must have both formative and summative aspects and should include participation from both the tutor and students. Evaluation strategies used in problem-based programs are presented in Chapter 9. A variety of types of media may be used in an evaluation system, such as computer, video, print, and standardized patients.

SPECIFIC FACILITIES TO SUPPORT THE PBL MODEL

As we have seen, the number and kind of learning resources to support learning in the PBL Model is extensive. These resources can be organized and made available to students in a number of specific facilities, and four will be looked at in detail, namely, an anatomy laboratory, a clinical skills laboratory, a library, and a computer laboratory.

Anatomy Laboratory

The same principles apply in developing an anatomy learning resource for students in PBL programs as apply in developing other learning resources for these students. The resources need to be readily accessible to the students throughout their education, user friendly, and designed to support self-directed and small group learning. Most importantly, they need to be designed to meet the learning needs of the students. Students will quickly come to recognize whether a resource satisfies their needs. If it does, it will become appreciated and effectively used by the students. Conversely, if it fails to help the students with their learning needs, the students will abandon their efforts to use the anatomy resources for learning and turn to other sources for information. Ideally the resources should be sufficiently flexible and adaptable to a range of uses and easily meet the needs of a variety of users.

An anatomy resource learning area designed to meet the learning needs of students in a PBL program is quite different from a traditional anatomy dissection lab. For these reasons the planning of an anatomy learning resource area should begin with the planning of the curriculum, and be included in any discussion of ongoing program changes.

Linking the learning of anatomy with the learning of related content, including the basic sciences such as physiology, histology, embryology, and pathology, or clinical content such as physical examination, enhances learning in both areas and facilitates the application of this knowledge to clinical practice.

Materials

The challenge of developing anatomy learning resource materials can appear to be a daunting one. The subject content is large, and commercially available resources are often costly. Simple basic resources developed by

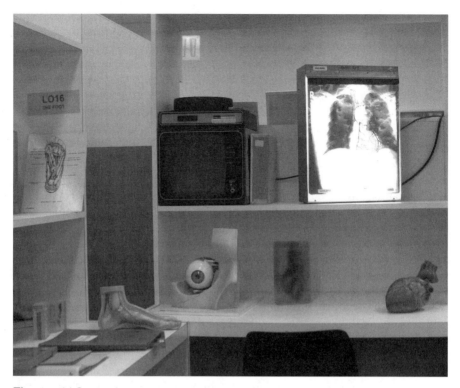

Figure 11.2   Types of Resources in an Anatomy Laboratory

faculty, although less "classy," are often very effective in helping students to learn and understand functional morphology. It is acceptable to be creative and practical. If it works, use it. Although excellent resources can be developed by faculty, the cost in faculty time may be an issue.

There are a number of properties to consider when selecting or developing learning resources. They should be attractive and interesting so that they readily engage the students, and include a range of different types of material that stimulate learning through the visual, tactile, and auditory senses. A specimen or model that is movable and that can be picked up, examined, and passed around among a group of students is far more likely to stimulate discussion and good learning than a resource in a fixed display in a glass case. Observe the students working with resources and note which are used by the students and which tend to gather dust.

A range of different types of resources can be used in an anatomy lab including models, encased specimens, charts, diagrams, scripts, articles, and X rays. These materials can be organized in modules designed to help students learn about an organ, region, system, or concept. An example is shown in Figure 11.2.

Dissected specimens that can be examined and studied by students are an excellent learning resource. The process of dissection is difficult, requires considerable skill, and can be very time-consuming. However, material prepared by a skilled dissector can be stored in moistening fluid and studied by a large number of students over a long period of time. For example, because students in PBL programs access resources when they have a "need to know," and are not restricted to prescheduled laboratory hours, a single heart can be studied by individual students or small groups at times that are convenient for them. If the material is handled carefully it will remain in good condition for many years. The more senior students tend to be the most careful in handling and caring for the specimens, probably because they recognize their value as a learning resource, and they often assume some responsibility for teaching and monitoring the incoming students to ensure that they provide good care for the material.

Reference texts are a valuable resource in the lab. Designated "working atlases" can be used by students while they are working with specimens. The working atlases should have illustrations that closely match the material the students are studying. Photographs of the lab specimens with the key structures labeled are ideal. This helps increase confidence in new students and encourages self-directed learning because they can be certain that they are identifying structures correctly.

The lab should contain a number of well located or portable blackboards and colored chalk, or white boards and various colored pens so students can illustrate and discuss the material they are studying. X ray viewing boxes are another useful resource since they enable students to view actual films. Larger viewers are useful for groups of students and allow comparison of several films at a time. Large high-resolution computer screens can be used to provide excellent high-quality radiological images, as well as other digital-based images.

The living human body is an invaluable resource for studying functional human anatomy, so students can be encouraged to observe and study their own structures in action. This is an excellent approach when studying the hand or peripheral pulses. Standardized patients can also be useful for learning surface anatomy and for practicing clinical skills. If students become accustomed to observing and studying the living body they tend to become more observant and are better able to relate their learning directly to patients.

Other resources that can be located in the anatomy lab include stethoscopes, sphygmomanometers, and ophthalmoscopes. These enable students to study the anatomy at the same time as they are practicing clinical skills. Locating this equipment in the anatomy lab provides a strong link between the learning of anatomy and its clinical application (Groves, Crowe, Stratford, and Binkley, 1993). The "linking" of anatomy and clinical skills enhances and increases the efficiency of learning.

Evaluation of the learning resources and the way in which they are used by students is essential to ensure that the resources meet the learning needs of the students, and that the resources are revised and upgraded as needed. Feedback from students is invaluable, since they are the learners and need to be listened to. If students know their input is valued they will be more willing to provide useful evaluation of resources. It is also important to observe students. Watch what they do, what they use, how they use it, and how long it is used. When they leave the resource area do they appear frustrated and confused, or happy and satisfied?

Resource Faculty

Although the faculty involved in teaching anatomy may have a range of different backgrounds, from the basic scientist to the practicing clinician, it is critically important that they are enthusiastic and supportive of PBL and have a solid understanding of the approach. Teachers who do not under-stand PBL may feel much more comfortable continuing to teach using the more traditional and familiar didactic format. They need to maintain and reinforce PBL to avoid conflicting approaches that can be counterproductive and frustrating to students. Ideally, clinical and basic science faculty will work as a team with faculty to provide a stimulating environment and role model for student learning.

In a PBL curriculum students will access the anatomy resources, both material and faculty, when they have established a "need to know," so they come with a desire for particular information and an understanding of how they will apply this new information. Therefore, if laboratory or faculty resources sessions are scheduled, it is important that they occur after students have encountered a patient problem and identified their learning objectives.

Organization of Resources

The organization of the resources within the laboratory area will affect the way in which the students use the resources. If models and text-based resources are located in one room while specimens are located in another, students will be less likely to integrate the learning from both types of resources. On the other hand, if related materials are located in the same area of the lab, or in close proximity to each other, students will be more likely to use the range of resources, perhaps even reviewing several types of resources at the same time. For example, in studying the heart it can be useful to have skeletal material (for surface land marking), models, X rays, dissected specimens, an atlas, and a live subject collected together in the study area. Students then have immediate access to those resources that best fill their learning needs. In addition, using the different resources will enhance and reinforce learning. This is also an ideal environment for students to learn and practice surface anatomy and clinical skills (Groves et al., 1993). Linking the learning of anatomy and clinical skills facilitates student learning and enables them to more easily grasp the relevance of an understanding of functional morphology to clinical practice.

Physical Requirements

The amount of space required to set up an anatomy learning resource area will depend on the number of users and the amount of learning resource material. Although a large area can accommodate more resources and more learners, even small areas, when used efficiently, can be developed to provide very functional resources for students in PBL programs. It is important that a resource area provide a warm and inviting atmosphere for learners. The room should be designed to support visual, auditory, and tactile learning. It should be well-lit, colorful, and bright. Carpeting on the floors creates a good acoustic environment for multiple users, and allows several small groups to carry on discussions without interfering with each other. A room with hard surface flooring will become noisy when even a small number of users are talking. If specimens are used in the area the room needs to be well-ventilated and handwash sinks made available in the lab. Numerous well-placed electrical outlets increase the flexibility of the lab area and ensure there are outlets located where needed to plug in equipment such as X ray viewers, audiovisual equipment, and computers.

Access to Anatomy Resources

Physical access to the laboratory is not the only concern for students using the resource. Some students may experience difficulty psychologically in accessing and using the anatomy resources because they include human material. In some cases the experience can be extremely stressful, interfere with learning, and develop into a serious problem (Finkelstein and Mathers, 1990; Abu-Hijleh, Hamdi, Moqattash, Harris, and Heseltine, 1997). This is probably a new experience for most students, and it is probably the first time they have seen human specimens. The process of dissection goes against a most fundamental human drive to protect and preserve the human body. To help students become comfortable using the anatomy resources, it is extremely important that all students receive an orientation to the laboratory. An orientation to small groups of students at a time, conducted in a gentle, sensitive, and supportive manner, is suggested. Each year students, family, and faculty are invited to attend a memorial service for the those who have donated their bodies to the school of anatomy.

Students in PBL programs need ample access to their learning resources so making the anatomy learning area accessible during extended hours in the evenings and during the weekends is helpful. Monitoring cameras and an electronic card key access system for the anatomy laboratory can allow students to access the resources in the evenings and on weekends while maintaining security of the area. This ensures that when students have a morphology learning issue they can easily access the appropriate resources in a timely fashion and enables them to revisit important material as they build their knowledge and skills.

Support

The number of staff needed to develop and maintain the anatomy learning area will depend on the size of the resource area and the number of users. If it is a large facility, it may be feasible to employ staff to produce and maintain the learning resources. Skills and training in art and computers are very useful for someone in this position. In smaller facilities it may be possible for an individual to assume responsibility for anatomy learning resources as well as other areas. If specimens are to be used in the laboratory, a trained dissector is needed to prepare good quality specimens, and to ensure that they are maintained and cared for properly.

Clinical Skills Laboratory (CSL)

As has been pointed out, ideally the clinical skills and anatomy teaching units should be located in close proximity. The educational aspects of teaching clinical skills to nurses will not be discussed here; rather the physical space and set-up of a CSL for a self-directed learning program will be described.

Physical Space

A clinical skills facility should simulate, as far as possible, the areas in which the students will be working. In many cases this would be a hospital setting, and rooms should be set up to mirror the clinical setting. Decisions on the number of rooms needed, probably between six and twelve, should be based on the number of people using the area, which often includes students from other disciplines such as medicine and other health professions, and possibly hospital staff for staff development sessions. Once learning objectives for clinical skills teaching have been developed, it will be easier to plan the space around these needs.

Some of the rooms can simulate a clinical examination room with either wall-mounted or mobile diagnostic equipment available, while others might be demonstration areas for various procedures to be taught and practiced, such as intravenous starts and monitoring, suturing, oxygen, and suctioning. Alternatively, the area could be set up with various organ systems in specific areas, with students going from one specific area to another to learn about physical assessment of particular systems.

In addition to these clinical teaching rooms, there needs to be office space for the staff and instructors. A comfortable area for students waiting to perform return demonstrations, evaluation sessions, or patient interviews is also desirable. Bathrooms, or at least sinks for hand-washing, need to be available, along with plenty of storage space for supplies and manikins and models. The area should be secure with several lockable areas available for storage.

The CSL may also need to house staff involved with the standardized patient (SP) program which is often closely related to the skills laboratory. The advantage of SPs is that they are trained to reproduce exact behaviors and symptoms of an illness repeatedly and consistently. This enhances student learning, and gives them confidence in dealing with patient encounters at least in the first years of nursing school. (See Chapter 12 for more details.) Staff who administer this program and patient trainers need office space as well.

A minimum of 1,000–1,500 sq m is suggested for a well-developed CSL and descriptions and layouts of clinical skills laboratories can be found on the World Wide Web, for example, the Clinical Skills Centre at St Bartholomew's Hospital in London, England (http://www.clinicalskillscentre.ac.uk/) and the Harrell Professional Development and Assessment Center at the University of Florida (http://www.med.ufl.edu/medinfo/harrell/harrell.html).

Resources

Having diagnostic equipment available in each room is useful, even though students often purchase their own. A box containing items such as stethoscopes, tape, gloves, and tongue depressors can be kept in each room. Manikins or models can be purchased for use in practicing skills such as intravenous insertion and monitoring, suturing, tube placement, wound care, catheterization, naso-gastric insertion, and dressing changes. Heart sounds or blood pressure simulators are sometimes included. The models are usually quite life-like and although they do not necessarily have the tactile simulation, they do provide students with a good practice environment. In addition, models that can be used to assist in teaching the pelvic or rectal exam are extremely important and serve to give students more confidence in their examination skills. While all of these are expensive acquisitions, they are essential for the comfort of students practicing these skills for the first time, and to give them confidence when they encounter a "real" patient. Preventative health teaching models such as testicles and breasts are valuable, as well as kits to emphasize hand-washing and infection control.

Wall posters and an atmosphere that is colorful and conducive to learning, as well as a staff member who has good rapport with the students are all essential for a well-functioning well-used skills area.

It would also be ideal, if the laboratory is not located near the library, to have a small resource room which could house computers for CD-ROM resources on physical assessment such as blood pressure and auscultation of heart and lung sounds. Some anatomical models and charts could also be available, together with videos demonstrating physical assessment and a playback machine.

Video cameras for closed-circuit television, wall-mounted in each room with two-way microphones and linked to a central A/V monitoring control area are also useful. Sound-proofing of each room may also be necessary. In smaller schools or those using a low-tech approach due to funding constraints, using portable cameras and one-way audio system may suffice for evaluative purposes. One-way mirror windows may be installed between two rooms if students are to be evaluated during interviewing or physical examination sessions.

Staffing

A clinical instructor who has a sound base of clinical nursing experience is necessary to supervise hands-on practice and to direct students to other resources. To support self-directed learning, the instructor can also help students who want to learn procedures and techniques on an ongoing basis. The instructor may also provide one-on-one remedial sessions when necessary to help the students gain more confidence or identify knowledge gaps by reproducing some clinical scenarios around which they need additional help. If the area is to be used by several disciplines, having a clinical instructor who could help all of these students would be an ideal situation.

Another staff member, either clerical or secretarial, is useful to order supplies, to hand out equipment for loan to users, to book rooms for individual study or practice and group sessions, and generally to facilitate teaching in the laboratory. This person could administer the laboratory in conjunction with either a faculty director or with a committee formed of representatives from the various programs using the laboratory.

Access

In some curricula, clinical skills are integrated with clinical courses in a way that requires students to attend scheduled sessions in the laboratory. These sessions can include demonstration, practice, and return demonstration evaluated by the instructors. However, students will often choose to visit the CSL on their own to practice other skills and gain more confidence. Therefore, it is important that the laboratory be available for students to use when needed, either individually or in pairs without their tutor, or in tutorial groups, to practice their clinical skills with an instructor.

Use of the area by students in the evening and on weekends greatly enhances the self-directed learning of these skills in a PBL environment, but staffing and security issues often hamper this. In fact, in a well-developed facility a security system using cameras and observation monitoring of the entrances may be needed.

Funding

Sufficient funds for an operating budget is a requirement for a well-developed CSL. Various teaching and clinical supplies need to be purchased; state-of-the-art diagnostic equipment should be available so that students learn on the equipment they will be using in the future. Sometimes infusion pump companies or similar resources will loan expensive pieces of equipment to programs on a semipermanent basis and this is an avenue worth exploring.

Integration of Clinical Skills Resources into the Curriculum

The person, or groups of people, administering the laboratory need to be proactive in promoting its use as a self-directed resource for practice, as well as for scheduled teaching sessions. It is probable that the teaching will be done in this area by many instructors affiliated with various educational programs and clinical areas in the adjoining hospital sites. Therefore, guidelines for use of the laboratory and of the equipment and supplies along with a list of recommended multimedia resources for both clinical and communication skills would be useful. Input is vital from the various teaching faculty and those who instruct in the laboratory, to keep equipment technically up-to-date and to provide suggestions for new models or manikins.

The CSL is a valuable resource for learning and testing professional skills which encompasses history-taking and communication skills and physical assessment.

Library

While a well-resourced and staffed library is a necessity in any educational setting, use of the problem-based, self-directed, and small group learning approach adds some extra requirements. Several studies (Saunders, Northup, and Mennin, 1985; Anderson, Camp, and Philp, 1990; Marshall, Fitzgerald, Busby, and Heaton, 1993) have shown that medical students in a PBL curriculum make greater use of the library, up to five to ten times more, than their counterparts in a conventional curriculum (Anderson et al., 1990, p. 79). It can be assumed that nursing students in a problem-based learning environment will use the library in a similar manner.

LaBeause (1999) provides a checklist of questions to be raised when planning a library for a PBL curriculum, centering around six issues (LaBeause, 1999, 314–316):

- User issues, including the degree to which PBL will be implemented
- Facilities and equipment issues, including seating and computer availability
- Library collections and resources issues, including a reserve collection
- Services issues, including hours of operation and circulation policies
- Staff issues, including the role of librarians in PBL
- Budget issues, including funding and cost recovery

Collections

The nature of nursing already requires that students access resources in a wide variety of subject areas (Pravikoff and Hawkes, 1997). The learning issues raised by the problem scenarios may also result in the search for information on a broad range of subjects. Library staff need to work closely with curriculum planners and problem developers to ensure that suitable and current resources are available to meet the learning objectives. In many cases, students will have to use the collections of other libraries in their institution or even outside their own institutions, such as public, school, and hospital libraries.

In addition to the regular collection of books and journals, the library may also put recommended or required resources from problem reference lists on reserve, that is, in a restricted access area with limited loan periods. If the students are not required to purchase textbooks, which is generally the case in a PBL curriculum, multiple copies of current texts might also be included in the reserve collection.

Self-directed learning necessitates a variety of formats, including print, multimedia, and electronic, to suit students' preferred learning styles. Therefore, libraries need to build a collection of audiovisual and computer resources along with the necessary viewing equipment.

Space Requirements

Since students in a PBL environment spend a great deal of time in the library in order to search for information to answer their learning issues, sufficient study space is a major issue. In addition to individual study tables or carrels, libraries should plan for group study rooms to meet the requirements of small group learning. While large tables in an open area can be used by groups, this can result in unacceptable noise levels. If the library includes a multimedia or computer resources area, group viewing rooms will also be valuable.

As students develop their information management skills, a library training room becomes an important consideration. The seating arrangements should be flexible to allow for demonstrations, group discussions, and individual work. Equipment requirements include a computer with a projection unit, an overhead projector, and a white-board. Computer workstations for hands-on practice are highly desirable for self-directed learning; however, costs of purchasing, maintaining, and upgrading equipment may be prohibitive for the library, and a shared institutional computer training facility may be more economically viable.

The Role of the Library in Curriculum Development

The importance of the library in developing and implementing an information management skills program is described in Chapter 5. Many nursing programs have worked with library staff to integrate knowledge management and information literacy into their curricula (Francis and Fisher, 1995; Layton and Hahn, 1995; Curtis, 1996; Bird and Roberts, 1998).

Including librarians on curriculum planning committees is very useful, since they can act as resource people for information literacy learning issues, and as cotutors for small group learning, particularly for courses dealing with critical appraisal and evidence-based nursing.

Access to Resources

The library catalogue continues to be a major tool to assist students in locating learning resources, particularly in a self-directed curriculum. As well as providing access to library holdings, the catalogue can also include resources held in other locations, for example, anatomy laboratory modules. In this way, students looking for resources to answer their information needs around a particular subject will be alerted to a wide variety of material.

In addition to providing printed indexes, the library is often the institutional contact for providing access to databases. In the nursing field, *Cumulative Index to Nursing and Allied Health Literature* (CINAHL) is an essential resource. Increasingly, more and higher quality resources are being distributed through the World Wide Web. By licensing Web-based resources such as textbooks and databases, the library can make access to current material more widely available and in a format that many students find appealing. The library can also create Web pages of evaluated resources to help students locate useful information. Any type of electronic resource will require that computer workstations be available.

As electronic resources become more prevalent and useful, access can become more decentralized, with distributed workstations in tutorial rooms. Access can also be expanded to clinical areas, so that students can transfer the information-seeking skills learned in the PBL setting to the clinical setting. Many students now have computers in their homes and student residences, making ready access to learning resources even more viable. No longer will students be required to go to the library in person to access their learning resources; the "virtual" library will come to them.

Computer Laboratories

As computer technology becomes ever more pervasive in the educational and clinical setting, students need ready access to electronic resources. Most educational institutions provide computer laboratories for students, allowing access to communication tools such as e-mail and electronic conferencing; utility software such as word processing and graphics, presentation and statistical packages; and Web access to course materials and other resources. In addition, equipment may be available for printing and scanning documents.

Drury (1997) describes the process of planning a computer learning laboratory for nursing students. Factors to be taken into consideration include space availability, commitment to technological support, ongoing financial commitment to the acquisition of equipment, payment for expert involvement and faculty training and support. The following suggestions provide a useful checklist for planning any computer facility (Drury, 1997, <cac.psu.edu/~dxm12/compart3.html>):

- Size of cohorts and actual laboratory specifications
- Environmental concerns: making the laboratory conducive to learning
- Ergonomic concerns: making the laboratory comfortable and efficient for students
- Security aspects: protecting the property and ensuring safe operation
- Security of information transmission: ethical consideration for student and faculty confidentiality
- Storage and other space needs
- Institutional support: immediate and ongoing
- Computer technology support: taking responsibility for the laboratory's functioning

While centralized computer facilities are easier to control in terms of security and to support in terms of equipment and user assistance, computer workstations in tutorial rooms, the anatomy laboratory, the clinical skills laboratory, and the library increase accessibility and enhance learning.

INTEGRATION OF RESOURCES

Whenever possible, educational institutions should integrate learning resources, both in the physical sense of setting up a learning resources center and in the curricular sense of making them an essential element in the planning and implementation of problem-based learning.

The centralization of resources into a learning resource center is an ideal, allowing for the integration of the anatomy and clinical skills laboratories with library, multimedia, and computer resources.

Locatis, Weisberg, and Spunt (1997) point out that computer technology trends are eroding the differences between traditional teaching laboratories and other library/information services, and that "modern resource centers and teaching laboratories should be integrated, both physically and functionally with each other and with other information resources in health professions schools" (p. 280).

If resources are not centrally organized and managed, there will be a need for strong coordination within the institution. Support structures will need to be in place to ensure that students are aware of all of the learning resources available. These can be provided by a formal learning resources office or by a learning resources committee with representatives from the educational programs and the various learning resources facilities.

CONCLUSION

As we have described, a wide range of learning resources and facilities are required to support a problem-based, self-directed, small group learning environment. These can be expensive in terms of financial, staff, and space requirements. Careful selection of resources and their organization and accessibility are important considerations when planning and implementing a PBL program.

It is important to recognize that students in PBL programs have special learning resource needs. In the optimal situation, the resources will be designed to meet the specific learning needs of the students; located adjacent to or integrated with other learning resources to facilitate integrated learning; accessible to students when they are needed; available in a learning environment that is inviting; and designed to encourage observation, handling, and discussion. Learning resources, along with well-designed PBL problems and effective and enthusiastic faculty, are essential for successful use of the PBL Model of education.

REFERENCES

Abu-Hijleh, M. F., Hamdi, N. A., Moqattash, S. T., Harris, P. F., and Heseltine, G. F. (1997). Attitudes and reactions of Arab medical students to the dissecting room. *Clinical Anatomy, 10*(4), 272–278.

Anderson, S., Camp, M. G., and Philp, J. R. (1990). Library utilization by medical students in a traditional or problem-based curriculum. In W. Bender, R. J. Hiemstra, J. A. Scherpbier, and R. P. Swierstra, (Eds.). *Teaching and Assessing Clinical Competence.* Groningen: BoekWerk.

Barrows, H. S. and Tamblyn, R. M. (1980). *Problem-based Learning: An Approach to Medical Education.* New York: Springer.

Billings, D. M. (1996). Designing nursing learning centers of the future. *Computers in Nursing, 14* (2), 80–81, 87.

Bird, D. and Roberts P. M. (1998). The role of library and information services in the modular curriculum. *Nurse Education Today, 87 (7),* 583–591.

The Clinical Skills Centre. [Online]. <www.clinicalskillscentre.ac.uk>

Curtis, K. L. (1996). Teaching roles of librarians in nursing education. *Bulletin of the Medical Library Association, 84* (3), 416–422.

Drury, R. M. (1997). Considerations in planning a computer learning laboratory for nursing students. *On-Line Journal of Nursing Informatics, 1*(2). <cac.psu.edu/~dxm12/conpart1.html>

Finkelstein, P. and Mathers, L. (1990). Post-traumatic stress among medical students in the anatomy dissection laboratory. *Clinical Anatomy, 3,* 219–226.

Fitzgerald, D., Flemming, T., and Bayley, L. (1999). Problem-based learning and libraries: The McMaster experience. In J. Rankin (Ed.), *Handbook on Problem-Based Learning.* New York: Forbes for Medical Library Association.

Francis, B. W. and Fisher, C. C. (1995). Multilevel library instruction for emerging nursing roles. *Bulletin of the Medical Library Association, 83*(4), 492–498.

Groves, H., Crowe, J., Stratford, P., and Binkley, J. (1993). Clinical skills in the anatomy laboratory: Linking the learning. In [Programme of the] International Conference on Student Centered Education in conjunction with the 8th Biennial General Network Meeting, Sherbrooke, Canada, August 22–27, 1993, p. 145.

Harrell Professional Development and Assessment Center (August 27, 1995). [Online]. <http://www.med.ufl.edu/medinfo/harrell/harrell.html>

Houston, M. S. (1993). The process of developing a computer-assisted instructional program. *Nurse Educator, 18*(3), 14–17.

Howard, B. (1990). Nurse education and convergent information technologies. *Nurse Education Today, 10*(2), 145–150.

LaBeause, J. H. (1999). Implications of a problem-based learning curriculum for health care libraries and librarians: Practical applications in preparing for change. In J. Rankin (Ed.), *Handbook on Problem-based Learning*. New York: Forbes for Medical Library Association.

Layton, B. and Hahn, K. (1995). The librarian as a partner in nursing education. *Bulletin of the Medical Library Association, 83*(4), 499–502.

Locatis, C., Weisberg, M., and Spunt, D. L. (1997). Learning resources centers, computer laboratories, and clinical simulation laboratories. In D. L. Moore (Ed.), *Guide for the Development and Management of Nursing Libraries and Information Resources*. New York: National League for Nursing.

Marshall, J. G., Fitzgerald, D., Busby, L., and Heaton, G. (1993). A study of library use in problem-based and traditional medical curricula. *Bulletin of the Medical Library Association, 81*(3), 299–305.

Pravikoff, D. S. and Hawkes, W. G. (1997). Introduction: Information resources and services for nursing. In D. L. Moore, (Ed.), *Guide for the Development and Management of Nursing Libraries and Information Resources*. New York: National League for Nursing.

Rizzolo, M. (1990). Factors influencing the development and use of interactive video in nursing education. *Computers in Nursing, 8*(4), 151–159.

Saba, V. K. (1988). Taming the computer jungle of NISs. *Nursing & Health Care 9*(9), 486–491.

Saunders, K., Northup, D. E., and Mennin, S. P. (1985). The library in a problem-based curriculum. In A. Kaufman (Ed.), *Implementing Problem-Based Medical Education: Lessons from Successful Innovations*. New York: Springer.

Saranto, K. and Tallberg, M. (1998). Nursing informatics in nursing education: A challenge to nurse teachers. *Nurse Education Today, 18*(1), 79–87.

Tallberg, M. (1995). Computers in nursing education. In D. M. Modly, et al. (Eds.), *Advancing Nursing Education Worldwide*. New York: Springer.

van der Vleuten, C. P. M. and Swanson, D. B. (1990). Assessment of clinical skills with standardized patients: State of the art. *Teaching and Learning in Medicine, 2*(2), 58–76.

Wilson, M. (1999). Using benchmarking practices for the learning resource center. *Nurse Educator, 24*(4), 16–20.

Standardized Patients as an Educational Resource

Andrea Baumann and Elizabeth Rideout

A standardized patient (SP) is a healthy person who has been carefully trained to simulate the historical, physical, and emotional features of a patient with sufficient realism to prevent detection by experienced clinicians.

This chapter will provide an overview of the valuable educational resource of using standardized patients (SPs) that is closely associated with the Problem-Based Learning (PBL) Model, but is equally applicable in any approach to student learning. A brief history will be presented and the advantages and disadvantages of using (SPs) will be outlined. The process of selecting and training an SP will be presented and examples of the use of an SP in a learning and an evaluation session will be provided.

HISTORY OF STANDARDIZED PATIENTS

The first reported use of a standardized patient was in 1963, at the University of Southern California, and the "inventor" of this educational resource was none other than Howard Barrows, also a founder of PBL (Barrows and Abrahamson, 1964). Barrows, a neurologist and medical educator, was searching for a method of evaluating the assessment skills of medical residents. The struggles Barrows faced in achieving acceptance of his invention are well-documented in the entertaining and comprehensive history of the SP presented by Wallace (1997), who also acknowledges other persons such as pediatrician Paula Stillman who helped to establish the SP as a credible teaching methodology and a reliable evaluation tool. The outcomes of their efforts are evident in the adoption of SPs in the teaching and evaluation of medical students in 111 of 138 North American medical schools that responded to the AAMC survey sent to all 142 schools (Anderson, Stillman, and Wang, 1994), and in the use of SPs as part of licensing examinations in medicine and physiotherapy in both the United States and Canada (Conn and Cody, 1989; Reznick, Blackmore, Dauphinée, Rothman, and Smee, 1996). Although there are fewer reports of the use of SPs in nursing, there are examples of SPs being used in teaching and evaluation at the baccalaureate level (Janes and Cooper, 1996) and the graduate level (O'Connor, Albert, and Thomas, 1999) as well as in the Nurse Educational Assessment Program (NEAP) that serves a quality assurance function (Parsons, Baumann, and Boblin-Cummings, 1997).

Although the most common use of SPs continues to be teaching or evaluating the skills and abilities of interviewing, counseling, physical examination, and clinical decision making, their use is also reported in research. For example, SPs have been used to evaluate the practice of health professionals in the community. Woodward, Hutchison, Norman, Brown, and Abelson have reported the use of SPs to determine the extent to which family physicians incorporate preventive care in their practice (1998) and the degree of variation in physicians' charges for health care encounters (1998). A similar use of SPs is reported by Carney and Ward (1998) who compared the HIV preventive practices of community-based nurse practitioners and physicians. Other research with SPs has focused primarily on the psychometric properties of their use. Investigators have explored such questions as the relationship between checklist and global rating scores, and between SP and faculty ratings, when SPs are used for performance evaluations (Regehr, Freeman, Robb, Missiha, and Heisey, 1999); and the reliability and validity of using SPs to evaluate the interpersonal skills of foreign-trained physicians (Boulet et al. 1998).

ADVANTAGES OF USING STANDARDIZED PATIENTS

The numerous advantages of using SPs in place of real patients for learning and evaluation include:

- *Availability.* Once a scenario is established and the patient trained, the SP is available at any time and any place. Therefore, it is not necessary to rely on the possibility of finding the appropriate patient to demonstrate a situation or to be available to evaluate a particular skill or ability.
- *Reliability.* Experienced SPs who are well-prepared are able to repeat a situation a number of times, maintaining the same presentation of symptoms, signs, and psychosocial aspects of the case. This ensures the experience remains the same for all students, a particularly useful feature when using SPs for evaluation purposes (Colliver and Williams, 1993; Swartz, Colliver, Robbs, and Cohen, 1999).
- *Adaptability.* Unlike an encounter with a real patient, SPs can be interrupted during an encounter and students can discuss any details of what is happening, including aspects of the patient assessment and any feelings of uncertainty the student may be having, in front of the SP.
- *No time restriction.* SPs are generally booked for a specific time period, during which students need not feel time pressures and can take as long as

necessary to interview, examine, or counsel a patient. They can use a variety of approaches to elicit information or perform a physical examination, to determine which is most effective. They can stop and repeat a section to improve performance and reinforce learning, whether it is at the beginning, middle, or end of an encounter.

- *Acceptability to students.* Students are sometimes reluctant to ask particular kinds of questions, to perform some aspects of a health assessment or to explore sensitive issues with real patients. Students appreciate the opportunity to practice new skills and strategies with SPs, since they need not fear harming the patient. Although they often describe the experience of interacting with SPs as stressful, they also value the opportunity to practice in an environment that is controlled.
- *Accurate feedback.* Well-prepared SPs provide useful and accurate feedback in a manner that is helpful and acceptable to students. The SP gives feedback on their own feelings of comfort and security during the interaction as well as on the level of concern and interest expressed by the student. They comment on the clarity of questions used in an interview and the approach to physical assessment, such as a touch that is too gentle or too harsh. In a summative evaluation situation, they are often involved in the decision regarding student performance, and have been found to be as accurate and reliable as faculty evaluators (Vu et al. 1992).

DISADVANTAGES OF USING STANDARDIZED PATIENTS

The disadvantages of SPs are few, and most are related to the costs associated with a fully developed SP program, which are considerable. There is generally an administrator who maintains information on the scenarios and the SPs who portray them, books the SPs, arranges their payment, and monitors their performance through feedback from the users of the service. Large scale SP programs often employ a trainer, who works with the SPs to develop their patient roles and assists them to become proficient at providing accurate and useful feedback. Of course, the largest cost is the payment of the SP, who receives remuneration for training sessions as well as the sessions with students. All these costs will vary with the size of the SP program and the rate of payment for the various individuals involved. Suffice it to say, unless there is a strong spirit of volunteerism in the educational program planning to maintain an SP program, there will be considerable financial cost.

Other potential disadvantages of using SPs are: (1) there may be some conditions and situations that cannot be simulated; (2) the circumstances in which the SP is encountered is often unrealistic, and students comment on such things as the room setting and the presence of other students and the tutor; and (3) although students generally find interaction with SPs a valuable learning experience, they also find the experience stressful.

RECRUITMENT AND TRAINING OF STANDARDIZED PATIENTS

The first step in this process is the clarification of goals for using an SP, which might be learning particular skills and abilities, providing formative evaluation, or determining summative evaluation.

The creation of patient scenarios in which SPs will be used is the next step. The scenario is central because it is the real-life situation that the SP will enact. (The process of developing scenarios and problem packages is described in detail in Chapter 7). Any problem package includes data that describes the particular patient in detail. However, when devising a problem package for which an SP will be used, there must be extensive detail. As O'Connor et al. (1999) says: "To be convincing, the SP has to respond with the same certainty a true client would to *any* question—and obviously students will ask a variety of unique questions. For example, if a patient is employed, s/he has to be prepared to respond to any interviewer who asks details of the workday—its stresses, exposure to hazards, perhaps relationships with bosses or co-workers and the like" (p. 243). Therefore, the patient data for the SP must be complete and presented in a way that allows the SP to feel comfortable being that patient. It is useful to organize the patient scenario and the accompanying patient data under headings such as demographic data, presentation/reason for the appointment, current difficulties and/or symptoms, past history of similar difficulties, history of other health concerns, current lifestyle and social history, and affect/behavior during the encounter. When physical findings are a part of the scenario, they too must be made explicit.

It is the patient description and patient data that will lead to the choice of the individual to portray the patient scenario. If there is an SP program, that office recruits potential SPs and they will select the particular individual for your use from their roster of "patients." Otherwise you may approach a number of possible sources, including local actors, friends, and neighbors, to find an SP. The Retirees Association of the college or university where your school is located is often a good source of SPs to depict older individuals. Stillman (1993) advises that good choices for an SP role are people interested in helping students learn, who do not idolize health care workers, and are not seeking to obtain assistance with their own health issues.

The next step in the process is the training of the SP to enact the patient scenario. This is done by staff of the Standardized Patient Program, if one exists. If not, the faculty member who will use the SP can do the training.

Essentially the training consists of much the same process as an actor learning a new role. The key facts of the scenario are committed to memory and the important issues are discussed with the trainer, the faculty member who wrote the case, and other SPs who may be portraying the same scenario. In some situations, meeting actual patients with similar health problems and concerns will be useful. For example, several scenarios were developed for an Objective Structured Clinical Examination that was part of the evaluation of a curriculum in Pediatric Oncology Nursing. Members of the group Parents of Children with Cancer attended the training sessions and gave valuable insights into the realism of the scenarios and the scripted responses of the children. If physical signs are a part of the scenario, someone skilled in physical assessment should work with the SP to ensure the signs are portrayed correctly. SPs are able to simulate a wide variety of signs: increased and decreased deep tendon reflexes, decreased breath sounds suggestive of a pneumothorax, weakness on one side, and difficulty swallowing to name a few.

Once the SPs have learned the scenario, a "dry run" is conducted, where the SP is interviewed and/or examined by a skilled practitioner who is often a faculty member involved in the course for which the SP will be used. If more than one SP will be playing the role, it is helpful for them to observe one another and to discuss any variations in their portrayal. Final details of the scenario can be determined at the "dry run" and any required additions or deletions made.

In addition to learning the scenario and their portrayal of it, SPs need to learn about giving feedback. This is given face-to-face in situations where students are learning and practicing new skills and obtaining formative feedback. In situations of summative evaluation, SPs are also called upon to evaluate student performance, although they might not give verbal feedback to the student. Therefore the training session must convey to the SP the pertinent issues in the scenario to be addressed by students, as well as the process of giving relevant feedback in an acceptable manner. SPs are informed that they should focus their feedback on how it felt to be the patient. Areas to be addressed include:

- Did the student convey caring and concern to the SP?
- What was the body language of the student?
- Were the questions asked clear and specific, or rambling and nonconcise?
- Was the interview rushed or too slow?
- Did the student have mannerisms that interfered with establishing a relationship and the open exchange of information?
- Did the student pursue the areas that were of concern and interest to the patient and follow any cues given by the patient?

SPs also give feedback on the physical assessment component of any scenario. They are instructed not to comment on the expected findings and whether or not the student obtained them. Instead they are to focus on what it felt like to be the patient.

- Was the examination organized?
- Was the SP's privacy respected?
- Did the student convey concern for the patient in the performance of the assessment?
- Was the touch of the student too gentle, too rough, or just right?

Once SPs are trained, they are ready for the teaching or evaluation session for which they have been prepared. The faculty member conducting the session should meet the SP just before it begins to reinforce the purpose of the encounter and the level of students with whom the SP will be working. Once the session is completed the SP also receives feedback about their performance in the role. This feedback is shared with the SP and returned to the SP administrator. (See Figure 12.1 for a sample feedback form.)

PREPARING THE STUDENT FOR INTERACTION WITH A STANDARDIZED PATIENT

Although the first interaction with an SP may be in a large group where a particular technique is being demonstrated or in a summative evaluation situation, most often students will encounter SPs in a tutorial as part of a clinical laboratory experience or in a PBL class, and it is for this latter experience that students generally require some orientation.

First, it is important to be clear about the purpose for which the SP will be used. As we have already described, the SP may be used to learn interviewing, counseling, and/or physical examination skills. Students should be encouraged to develop any specific objectives for their interaction with the patient, and be provided with time to do some advance preparation before their meeting with the SP. Usually when the tutorial group makes the decision to use an SP, they discuss and plan one week and book the patient for the following week. The time allotted for their interaction with the SP should also be clarified at the planning session. Usually in a three-hour class, some time is used at the beginning and end of the class for planning and the SP is booked for about two hours.

The tutorial group generally meet in a regular classroom or a clinical skills laboratory. Since the class setting is of course simulated, the location for the interaction with the "real patient" should be clarified, whether it be a hospital room, the patient's home, the Nurse Practitioner's office, or the office of the School Nurse. Often the student–SP interaction takes place in one area of the classroom while the rest of the class watches. Another approach is to use rooms with two-way mirrors, where the group watches from one side while the student and SP are on the other side.

Quality Report

Simulator Name: _____ Date: _____

Simulation: _____

User's Name: _____   Supervisor [   ]   Learner [   ]

Program: _____

Rating Scale: 1 = Needs to be retrained   2 = Needs to be reviewed
               3 = Few minor changes necessary 4 = Good
               5 = Excellent

1. Please rate the quality of this simulator using the above scale.
                                          Low   High
   a. Realism of the simulator   1   2   3   4   5
   b. Clinical signs shown by simulator   1   2   3   4   5
   c. Feedback given by simulator   1   2   3   4   5

(If you gave this simulator a 3 or below in Question 1, please identify the
specific "problem areas" that should be reviewed with the simulator for realism
or consistency).

Comments: _____

2. Was the simulator suitable for your particular goals?   Yes [   ]   No [   ]

3. The simulator feedback covered:
   a) Interpersonal qualities _____   b) Professional manner _____

Comments: _____

4. If I had this simulation again, I would recommend the following
   improvements:

   _____

   _____

5. Did the simulator arrive ON TIME?   Yes [   ]   No [   ]

Date: _____   Signature: _____

Figure 12.1 Standardized Patient Feedback Form
© School of Nursing, McMaster University.

There are a variety of ways the interview or examination can be conducted within the tutorial. During the early development of interviewing and physical examination skills it may be productive to have the whole group (usually a maximum of ten students) involved in asking questions and suggesting and practicing the physical examination skills. However, students often find it more effective if one student at a time takes on the role of interviewer/examiner. Whichever approach is taken, it is important that the student know the interaction can be stopped at any time, using a period of "time-out," which distinguishes interaction time with the SP from discussion time. The group should develop some sort of hand signal to indicate that a "time-out" has been called, which usually occurs when issues, techniques, direction, or reactions need to be discussed or clarified. Most often a "time-out" is called by the student who wants direction about where to go next in the interview or examination, although it may be decided in the planning that any group member, including the tutor, can call the "time-out." During discussion the SP remains quiet, in suspended animation, and does not participate. Once the student and group are ready to proceed, they call "time-in," the SP resumes the role, and the interview or examination proceeds.

Students need to be told clearly that SPs have been trained to anticipate that the treatment they receive while in the simulation will be the same as they would receive if they were actual patients. Respectful and professional behavior on the part of the students is an expectation. An important feature for students' use of SPs is the opportunity to receive objective feedback from the patient's point of view. This feedback to the student is an essential part of the process and takes place at the end of each session. Generally a feedback session begins with the student doing a self-evaluation of what they did well and their areas for improvement. The SP is then asked to give feedback, followed by the group members who share their observations of the interaction. The SP is also given verbal as well as written feedback on their portrayal of the SP.

The preparation of students for encounters with SPs for the purpose of summative evaluation is less extensive but has some of the same features. The purpose of the evaluation, the time available, and the setting of the interaction should be discussed. The criteria for evaluation usually take the form of checklists that describe the specific behaviors expected of students. These checklists may or may not be shared with the students. The disadvantage of sharing them is the tendency for students to then "study to the checklist" rather than focus their preparation on learning the skill or ability on which they will be tested. On the other hand, faculty should adhere to the "no surprises" guideline (as described in Chapter 9 on student evaluation) and ensure that the general, if not the specific, expectations are made explicit.

EXAMPLE OF A STANDARDIZED PATIENT SCENARIO

As we have noted above, SPs are a useful adjunct to learning interviewing, counseling, and physical assessment skills. They are also an important part of an Objective Structured Examination (OSCE), used for evaluation purposes.

Table 12.1   *Example of a Scenario with Standardized Patient*

Angie is a fourteen year old who was diagnosed with a brain tumor four months ago. Angie had surgery and was treated with chemotherapy and radiation. You are a student nurse in the Oncology Clinic and Angie has come for her regular follow up visit.

Angie is due to return to school. During a regular visit to the clinic, Angie asks you how she can go to school with a bald head, she still gets exhausted really easily, and she is not sure how many people will know what has happened to her. Besides, she is enrolled in a new school now that she is entering ninth grade.

The scenario presented in Table 12.1 could be used for either purpose. The scenario as presented might be part of a problem package for use with intermediate level students exploring issues of cancer care for adolescents, in which case Angie would be available as a resource for students to practice interviewing and counseling with an adolescent. Perhaps a second scenario of the problem package would see Angie return to the clinic with her parents, when the focus would be learning about and practicing a family assessment.

On the other hand, this patient scenario might be one station within an OCSE for intermediate level students, used to evaluate the students' therapeutic communication skills. In this instance, the student would be expected to interview the SP within a specified time frame, to begin to establish a therapeutic relationship and to conduct an initial assessment. The students would be evaluated against preset criteria and a judgment made of the students' performance.

The importance of realism of presentation is equally important whether the SP is being used to learn new skills or for summative evaluation. Instructions for training an SP must be sufficiently detailed and an example of the information used to prepare Angie are presented in Table 12.2.

CONCLUSION

The benefits of using standardized patients as an educational resource within any program are considerable, and their use in PBL curricula has been described since the introduction of the educational approach. Although there are considerable costs associated with establishing and maintaining an SP program, in our experience the benefits far outweigh those costs. O'Connor et al (1999) concur: "We have found SPs a versatile and valuable strategy for teaching and evaluation. Developing and producing scenarios— and then orchestrating the experience—requires human and financial resources, but our judgment is that the effort and expense are well worth the cost" (p. 246).

Table 12.2   *Instructions for Standardized Patient*

Simulation:	Teenager (Angie) returning to school after surgery for a brain tumor, chemotherapy, and radiation.
Age:	14 years old
˙Setting:	Clinic visit
Background:	

It has been four months since your surgery to remove a brain tumor. You were in hospital for two months and you have been two months at home since your surgery, chemotherapy, and radiation treatment. You have been told the surgery went well and you should be OK but still you don't want to talk about it and certainly not tell everyone. You get very tired. The longest time you have been out of the house is about four hours to go shopping and have lunch or to come to the clinic. You went to the movies with your girl friend once and afterwards were tired out.

Now you have been told you can go back to school. You are going to go to Westdale High School which you chose because it is big. Now you are scared because you only know two friends from your grade eight class who will be going to Westdale. They live close by and they have come to visit several times. Most of the other people from your grade eight class have chosen a different high school.

Your aunt took you shopping for a wig and you wear it but you think it does not look real. You are sure that everyone will look at you funny and ask all kinds of stupid questions. Also your father and mother have been really fighting a lot lately and your mother can't seem to concentrate and listen to you. Your aunt is good to talk to but she lives in Toronto and you only see her occasionally.

You feel really lost and alone and want direction on how to deal with school. Your worst fears are being teased, being asked a lot of questions, failing because you are too tired to study, not making any friends because you look so funny, not having energy to do any outside activities. You really don't want to talk about your Mom and Dad's fighting because you think you caused their problems when you got sick.

Props:	Wear a hat over your natural hair which will be the wig.
Affect:	Appear withdrawn, fatigued, and fidget.

REFERENCES

Anderson, M. B., Stillman, P. L., and Wang, Y. (1994). Growing use of standardized patients in teaching and evaluation in medical education. *Teaching and Learning in Medicine, 6*, 15–22.

Barrows, H. S. and Abrahamson, S. (1964). The programmed patient: A technique for appraising student performance in clinical neurology. *Communications, 39*, 802–805.

Boulet, J. R., Ben-David, M. F., Ziv, A., Burdick, W. P., Curtis, M., Peitzman, S., and Gary, N. E. (1998). Using standardized patients to assess the interpersonal skills of physicians. *Academic Medicine, 73*(10), S94–S96.

Carney, P. A. and Ward, D. H. (1998). Using unannounced standardized patients to assess the HIV preventive practices of nurse practitioners and family physicians. *Nurse Practitioner, 23*(2), 56–58, 63, 67–68.

Colliver, J. A. and Williams, R. G. (1993). Technical issues: Test application. *Academic Medicine, 70*(12), 1062–1064.

Conn, H. L. and Cody, R. P. (1989). Results of the second clinical skills examination of the ECFMG. *Academic Medicine, 62,* 448–453.

Hutchison, B., Woodward, C., Norman, G. R., Abelson, J., and Brown, J. A. (1998a). Provision of preventive care to unannounced standardized patients. *Canadian Medical Association Journal, 158*(2), 185–193.

Janes, B. and Cooper, J. (1996). Simulations in nursing education. *Australian Journal of Advanced Nursing, 13*(4), 35–39.

O'Connor, F. W., Albert, M. L., and Thomas, M. D. (1999). Incorporating standardized patients into a psychosocial nurse practitioner program. *Archives of Psychiatric Nursing, 13*(5), 240–247.

Parsons, M., Baumann, A., and Boblin-Cummings, S. (1997). Issues involved in conducting a nurse educational assessment program. *Canadian Nursing Management, 2,* 6–7.

Regehr, G., Freeman, R., Robb, A., Missiha, N., and Heisey, R. (1999). OSCE performance evaluations made by standardized patients: Comparing checklist and global rating scores. *Academic Medicine, 74*(10), S135–S137.

Reznick, R. K., Blackmore, D., Dauphinée, W. D., Rothman, A. I., and Smee, S. (1996) Large-scale, high-stakes testing with an OSCE: Report from the Medical Council of Canada. *Academic Medicine, 71,* S19–S21.

Stillman, P. L. (1993). Technical issues: Logistics. *Academic Medicine, 68*(6), 464–470.

Swartz, M. H., Colliver, J. A., Robbs, R. S., and Cohen, D. S. (1999). Effect of multiple standardized patients on case and examination means and passing rates. *Academic Medicine, 74*(10), S131–S133.

Vu, N. V., Marcy, M. M., Colliver, J. A., Verhulst, S. J., Travis, T. A., and Barrows, H. S. (1992). Standardized (simulated) patients' accuracy in recording clinical performance checklist items. *Medical Education, 26,* 99–104.

Wallace, P. (1997). Following the threads of an innovation: The history of standardized patients in medical education. *Caduceus, 13*(2), 5–28.

Woodward, C. and Gliva-McConvey, G. (1995). The effect of simulating on standardized patients. *Academic Medicine, 70*(5), 418–420.

Woodward, C., Hutchison, B., Norman, G. R., Brown, J. A., and Abelson, J. (1998). What factors influence primary care physicians' charges for their services? An exploratory study using randomized patients. *Canadian Medical Association Journal, 158*(2), 197–202.

Problem-Based Learning in Master's Degree Education

Constance M. Baker

Health care delivery has been revolutionized around the world by the global knowledge explosion, technological advances, economic changes, and demographic shifts. The dramatic transformation of health care delivery necessitates a dramatic transformation in nursing education. The demand for evidence-based practice and data-driven outcomes requires nurses who can engage in critical thinking and clinical reasoning. Indeed, skills in critical thinking and clinical judgment are the first priority in the latest position statements on nursing education by the American Association of Colleges of Nursing (AACN, 1999) and the Canadian Association of University Schools of Nursing (CAUSN, 1998). In 1992, critical thinking was given impetus in the United States when accreditation criteria were revised by the National League for Nursing (NLN, 1992). Nursing faculty are also challenged to evaluate the current evolution of a market-driven health care delivery system, anticipate the consolidated network systems of the future, and attend to the curriculum consequences of such statements as Pew's "Twenty-One Competencies for the 21st Century" (Bellack and O'Neil, 2000).

Masters degree nursing education is recognized as the appropriate preparation for advanced professional nursing practice in primary care, clinical specialities, nursing administration, and nursing education. Further, it is in masters degree programs that nursing students are helped to merge their research knowledge and critical thinking skills to deliver evidence-based practice.

Clinical reasoning skills are increasingly cited as a crucial component of advanced nursing practice, with models such as Pesut and Herman's new OPT (outcome-present state-test) Reasoning Model being proposed as appropriate teaching tools (Pesut and Herman, 1999). One educational strategy to prepare reflective nurse clinicians to engage in critical thinking and clinical reasoning is problem-based learning (PBL).

This chapter summarizes PBL applications in nursing masters programs around the world. First, basic tenets of PBL for masters level education are presented, along with student and faculty characteristics. Second, specific nursing masters programs are identified, including those using PBL in inter-professional masters courses. Third, the research evidence on PBL outcomes in graduate nursing programs is assessed. Finally, the integration of problem-based learning and electronic technologies is projected for the future.

GRADUATE STUDENTS AND FACULTY IN PBL

Problem-based learning is a student-centered approach to education in which the faculty tutor creates a context where the student uses prior knowledge to solve real-life problems. Graduate students, like their under-graduate counterparts, often express concerns about moving from a passive learning environment and relinquishing previously effective academic behaviors, to an active learning environment where they must assume responsibility for their own learning and assume the requirements of active participation (Savin-Baden, 1997). Graduate students, who are usually older than undergraduates and employed in professional positions, are already facing considerable pressures in the transition from employee to student. Faculty need to orient graduate students to the new expectations of active and collaborative learning, and provide support when graduate students question requirements such as establishing their own learning goals and identifying their own resources. Business faculty using PBL in a Masters in Business Administration (MBA) program interpret student anxiety as a necessary motivating force to stimulate students' "need to know" so they actively pursue self-directed learning activities (Stinson and Milter, 1996).

The learner-centered nature of problem-based learning forces graduate faculty to address four aspects of learning: basic cognitive and metacognitive factors; motivational and affective factors; social and developmental factors; and individual differences in learning (Bonk and King, 1998). Faculty must consider how best to guide thinking, sustain motivation, foster social interac-tion, and acknowledge differences. Self-directed searching for new knowledge and collaborative problem solving within a PBL teacher-graduate student partnership should contribute to mutual respect and genuine caring. As partners in analyzing the PBL problems and critiquing the resources and literature, faculty can create a learning environment where graduate students experiment with new behaviors and engage in critical reflection (Roberts and Chandler, 1996), which can be formalized through the use of journals and faculty feedback. The care exhibited by faculty facilitating student learning is consistent with the definition of caring as "a nurturing way of relating to a valued other toward whom one has a personal sense of commitment and responsibility" (Swanson, 1991, p. 162). A learning community created in an academic course structured by PBL should be an empowering and caring community.

The dimensions of learner experiences in graduate PBL courses have been described in a model focused on three stances: personal, pedagogical, and interactional (Savin-Badin, 1997). The personal stance includes the means by which students discover, define, and place themselves within the PBL environment. The pedagogical stance refers to how students see themselves as learners and includes their prior learning experiences, their relationships between the self and the course content, and their personal reflections on the interaction of these aspects and the requisite disjunctions and paradoxes. The interactional stance refers to how the learner interacts with others in the PBL course environment and how they construct meaning in relation to one another. Faculty have unique opportunities in each of these three learner stances to demonstrate their beliefs that students have potential to learn, their awareness of students' striving efforts, their emotional presence in the teacher-student partnership, and their teaching and facilitation skills. Thus, faculty caring is demonstrated in graduate PBL courses through deliberate, rational, and knowledgeable acts of assisting students' goal achievement, a balance between scientific knowledge and humanistic teacher behaviors.

APPLICATION OF PBL IN NURSING MASTERS PROGRAMS

Problem-based learning has been used in medical schools for over 30 years, in some Canadian, Australian, and United Kingdom nursing schools for nearly 10 years, and has recently spread into other disciplines (Baker, 2000a). In nursing, Canada's McMaster University School of Nursing pioneered the use of the PBL Model in nursing education and has sustained its evolution with annual summer workshops that support nursing faculty development in the method (Drummond-Young, 1998). PBL has been adopted in nursing schools throughout Australia and in the United Kingdom, and in selected undergraduate courses in China, Japan, South Africa, Thailand, and the United States (Baker, 2000b).

The problem-based learning literature reveals that PBL is being implemented in nine different nursing masters specialities in 16 different universities in eight countries around the world (Table 13.1). Australia and the United States appear to lead the other countries with published reports on eight and seven masters degree programs, respectively. The 15 nursing masters programs in Australia and the United States are all located in universities where PBL had been implemented previously in the medical schools. Since these data come from the published literature found in various computerized search engines and university web pages, it may be incomplete.

Table 13.1 *Universities using PBL in nursing masters courses by academic specialty and country*

Academic Specialty	Australia	Canada	Ireland	Netherlands	Scotland	South Africa	United Kingdom	United States
Community Health	Griffith	Ottawa		Maastricht	Queen Margaret			Arizona, Kentucky
Nurse Midwives and/or Nurse Practitioners	Griffith Newcastle		Queen's				Thames Valley	New Mexico Southern California
Advanced Practice and/or Clinical Nurse Specialists	Newcastle Griffith LaTrobe Griffith				Queen Margaret			Hawaii
Administration/ Management and/or Nursing Education	Newcastle					Orange Free State Natal Durban		Indiana

Community Health Nursing

The predominant speciality using PBL is community health nursing with six masters programs in five countries reporting the use of PBL. Two community health nursing masters programs in the United States—the University of Arizona and the University of Kentucky—use the PBL Model. At the University of Arizona, case studies have been developed for community health (Fairbanks and Candelaria, 1998) and a unique interdisciplinary PBL practicum is being offered in a rural Arizona community (Slack and McEwen, 1997). Evaluation data indicate that this PBL practicum strengthens and enriches the PBL seminars. Nursing faculty at the University of Kentucky invested a year to integrate PBL into the MSN program in community health (King, Sebastian, Stanhope, and Hickman, 1997). A series of cases were developed to illustrate major themes in three core community health nursing courses (Sebastian and Stanhope, 1999), and curriculum development and evaluation issues are addressed in an instructor's resource guide (Stanhope & Sebastian, 1999).

The University of Maastricht in the Netherlands is unique in that "student-oriented PBL" is used in all the academic programs throughout the university, including the masters programs in community health (www.unimaas.nl/um/pbl). Faculty in Nursing Science have designed the master's curriculum around three themes: health existence, health determinants, and health interventions and offer multiprofessional tutorial groups.

Graduate nursing faculty at Australia's Griffith University (www.griffith.edu.au/school/nrs) use PBL in the public health nursing masters program. Griffith is, like McMaster University, a pioneer in the use of PBL and the source of some of the early and best writing on PBL in nursing (Alavi, 1995; Creedy and Hand, 1994; Creedy, Horsfall, and Hand, 1992). Nursing faculty at the University of Ottawa (Edwards et al., 1998) and at Scotland's Queen Margaret University (Dewar and Walker, 1999) collaborated with clinical experts in community health nursing to design PBL cases for graduate students and offer useful insights regarding tutor preparation. Thus, the literature reveals unique aspects of six community health nursing masters programs using PBL.

Nurse Midwives and Nurse Practitioners

Masters programs for nurse midwives and nurse practitioners are combined in this report because of their similarities in preparing nurses for autonomous practice. PBL methodology is used to deliver nurse midwifery programs in five universities in four countries. PBL began at the University of New Mexico's medical school in the mid-1970s, and now it is being used in graduate programs across several disciplines, including nurse midwifery and nurse practitioner (Urbina, Hess, Andrews, Hammond, and Hansbarger, 1997). The other four midwifery programs using PBL include two universities in Australia, Griffith and Newcastle, Queen's University in Ireland (Sinclair, Brown, and Jones, 1999), and Thames Valley University in London (Thomas, Quant, and Cooke, 1998).

Advanced Practice Nursing and Clinical Nurse Specialist

PBL is used in advanced nursing practice and clinical specialist programs in five universities in three countries. Nursing faculty at Australia's University of Newcastle have embraced the philosophy and methodology of PBL for all their degree programs—BSN through the PhD (www.newcastle.edu.au/department/ns/nursingweb). The advanced practice masters programs offered at both Australia's University of Newcastle and Scotland's Queen Margaret University appear to be similar to the clinical specialty format used at Griffith University in gerontological and mental health nursing, and Australia's LaTrobe University (Blackford and Street, 1999). Finally, at the University of Hawaii, PBL is used to prepare advanced practice psychiatric nurses to strengthen their critical thinking abilities (Inouye and Flannelly, 1998).

Nursing Education and Administration

PBL is being used in four masters programs focused on nursing's functional roles of education and administration. Two universities in South Africa have developed masters degree programs in nursing education using PBL. The University of Natal Durban offers a one-year masters degree in teacher preparation for nurses, both academic and community-based (Dana, 1997), and the University of Orange Free State has based their masters degree program in nursing education on PBL philosophy and methodology (Bitzer, 1997). PBL is being used in the nursing administration program at Australia's University of Newcastle.

At Indiana University in the United States, nursing faculty integrated four major courses in the nursing administration masters program, based on the model of PBL adopted for use in the Hahnemann School of Medicine (Baker, 2000a). The course objectives were retained for the four courses, and the required course content was embedded in ten PBL problems which were developed. Thus the course objectives and content for the program were retained, while the teaching methodology and scheduling were changed rather dramatically. The program is delivered over two academic semesters via the executive format of one weekend a month. The weekend begins with three hours of class on Friday evening, seven hours on Saturday, and four hours on Sunday. Between weekends students continue analyzing their learning issues with asynchronous computer conferencing and discuss aspects of the case related to application.

Table 13.2 summarizes a PBL case developed for nursing administration. Briefly, the chief nurse executive needs to persuade the hospital's top management team that acquiring "Magnet Hospital" designation is a cost-

Table 13.2 *Example of PBL Case Used in the Nursing Administration Masters Program*

Case Synopsis:

You are the chief nurse at Millennium Hospital, a 440-bed, acute care, nonprofit hospital located in a midwestern state. You and the four nursing directors have decided that the hospital is ready to apply for the American Nurses' Credentialing Center (ANCC) Magnet Nursing Service Recognition Program. How will you persuade the hospital's top management team to support this application?

Case Objective:

1. Analyze internal and external economic-political forces in macro strategic planning
2. Distinguish among theories of leadership relevant for top management teams
3. Contrast chief nurse executive roles on top management team (TMT) and on nursing team
4. Identify adaptations required to present vision of future to TMT-peers and nurse followers
5. Appraise hospital readiness to apply for Magnet Hospital Recognition Program
6. Synthesize research on Magnet Hospitals and nursing administration practice
7. Apply ANA's *Scope and Standards for Nurse Administrators*

Key Concepts:

Top management team
Leadership
Executive decision making
Marketing

effective strategy for marketing the hospital. The case expands and evolves through four scenarios: in the first scenario the chief nurse executive is participating in a meeting of the hospital's top management team; in the second she is giving feedback to her four nursing directors and designing strategy with them; in the third she is meeting with the hospital's chief financial officer; and in the fourth she is presenting nursing's plan to the top management team. Combined, the four scenarios provide the opportunity to analyze environmental forces influencing strategic planning, examine leadership theories relevant to nursing administration, assess criteria for "Magnet Hospital" designation, and explore factors influencing quality patient care. The key concepts of the case are: top management team, leadership, strategic long-term planning, executive decision making, and marketing.

Figure 13.1 presents a concept map (Daly, Shaw, Balistrieri, Glasenapp, and Piacentine, 1999; Edmondson, 1994), which outlines top management team (TMT), the concept mapped throughout the four scenarios in this case.

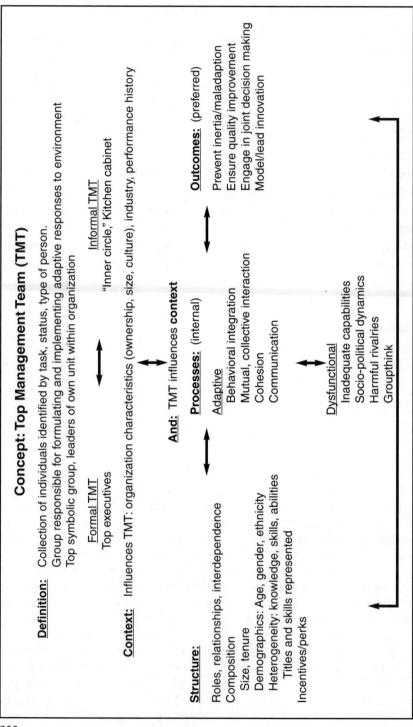

Concept: Top Management Team (TMT)

Definition: Collection of individuals identified by task, status, type of person.
Group responsible for formulating and implementing adaptive responses to environment
Top symbolic group, leaders of own unit within organization

Formal TMT
Top executives

Informal TMT
"Inner circle," Kitchen cabinet

Context: Influences TMT: organization characteristics (ownership, size, culture), industry, performance history

And: TMT influences **context**

Processes: (internal)

Adaptive
Behavioral integration
Mutual, collective interaction
Cohesion
Communication

Dysfunctional
Inadequate capabilities
Socio-political dynamics
Harmful rivalries
Groupthink

Outcomes: (preferred)

Prevent inertia/maladaption
Ensure quality improvement
Engage in joint decision making
Model/lead innovation

Structure:

Roles, relationships, interdependence
Composition
Size, tenure
Demographics: Age, gender, ethnicity
Heterogeneity: knowledge, skills, abilities
Titles and skills represented
Incentives/perks

Figure 13.1 Example of an Evolving Concept Map Created in the Nursing Administration Masters Program.

To supplement the PBL discussion, content experts presented a 90 minute "resource lecture" on the topic of strategic leadership, and the chief nurse's role on top management teams. Nursing administration faculty presented two one-hour skill labs focused on three issues: (1) conducting an organizational assessment and SWOT (strengths, weaknesses, opportunities, threats) analysis; (2) developing the plan and time lines for seeking Magnet Nursing Services Recognition from American Nurses Credentialing Center (ANCC); and (3) planning meeting agendas to communicate new goals and vision to TMT-peers and nurse followers.

This case was designed to structure nursing administration knowledge in a real-life context, motivate students' self-directed learning about Magnet Hospitals, encourage teamwork, and increase students' critical thinking skills. At the end of the fourth scenario, the PBL case objectives are distributed, learning is synthesized, and the process is assessed. Each PBL case is evaluated as part of the formative and summative evaluation plan. A web-based case evaluation format is being used to assess knowledge acquisition, communication skills, responsibility and respect, and self-awareness (Chaves, Chaves, and Lantz, 1998). Future evaluation plans include developing a critical thinking assessment.

In summary, problem-based learning is being used in at least 23 nursing masters programs in eight countries around the world. The literature suggests that programs are in various stages of maturation in relation to program development and evaluation. The range seems to be from some nursing schools, like Maastricht and Newcastle, where PBL has been adopted as a curriculum model for the entire institution, to other nursing schools using PBL in one or two masters courses. The literature is comprised almost entirely of case studies, with little indication of future projections for PBL expansion. Implementation issues are considerably different depending on the school's philosophy and stage of maturation. For example, launching PBL in one or two courses could be more difficult than launching an entire PBL program because a few course-based faculty are challenging the prevailing norms of a larger faculty group. Some of these themes need to be developed in future scholarship.

NURSES IN INTERDISCIPLINARY MASTERS COURSES

A critical step in meeting the interdisciplinary demands of delivering health care worldwide is participation in interdisciplinary education. Interdisciplinary professional practice and research require that health professional students observe and practice collaboration during their education. The "pure" model of PBL requires student-centered, interdisciplinary, small groups analyzing problems in a clinical context (Barrows, 1998). Interdisciplinary PBL promises to prepare students for work in real practice arenas by expanding their knowledge and experience of interaction with other health care students and faculty. The professional literature yielded 16 examples of nursing masters students participating in interdisciplinary problem-based learning in ten different countries. Table 13.3 shows that PBL is being used in seven public health masters programs in Australia, Brazil (Coelho-Filho, Soares, & do Carma e Sa, 1998), Canada (Batty, 1997), the Netherlands (Parsell and Bligh, 1998), South Africa (Iputo, 1997), and two in the United States, MCP Hahnemann University and the University of New Mexico (Urbina et al, 1997). In the United States PBL is being used in three other Masters programs related to public health: rural health (Slack and McEwen, 1997), allied health (Lary, Lavigne, Muma, and Jones, 1997), and gerontology (Silver et al., 1999). The four Universities offering interdisciplinary masters courses in social or physical sciences are Charles in the Czech Republic (Vrbova, Holmerova, and Hrubantova, 1997), Lingoping in Sweden (Parsell and Bligh, 1998), Bristol in the United Kingdom (Parsell and Bligh, 1998), and Baylor in Texas (Yeoman, Sebastian, and Richards, 1998). Finally, PBL is being used in two courses in women's health: a midwifery course at Queens in Ireland (Sinclair, Brown, and Jones, 1999) and a women's health course at Washington in the United States (Cain, 1993).

Interdisciplinary learning has been advocated by the World Health Organization since 1984 because the team approach is basic to delivering effective primary health care. In the United Kingdom, the Centre for the Advancement of Inter-professional Learning reports that the majority of interdisciplinary programs occurs at the graduate level (Parsell and Bligh, 1998). Similar professional organizations have begun in other European countries and offer faculty development programs, especially for faculty using PBL in interprofessional learning.

The aptitude of nursing faculty to adopt tutor roles in interdisciplinary PBL could be strengthened by seeking consultation and collaboration with health professional colleagues who are implementing PBL in education programs and clinical practicums. Nursing faculty who prepare nurses to practice effectively in "managed care" environments can seek help from colleagues in several medical schools where PBL cases are being used to prepare faculty tutors and to introduce students to managed care practices and principles (Phillips, Lee, Berman, and Madoff, 1997). There is scant literature on interdisciplinary PBL and faculty issues.

ASSESSING PROBLEM-BASED LEARNING OUTCOMES

Research on outcomes of PBL probably exceeds the assessment of any other instructional method and underlying philosophy. Medicine leads the other disciplines with well over 200 English language articles reporting evaluation

Table 13.3 *Universities Using PBL in Interdisciplinary Masters Courses by Country and Major*

Country	Allied Health	Gerontology	Public Health	Rural Health	Social/Physical Sciences	Women's Health
			Major			
Australia			Adelaide			
Brazil			Ceara			
Canada			Toronto			
Czech Republic					Charles	
Ireland						Queens
Netherlands			Maastricht			
Sweden					Linkoping	
South Africa			Transkei			
United Kingdom					Bristol	
United States	Wichita State	George Washington	Hahnemann New Mexico	Arizona	Baylor	Washington

research (Albanese and Mitchell, 1993; Vernon and Blake, 1993). A summary of the experimental evidence on the psychological basis of some of the PBL outcomes concludes that problem-based curricula may enhance transfer of concepts to new problems and clinical application, foster increased retention of knowledge, increase intrinsic interest in the subject, and strengthen self-directed learning skills (Norman and Schmidt, 1992). Synthesizing educational outcomes research in the health care disciplines is extremely difficult because of different definitions of PBL (Barrows, 1998), various forms of implementation—entire curriculum to single course units, a wide range of study designs/case studies to experimental designs, and multiple outcome criteria/standardized achievement tests to diaries and journals. (For a more extensive review of the literature on PBL outcomes, see Chapter 2.)

Most of the published evaluation research of PBL in nursing masters programs is qualitative and course-based and focused almost exclusively on student perceptions of the process and outcomes of participating in PBL. For example, one article reports that positive outcomes are achieved, but few data are presented to support the claim that students are more effective team members and have experienced "personal growth" (Slack and McEwen, 1997). The unique challenges and frustrations of using PBL in a traditional curriculum in a master's program in community health nursing are reported by Edwards et al. (1998) who also conclude that both students and tutors report an overall sense of satisfaction. In a demonstration project designed to enhance pediatric nurses' practice with children and families of non-English speaking backgrounds, participants in the master's level program were enthusiastic about the PBL approach but were frustrated with inexperienced tutors, scant library resources, and lack of definitive answers to problems (Blackford and Street, 1999). "Illuminative evaluation" methodology was used for an in-depth analysis of six masters students and the stakeholders in a work-based learning program and the results revealed gaps between PBL philosophy and PBL implementation (Dewar and Walker, 1999). Institutional and scheduling issues are presented as the basis for masters students' lack of enthusiasm about the virtues of PBL at the University of New Mexico's nurse practitioner and midwifery programs (Urbina et al., 1997).

In a quantitative pilot study, which compared student responses before and after completing two masters courses at the University of Hawaii, all students reported heightened interest in PBL, and increased critical thinking skills were noted among those students who scored the lowest prior to beginning the course (Inouye and Flannelly, 1998). A comparison study of 15 nurse practitioner students in PBL sessions and 13 nurse practitioner students in traditional lectures revealed that the PBL students scored higher in critical thinking and problem-solving skills (Khoiny, 1995). A combination of qualitative and quantitative measures are being tested in Kentucky's community health nursing masters program. Thus far, both formative and summative evaluation have been positive in a series of masters courses in community health nursing (King et al., 1997).

More evaluation studies are expected as PBL becomes more widespread in nursing masters programs. Besides students' outcomes, attention should be directed to issues related to the faculty and the institution. Assessing PBL outcomes is challenging because standardized elements often do not exist that can be replicated, measured, and compared. Educators in the health professions are challenged to prepare a different kind of graduate for the uncertainties of the twenty-first century, and PBL holds such promise even though the evaluation methods need refinement (Bruhn, 1997).

FUTURE OF PBL AND TECHNOLOGY IN GRADUATE NURSING EDUCATION

Educators in the health professions are challenged to design student learning opportunities related to computer technologies and information science. Health professionals are facing escalating information management challenges in clinical practice as computer technology permeates all aspects of patient care (Ball, Hannah, Newbold, and Douglas, 2000). Professional organizations and accrediting bodies have issued statements regarding preparation of contemporary nurses in computer technology [International Medical Informatics Association (IMIA), 1999; American Association of Colleges of Nursing (AACN), 1999]. Specifically, nurses must be able to use the information systems operating in their places of employment. Employers assume nurses' ability to use computer technology and electronic networks for communication with other professionals. Nurses should be able to search, retrieve, and organize information from a variety of computerized information sources. Nurses need to be able to seek information for decision making through expert systems and knowledge databases in patient care. The professional literature has many case studies of schools of nursing redesigning the curriculum to include more instruction in computer technology and information science (Chapter 5; Travis and Brennan, 1998).

Extraordinary gains in communication and information technology are influencing faculty's philosophy of teaching and learning, program delivery practices, and students' expectations (Diekelmann, Schuster, and Nosek, 1998). Both communication technology (electronic mail, listserv, electronic conferencing systems, chat rooms, coffee houses) and information technology (World Wide Web, search engines, online journals, web-based courses) are being used to deliver academic courses. Comprehensive efforts to assess the outcomes of web-based courses is underway and focuses on the interaction of the technology, educational practices, faculty support, and learner support (Billings, 2000), and some of that research is presented in Chapter 14.

Computer technology can be used in every step of the PBL process. In fact, business faculty at Ohio University in the United States offer the entire Masters of Business Administration (MBA) online using PBL and computer technology (Stinson and Milter, 1996). When the problem scenario is presented online, students are able to glean initial information from a computer-based case (Bresnitz, 1996). The students' self-directed study includes using the World Wide Web to access data about learning issues from professional organizations, governmental agencies, libraries, and other stakeholders involved in the learning issue topic. Students present their synthesized data reports through online electronic communication and the other students in the course critique the computer entries, determine whether or not their PBL hypotheses have been supported, and may reframe the learning issue. Concept mapping can be launched on the Internet by differentiating definitions, linking key characteristics, and applying information to hypothesis testing. Students can initiate their own learning synthesis in their computer entries with each other and faculty can stimulate the process by posing metacognitive questions on the computer. Web-based evaluation tools are being applied to all stakeholders in a PBL case: individual student, student peers, and tutors (Chaves, Chaves, and Lantz, 1998). Efforts are underway at Indiana University to assess students' critical thinking behaviors in their web-based discourse. Course evaluations are also conducted on the computer.

Computer technology is being applied to generate PBL cases and simulations, develop electronic study guides, create computer-based (virtual) student groups, and implement evaluation procedures. Curriculum development and management is being enhanced with specially designed computer tools (Field and Sefton, 1998). Computer simulations are being used as a research tool to document how students learn (Rendas, Pinto, and Gamboa, 1999).

Thus, there is considerable evidence that PBL is compatible with communication and information technology. A potential next step for nursing faculty is to create partnerships among schools of nursing and design on-line masters programs using PBL.

CONCLUSION

The knowledge explosion, technological advances, economic changes, and demographic shifts have increased the demand for advanced practice nurses who can critically analyze new information and engage in clinical reasoning within an interdisciplinary health care context. PBL is presented as an appropriate humanistic and caring pedagogy for an environment in great transition. The worldwide diffusion of PBL in nursing masters programs has been phenomenal; nine different nursing specialities are being offered in 16 different universities in eight countries. The learner-centered nature of PBL creates unique opportunities for nursing faculty to model interdisciplinary collaboration. The literature also presents nursing masters students in 16 universities located in ten countries as participating in interdisciplinary PBL courses. Contemporary research provides evidence that PBL can strengthen clinical reasoning, motivate learning, encourage teamwork and peer review, and enhance lifelong learning. The increased use of educational technology heightens the urgency to use PBL to design masters programs for distance learning.

REFERENCES

Alavi, C. (1995) *Problem-based Learning in a Health Sciences Curriculum.* London: Routledge.

Albanese, M. A. and Mitchell, S. (1993). Problem-based learning: A review of literature on its outcomes and implementation issues. *Academic Medicine, 68,* 52–81.

American Association of Colleges of Nursing. (1999). Position Statement: A vision of baccalaureate and graduate nursing education: The next decade. *Journal of Professional Nursing, 15,* 59–65.

Baker, C. M. (2000a). Using problem-based learning to redesign nursing administration masters programs. *Journal of Nursing Administration, 30*(1), 41–47.

Baker, C. M. (2000b). Problem-based learning for nursing: Integrating lessons from other disciplines with nursing experiences. *Journal of Professional Nursing, 16*(5), in press.

Ball, M. J., Hannah, K. J., Newbold, S. K., and Douglas, J. V. (Eds). (2000). *Nursing Informatics: Where Caring and Technology Meet.* New York: Springer-Verlag.

Barrows, H. S. (1998). The essentials of problem-based learning. *Journal of Dental Education, 62,* 630–633.

Batty, H. P. (1997). A multidisciplinary experiential course instructional methodology for academic clinicians. *Academic Medicine, 72*(5), 463–464.

Bellack, J. P. and O'Neil, E. H. (2000). Recreating nursing practice for a new century. *Nursing and Health Care Perspectives. 21*(1), 14–21.

Billings, D. M. (2000). A framework for assessing outcomes and practices in web-based courses in nursing. *Journal of Nursing Education, 39* (2), 60–67.

Bitzer, E. M. (1997). Programme evaluation in problem-based and community-based nursing education. *Curationis, 20*(1), 8–10.

Blackford, J. and Street, A. (1999). Problem-based learning: An educational strategy to support nurses working in a multicultural community. *Nurse Education Today, 19,* 364–372.

Bonk, C. J. and King, K. S. (Eds.) (1998). *Electronic Collaborators: Learner-centered Technologies for Literacy, Apprenticeship, and Discourse.* Mahwah, NJ: Lawrence Erlbaum.

Bresnitz, E. A. (1996). Computer-based learning in PBL. *Academic Medicine, 71*(5), 540.

Bruhn, J. G. (1997). Outcomes of problem-based learning in health care professional education: A critique. *Family and Community Health. 20,* 66–74.

Cain, J. M. (1993). Undergraduate and graduate education in women's health: Reconsidering faculty, setting, and content. *Women's Health Issues, 3*(2), 104–109.

Canadian Association of University Schools of Nursing. (1998). CAUSN Position Statements on Education. http://www.causn.org.

Chaves, J. F., Chaves, J. A., and Lantz, M. S. (1998). The PBL-Evaluator: A web-based tool for assessment in tutorials. *Journal of Dental Education, 62,* 671–674.

Coelho-Filho, J. M., Soares, S. M., and do Carma e Sa, H. L. (1998). Problem-based learning: Application and possibilities in Brazil. *Revista Paulista de Medicina, 116*(4), 1784–1785.

Creedy, D. and Hand, B. (1994). The implementation of problem-based learning: Changing pedagogy in nursing education. *Journal of Advanced Nursing, 20*(4), 692–702.

Creedy, D., Horsfall, J., and Hand, B. (1992). Problem-based learning in nursing education: An Australian view. *Journal of Advanced Nursing, 17,* 727–733.

Daly, B. J., Shaw, C. R., Balistrieri, T., Glasenapp, K., and Piacentine, L. (1999). Concept maps: A strategy to teach and evaluate critical thinking. *Journal of Nursing Education, 38*(1), 42–47.

Dana, N. (1997). Preparing educators for problem-based and community-based curricula: A student's experiences. *Curationis: South Africa Journal of Nursing, 20,* 41–43.

Department of Education, Employment and Training. (1994). *National Review of Nurse Education in the Higher Education Sector.* Canberra, Australia.

Dewar, B. J. and Walker, E. (1999). Experiential learning: Issues for supervision. *Journal of Advanced Nursing, 30*(6), 1459–1467.

Diekelmann, N., Schuster, R., and Nosek, C. (1998). Creating new pedagogies at the millenium: The common experiences of the University of Wisconsin-Madison teachers using distance education technologies. *Teaching with Technology Today* (Online journal). <http://www.uwsa.edu/olit/ttt/98.pdf>

Drummond-Young, M. (1998). Educating educators in problem-based learning. *The Canadian Nurse.* 47–48.

Edmondson, K. M., (1994). Concept maps and the development of cases for problem-based learning. *Academic Medicine, 69*(2), 108–110.

Edwards, N. C., Hebert, D., Moyer, A., Peterson, J., Sims-Jones, N., and Verhovsek, H. (1998). Problem-based learning: Preparing post-RN students for community-based care. *Journal of Nursing Education, 37,* 139–141.

Fairbanks, J. and Candelaria, J. (1998). *Case Studies in Community Health.* Thousand Oaks, CA: Sage.

Field, M. J. and Sefton, A. J. (1998). Computer-based management of content in planning a problem-based medical curriculum. *Medical Education, 32,* 163–171.

International Medical Informatics Association. (October, 1999). IMIA Recommendations on Education in Health and Medical Informatics. http://www.imia.org/wg1

Inouye, J. and Flannelly, L. (1998). Inquiry-based learning as a teaching strategy for critical thinking. *Clinical Nurse Specialist, 12*(2), 67–72.

Iputo, J. E. (1997). Does problem-based learning have a future in South Africa? *Medical Education Online.* <http://www.utmb.edu/meo/>

King, M. G., Sebastian, J. G., Stanhope, M. K., and Hickman, M. J. (1997). Using problem-based learning to prepare advanced practice community health nurses for the 21st century. *Family and Community Health, 20,* 29–39.

Khoiny, F. E. (1995). *The effectiveness of problem-based learning in nurse practitioner education.* Unpublished doctoral dissertation. University of Southern California, Los Angeles, CA.

Lary, M. J., Lavigne, S. E., Muma, R. D., and Jones, S. E. (1997). Breaking down barriers: Multidisciplinary education model. *Journal of Allied Health, 26*(2), 63–69.

National League for Nursing. (1992). Criteria and guidelines for the evaluation of baccalaureate and higher degree programs in nursing. New York: *NLN Publications* no. 15-2474.

Norman, G. R. and Schmidt, H. G. (1992). The psychological basis of problem-based learning: A review of the evidence. *Academic Medicine, 67,* 557–565.

Parsell G. and Bligh, J. (1998). Interprofessional learning. *Postgraduate Medical Journal, 74,* 89–95.

Pesut, D. J. and Herman, J. (1999). *Clinical Reasoning: The Art and Science of Critical and Creative Thinking.* Albany, NY: Delmar.

Phillips, R. R., Lee, M. Y., Berman, H. A., and Madoff, M. A. (1997). The Tufts Partnership for managed care education. *Academic Medicine, 72,* 347–356.

Rendas, A., Rosado Pinto, P., and Gamboa, T. (1999). A computer simulation designed for problem-based learning. *Medical Education, 33,* 47–54.

Roberts, S. J. and Chandler, G. (1996). Empowerment of graduate students: A dialogue toward change. *Journal of Professional Nursing, 12*(4), 233–239.

Savin-Baden, M. (1997). Problem-based learning, Part 2: Understanding learners stances. *British Journal of Occupational Therapy, 60*(12), 531–535.

Sebastian, J. G. and Stanhope, M. (1999). *Case Studies in Community Health Nursing Practice: A Problem-based Learning Approach.* St. Louis, MO: Mosby.

Silver, S., Turley, C., Smith, C., Laird, J., Majewski, T., Maguire, B., Orndorff, J., Rice, L., and Vowels, R. (1999). Multidisciplinary team dynamics in the production of problem-based learning cases in issues related to older adults. *Journal of Allied Health, 28*(1), 21–24.

Sinclair, M., Brown, G., and Jones, A. (1999). Project-based learning in midwifery education. *Practicing Midwife, 2*(2), 19–22.

Slack, M. K. and McEwen, M. M. (1997). An interdisciplinary problem-based practicum in case management and rural border health. *Family and Community Health, 20,* 40–53.

Stanhope, M. and Sebastian, J. G. (1999). *Instructor's Resource Guide to Accompany Case Studies in Community Health Nursing Practice: A problem-based Learning Approach.* St. Louis, MO: Mosby.

Stinson, J. E. and Milter, R. G. (1996). Problem-based learning in business education: Curriculum design and implementation issues. In L. Wilkerson and W. Gijslaers (Eds.), *New Directions in Teaching and Learning in Higher Education.* San Francisco: Jossey-Bass, 33–42.

Swanson, K. M. (1991). Empirical development of a middle range theory of caring. *Nursing Research, 40*(3), 161–166.

Thomas, B. G., Quant, V. M., and Cooke, P. (1998). The development of a problem-based curriculum in midwifery. *Midwifery, 14*(4), 261–265.

Travis, L. and Brennan, P. F. (1998). Information science for the future: An innovative nursing informatics curriculum. *Journal of Nursing Education, 37*(4), 162–168.

Urbina, C., Hess, D., Andrews, R., Hammond, R., and Hansbarger, C. (1997). Problem-based learning in an interdisciplinary setting. *Family and Community Health, 20,* 16–28.

Vernon, D. T. and Blake, R. L. (1993). Does problem-based learning work? A meta-analysis of evaluative research. *Academic Medicine, 68,* 550–563.

Vrbova, H., Holmerova, I., and Hrubantova, L. (1997). Multiprofessional education in social medicine and clinical ethics. *Shornik Lekarsky, 98*(4), 331–334.

Yeoman, L. C., Sebastian, R. V., and Richards, B. F. (1998). Inclusion of Allied Health students in a problem-based learning course. *Academic Medicine, 73*(5), 607–608.

Using Problem-Based Learning in Distance Education

CHAPTER 14

Otto H. Sanchez-Sweatman

Distance education is a broad term that encompasses a diversity of pedagogical strategies and tools, which have in common a geographical dissociation between students, teachers, and their peers. Although distance education has been used since the early twentieth century, it has received particular attention in the last decade, primarily because of revolutionary and exponential advances in computer-based technologies that have increased access to information and ease of communication. Additionally, the characteristics of learners have changed, from students who formerly relocated to pursue nursing education, with considerable lifestyle and workplace consequences, to adult learners who wish to pursue continuing education during and after their school years, without bringing about radical changes in their professional and personal life settings. This chapter will present a discussion of specific distance education tools, followed by a review of recent applications and evaluations of distance education strategies in nursing and medicine, with particular emphasis on those that encourage the outcomes associated with problem-based learning (PBL) approaches.

DISTANCE EDUCATION MODALITIES

In the past, most distance education tools served the purpose of providing information and thus promoted didactic, teacher-centered education. With new technologies and educational advances, distance education is now promoting creative and critical approaches to concepts as well as student-centered delivery. The "new generation" of distance education is going beyond access and convenience into a focus on the learner (Billings, 1999).

The emphasis has shifted to the use of interactive tools, such as multimedia, clinical databases, and simulated and actual case studies, as well as the always-improving communication tools, including asynchronous and synchronous group communication. It must be remembered that all of these contribute to the desired outcomes for nursing education; yet the technology

311

used should not distract from the educational goals, so that the tools do not become time-consuming and overwhelming technical challenges. Instead, the tools must be reliable and relatively simple to use.

There are three generations of distance education technology, namely, and in chronological order, written and recorded materials, telecommunications (or audio and video teleconferencing), and computers and Internet-based tools, and these are all still used in various modalities (Garrison, 1985).

Written and Recorded Materials

This modality was the first to be adopted for distance education, with its use first reported in the early 1900s. Although correspondence courses employing both printed material and audio recordings mark the origin of distance education, this format is not ideally suited for the learning process and outcomes of PBL since it does not allow quick interactions that facilitate discussion of concepts, cases, or clinical situations.

Telecommunications: Audio and Video Teleconferencing

Audio conferencing requires voice- or touch-activated multidirectional microphones to facilitate nondisruptive communication (Edwards, Hugo, Cragg, and Peterson, 1999). A significant disadvantage of audio conferencing is the lack of visual cues, which may be compensated by video conferencing, a more costly and technically challenging endeavor (Chandler and Hanrahan, 2000). Interactive television is purported to provide the closest resemblance to the traditional classroom (Fetzer, 2000), since it allows two-way video and audio, (i.e., real-time communication). Desktop videoconferencing has recently been used successfully in a case-based nursing course on women's health where students were linked between the United States and England (Waddell, Tronsgard, Smith, and Smith, 1999). However, there is some evidence that, when given a choice, students prefer the teaching effectiveness provided by traditional classroom sessions over videoconferencing (Fetzer, 2000; Yucha and Princen, 2000). Audio and audiovisual conferencing are also technically complex since they require the availability of expensive equipment, and depend on the availability, reliability, and integrity of telephone communication systems and Internet networks.

Computers: Internet-Based Tools

These modalities, roughly classified as information technology (IT) tools, are undergoing continuous development and improvement, and access to up-to-date communication and computer technology is expanding exponentially. As a result, students and faculty members are becoming increasingly comfortable with the technology and its use.

Course Web Pages

This is the first step in the development of an online support for a course, since a web page will display the Internet-based tools to be used in an online course. Web-page design is easily achieved by careful planning of the elements and hyperlinks to be embedded into the homepage, which is the opening entry page to the course website. A web page can be used as the primary tool to deliver "web-based" courses or as an accessory tool for "web-enhanced" courses. A unique advantage of course web pages is that, since they are posted on the World Wide Web (WWW), they have the potential to provide global access to the course materials. In nursing, this has encouraged the development of international and multi-institutional course and educational programs (Kirkpatrick, Brown, and Atkins, 1998; Kirkpatrick and Brown, 1999). Also, hypertext can be used, which is defined as a nonlinear and multidimensional format in which words are linked by associations and displayed as hyperlinks in web pages (Tripp and Roby, 1990). This allows students to perform more individualized information retrieval, given that this information structure permits access to different information sources (Gillham, 1998).

In terms of content, course websites can include pre-course materials in the form of modules or interactive self-assessment questionnaires, that will allow the students to test their prior knowledge required for the course, as well as pointing out to them the areas requiring review. This application of web-based courses is particularly congruent with PBL. Elements of a web page can be divided into information tools, pointing to resources and course materials, and communication tools, such as person-to-person electronic mail, asynchronous computer conferencing sites, and synchronous online tools.

One challenge in the use of the Internet is the wealth of information available. Students can easily be overwhelmed or use unreliable sources of information. In this sense it is very important that course faculty and students learn to evaluate the quality of the content provided on websites in order to become selective. This is accomplished by creating guided virtual learning modules, identifying specific search strategies, and providing interactive games that will lead the learners into preselected useful and valid resources (McGonigle and Mastrian, 1998). It is also useful to provide criteria students can use to critique various sites and the information provided (Jadad and Gagliardi, 1998; Kim, Eng, Deering, and Maxfield, 1999).

Person-to-Person Electronic Mail (E-mail)

E-mail is used as a dominant means of communication and as a tool for case study discussion that may be individualized for task development on a one-to-one basis between a student and a tutor (Todd, 1998). This is the most effective tool to deliver fast feedback. However, it is time-consuming, and faculty need to take care to negotiate ground rules with students about when e-mails will be answered and in what format. Ideally, responses should be prioritized, and any e-mail discussions that can benefit more than one student should be posted into other course tools for access to all students. Obviously, this must be done after an informal agreement between the student and faculty member to make it public.

Asynchronous Computer Conferencing

Asynchronous Computer Conferencing includes e-mail listservers, working as group electronic mail, and discussion or online newsgroups or web-boards, allowing group messages to be posted for student and faculty access at any time. These tools provide a high degree of time flexibility for posting messages, and they are being recognized increasingly as one of the most important discussion methodologies on Internet-based distance education. One advantage of newsgroups over listservers, is that the former stay posted on the server for retrospective reading and follow-up. Additionally, newsgroups provide a discussion forum absent in a lecture-based course. Students may use asynchronous computer conferencing as a way of interacting and exchanging ideas and information, which is not achievable in more traditional course settings. Also, messages and their replies may be "threaded" to each other, so that any observer can follow the discussion on one particular topic. This is particularly useful for discussions of PBL problems, since it encourages students to contribute and build upon other comments, rather than providing isolated contributions. The messages in this tool are better documented and more planned, as compared with synchronous discussion methods. Additionally, the fact that they are performed online allows the students to actually hyperlink to useful World Wide Web resources. The role of the faculty member in this instance is to verify the resources posted as to their quality and usefulness, quickly dismissing any source that might be confusing to the students. As in face-to-face tutorial sessions, other roles of faculty include facilitating discussions and monitoring group process.

Asynchronous computer conferencing was used recently in a successful international case-based course for nursing graduate students (Iwasiw et al., 2000), in which this methodology was effective in allowing international discussion of case studies at the graduate level, and within the context of a course for credit.

Synchronous Online Tutorials

Such tutorials, better known as "chat sessions," closely replicate real-time interactions in a PBL tutorial. These sessions are better performed in a text-only basis, which distinguishes them from "netMeeting" formats, in which audiovisual, live, online connections are used. The text-only format substantially decreases technical difficulties, since it does not require broad bandwidth connection networks. The tutorial sessions are scheduled and may be used to discuss problems with formats very similar to the traditional PBL approach. Synchronous online tutorials provide effective means of eliminating the feeling of isolation felt by students taking distance-based courses, in that they allow students to interact directly and in real-time with their peers and the faculty member.

Compact Disks

The technology of compact disks provides the unique advantage of a high capacity for data storage, which allows access to software containing multimedia tools, such as text, audiovisual, and graphics that cannot be stored and effectively delivered using Internet-based tools. For these reasons, compact disks are the main instrument used to provide interactive multimedia learning modules. In this context, multimedia is enriched by the use of digitized images and videos, together with audio tools, delivered in an interactive bidirectional fashion. The major drawbacks of this technology involve their development and upgrading. These two essential activities in multimedia technology require a creative, well-planned, and interdisciplinary team effort that involves faculty time as well as substantial financial commitments (Ribbons, 1998a). Their main advantage is their interactivity, which promotes active learning and allows students to be engaged with the course material. In this sense, compact disk technology allows access to large amounts of information. They also can be used to provide exposure to interactive graphics, games, and simulated classes or clinical settings.

COMFORT OF STUDENTS AND FACULTY WITH COMPUTER USE

Certainly as the discussion above indicates, the focus in distance education has shifted to the wide and ever-increasing range of computer-based applications. Lifelong learning is viewed as a pivotal outcome in nursing curricula, and college and university programs have identified the need for students both on-campus and off-campus, to develop the skills that will transform them into lifelong learners. In this context, increasing access to computer technology is providing educators with a unique opportunity to facilitate this goal.

Several recent studies have explored questions related to the use of computer technology in nursing education. To determine the prevalence of the integration of information and computer technology in undergraduate and graduate nursing educational programs, Carty and Rosenfeld (1998) performed the most comprehensive survey of nursing schools thus far. Their study, which included 190 accredited nursing schools in the United States, found that by 1996 the majority of faculty members and students had access to computer-based resources, including local and Internet-based networks, as well as to library databases such as CINAHL and MEDLINE. However, less than one-third of the schools surveyed had incorporated informatics into the curriculum or into specific courses.

Familiarity with computer technology and skills was evaluated by Sinclair and Gardner (1999) in cohorts of students who entered nursing programs in the United Kingdom during 1997 and 1998. Most students had prior training in computers and, although the levels of perceived competence were relatively homogeneous, knowledge and confidence in the use of computers were not. For this reason, the authors recommended that nursing programs should support a consistent training approach for all entrants. In another recent study, Bachman and Panzarine (1998) evaluated a course designed to increase Internet use by nursing students. Students who took the course made increased use of e-mail and "chat groups" to communicate with peers compared to a control group. Furthermore, students who completed the course also increased their computer knowledge and skills significantly, and improved their use of the Internet for health information, when compared to the control group. Moreover, a recent cross-sectional survey of nursing faculty members in baccalaureate programs in the New England region of the United States found that teachers with high computer literacy skills were more likely to integrate them into the curriculum and their teaching practices (Austin, 1999). These findings suggest that, although computer technology is available within nursing educational programs, its implementation continues to be approached with some caution. The need for specific programs to increase the knowledge and skills of students and faculty in the use of information technology is also a consistent finding. Given the stage of development of computer technology use in nursing education generally, to what extent is it used in distance education and with what results?

SATISFACTION AND EFFECTIVENESS WITH USE OF DISTANCE EDUCATION MODALITIES

The level of satisfaction with distance education, and the effectiveness of printed and computer-mediated distance education in nursing and medicine courses have been examined over the last two decades. This analysis has only recently started to include the potential of distance education technologies to support and promote elements inherent in the PBL philosophy, to clarify and improve upon them thereby increasing their sense of mastery within a self-directed learning, information retrieval skills, group communication and group decision making. For this reason, the literature reviewed below has been published in the last decade, as the quality and quantity of research and publication related to the use of newer distance modalities continues to grow rapidly. As well, the studies included all have a problem-based (or case-based) component in the educational intervention being assessed.

Satisfaction with Distance Education Modalities

Ryan, Carlton, and Ali (1999) explored the responses of nursing students enrolled in a graduate program to a variety of instructional modalities. The options included on-campus classes that used group discussions, lectures, student presentations, and videotapes, and off-campus WWW modules which covered about 50 percent of the course content and comprised electronic discussions and quizzes. The participants completed a questionnaire at the end of the course. The nurses rated the classroom-based modules significantly higher than the distance education modules with regards to the content covered, student interaction and participation, and communication skills. By contrast, Edwards et al. (1999) used a pre/post questionnaire to investigate changes in learning preferences, satisfaction with PBL and the ability to problem-solve among 30 nursing students, 9 enrolled in a distance format and 21 on-campus. They found that audio conferences were effective in delivering PBL approaches, as long as the students worked in groups who were together physically, which encouraged active discussion off- and online.

Coulehan, Williams, and Naser (1995) assessed the satisfaction level of second-year medical students who used an electronic-based discussion format to learn about ethical and social issues embedded in a series of case studies. They found high levels of satisfaction among the students, who reported that e-mail provided better opportunities for "quiet, passive and/or nonconfrontational" students to participate. They also noted that the printed and posted electronic messages gave more time for students to organize their information and thoughts, and deliver them in ways that improved their writing skills. When asked if they would participate again in a course using this format, they ranked their experience as 8.8/10 and indicated it was more educational than small group discussion (8.1), lectures (5.1), and formal papers (5.0).

Mooney, Bligh, Leinster, and Warenius. (1995) piloted a PBL oncology module, developed as a hypertext tool, that allowed undergraduate medical students to interactively self-assess their knowledge and clinical reasoning. In this pilot study, the authors assessed the level of satisfaction with the distance format and found students responded very positively to it. They did not evaluate educational outcomes of their approach.

Effectiveness of Distance Education

Studies of the effectiveness of distance education have traditionally compared the educational outcomes of students using distance modalities with those enrolled in courses offered in a regular classroom or tutorial. Reviews of this literature have provided mixed results. There seems to be a general agreement that most studies have not found significant differences in students learning outcomes and fulfilment of course objectives with distance-based course formats, and that these observations appear to be independent of the type of distance education technology used (Billings, 2000). However, it is clear that there are not enough rigorous published studies yet to safely confirm these notions.

For example, in nursing, various studies have addressed the effectiveness of distance education in maintaining and promoting characteristics existent in face-to-face PBL approaches. Yucha and Princen (2000) reported that nursing students taking an Internet-based pathophysiology course did not differ from students taking the course in a traditional classroom in their grades achieved, the time spent on each module, or their attitudes about the module. In a study with a clinical application as the outcome, Madorin and Iwasiw (1999) used a pre/post design to assess the effectiveness of a computer-based questionnaire compared to a computer simulation in changing the level of confidence of second-year baccalaureate nursing students to perform a number of surgical nursing skills. They found a statistically significant increase in the performance of the students who used the computer simulations. These students reported higher levels of confidence and were noted to monitor surgical drains/tubes more frequently. The authors concluded that computer simulations of issues related to the monitoring and care of surgical drains is an effective teaching strategy.

In a study of physicians practicing in rural areas in three African and Asian countries, Engel et al. (1992) analyzed the effectiveness of problem-based printed modules when compared with modules containing conventional structured information. Their study evaluated the use of the clinical problem format, offered through distance education, for improving reasoned decision-making skills. The authors found no differences in outcomes between the two print formats. They interpreted these findings as an endorsement that distance education can be used to promote PBL activities in medical students and physicians who are limited in their ability to travel to pursue continuing education.

Computer-based learning has also been shown to strengthen the information retrieval skills of students, which is a desired outcome of nursing education in general and problem-based approaches in particular. Distance-based student groups have reported a high degree of satisfaction regarding their acquisition of information retrieval skills, as well as their use of online discussion groups, when compared with on-site student groups. Colling and Rogers (1999) recently evaluated the use of Internet resources by undergraduate nursing students using a case-based assignment that asked them to use and evaluate websites relevant to a chosen clinical situation. The authors found that the majority of students and faculty involved considered the assignment beneficial, as they found Internet resources to be useful in providing up-to-date and applicable clinical information.

Faculty Perspectives of Distance Education

From the faculty perspective, there are some issues of concern when using distance education formats in courses traditionally offered on campus, namely, the degree of course redesign needed, and hence the time and effort required to develop the learning tools. These concerns were identified in a recent study by Yucha and Princen (2000), who assessed the effectiveness of a graduate distance-based pathophysiology module. They found that the development of one module with case studies was time-consuming for both the instructor and the technical support personnel. In their study, most of the time was spent searching and evaluating the usefulness of Internet resources to be used by the students, as well as reformatting the course material to Internet suitability. Use of PBL formats would obviate some of this effort and time, since the searching for and selecting of resources is performed mainly by the group of students. Also, the recent availability of word-processing software that allows easy reformatting into Internet-suitable documents may decrease the time and effort required in the near future.

Regarding course redesign, a somewhat prevalent notion is that the use of computer-based distance education tools requires drastic redesign of the course content (Carlton, Ryan, and Siktberg, 1998). In this sense, it is becoming clear that the only major change is in the delivery format of that content and a re-configuration of learning activities (Billings, 1999), that may be enriched by the use of more interactive information and communication tools. This provides the students with a wider range of learning tools, which increases the potential of better adapting to each their individual learning needs.

To summarize, the studies discussed above emphasize the notion that the educational philosophy of student-centeredness must be preserved in distance education modalities. In these, as in any other learning strategy, the priority must be educational and not technocentric. The goal is not to use technology only "because it is there," but to apply it to enrich and comple-ment the learning experience. In this sense, Ribbons (1998b) highlighted that distance education technology, like any other educational strategy, must still encourage the development of critical thinking skills. Distance education tools can be used for this purpose, as they can be delivered in a student-centered fashion by using strategies that facilitate preservation of these prin-ciples, including interactive multimedia and discussion of case studies during real-time synchronous online sessions and/or asynchronous discussion groups. On the other hand, it is important to limit the use of techniques that do not encourage interactive participation such as audio- and videocassettes, which provide information to students, who may or may not remain passive to this information. Problem-based learning can be integrated into distance education modalities, and has proven to be successful in undergraduate and postgraduate nursing students. For instance, Rogerson and Harden (1999) describe a seven-year experience of developing Internet-based courses that use as major tools online clinical scenarios, organized as learning modules, which are followed by clinical and professional challenges to the students, who are subsequently followed up and evaluated with online assessment tools. Other examples of learner-centered distance education formats have been recently reported for community health nursing (Blakeley and Curran-Smith, 1998), nurse practitioner education (Wambach et al., 1999) and nursing doctoral programs (Milstead and Nelson, 1998).

ADVANTAGES, DISADVANTAGES, AND CHALLENGES OF DISTANCE EDUCATION

The implementation of distance education formats in courses and programs can be challenging and include the need for a shift in the attitudes toward the use of distance education tools by students and faculty, which often occurs empirically. Although there are many technologies available, the challenge is to select those that will best facilitate fulfilment of course objectives. In addition, they need to be easy to operate and accessible by all students, avoiding any technological distractions, such as time delays, slow download times, or incompatible file formats or softwares. These issues highlight the importance of faculty and student development, and technical support, when implementation of distance-based course delivery is considered.

Advantages of Distance Education

Perusal of the recent literature identifies general advantages provided by the use of distance education technology with a PBL approach:

- Distance education provides the ability to deal with a wide range of learning needs (Stanton and Grant, 1999), since several distinct tools can be provided to adapt to different learning strategies and needs of students.
- With the use of online asynchronous discussion groups, students can participate in discussions any time and from any place. Thus the Internet-based systems are flexible in terms of study time, pace, and place (Rogerson and Harden, 1999).
- One of the reasons for the recent expansion of distance education is that it increases access to education for students, especially for those who are geographically or personally unable to leave their community. Distance education is meant to serve potential students who would not consider furthering their education if relocation or work-withdrawal was a factor. In this sense, distance education allows these students to remain at their sites, with their families, and still obtain higher education.
- The use of distance education technologies develops computer skills and familiarizes students with communication and information tools that they can later use for professional continuing education. Indeed, the skills developed during distance-based courses, such as intelligent processing of information retrieved from databases, will not only benefit the course outcomes, but will also guarantee that students can use these skills as lifelong learners.
- Distance education strategies encourage online team building and collaboration with peers, since it assures formation of communities of learners for long-term interaction and exchange of information and ideas. An electronic classroom can be designed to support student empowerment whereby students engage in group discussion, reflect, and

rework their ideas within a supportive community of learners (Davie and Wells, 1991).

Disadvantages and Challenges of Distance Education

There are also challenges and disadvantages related to the use of distance education modalities to complement or replace on-site PBL:

- There is a lack of visual and nonverbal cues, which are important in faculty-student and student-student interactions, especially when discussing case studies and complex concepts. They are also important when giving feedback to students, especially to those who are not performing well. In these situations, electronic communication is not sufficient to provide the nonverbal information that is an essential part of communication concerning the problems or concerns of students and faculty.

- As mentioned above, in some studies, students have mentioned that distance education formats, at times, may limit the amount and quality of feedback of their work, progress, and performance by the course instructors (Edwards et al., 1999). In contrast, other studies have argued that e-mail is a rapid and effective way of providing feedback to students (Coulehan et al., 1995).

- Students may feel geographically and academically isolated from their classmates and the educational community. In this regard, Edwards et al. (1999) observed that students who formed small subgroups and studied regularly together performed better than those working in complete isolation.

- Due to the lack of scheduled course activities, students taking distance education courses must have strong time-management skills to cover the course materials by themselves. Consequently, students must be task-oriented and good at work-time scheduling. For a distance-based course, time commitment and expectations are suggested by the course professor, but are just theoretical, and must be applied by the students by themselves.

CONCLUSION

It is clear that distance education is evolving at a rapid pace with the advent of computer-based technologies and increasing access to them by students and teachers. As more systematic research studies evaluate the use of distance education learning tools in nursing education, knowledge gaps regarding the effectiveness of these tools in educational outcomes, interdisciplinary communication, and caring attributes will be clarified (Mallow and Gilje, 1999). In the context of Internet-facilitated nursing courses delivered using problem-based learning, new educational models have recently been proposed. Specifically, Giani and Martone (1998), in an attempt to integrate PBL and Internet-based tools as dynamic knowledge network models, have identified the Internet as a useful repository of structured information, as well as a valuable communication tool in synchronous and asynchronous fashions. Additionally, Billings (2000) has proposed a universal framework for assessing outcomes and teaching/learning practices with computer-based technologies. Among the elements identified in this conceptual framework and that may be assessed both quantitatively and qualitatively, there are many that are common with the PBL evaluation. These include educational outcomes such as: the degree of active learning, critical thinking, and creativity; communication outcomes, including tutor-student feedback, student-student and student-tutor interaction; and technical outcomes such as accessibility, convenience, student satisfaction, faculty and student technical support, familiarity with technology, and financial support. The future of distance education and its use in problem-based education will largely depend on research addressing the pedagogical effectiveness of these modalities. Since the technology for distance education is available now and will continue to improve, it will be up to academics and students to determine if it will be used effectively as a learning tool in the rapidly evolving field of nursing education.

REFERENCES

Austin, S. I. (1999). Baccalaureate nursing faculty performance of nursing computer literacy skills and curriculum integration of these skills through teaching practice. *Journal of Nursing Education, 38,* 260–266.

Bachman, J. A. and Panzarine, S. (1998). Enabling student nurses to use the information superhighway. *Journal of Nursing Education, 37,* 155–161.

Billings, D. M. (1999). The "next generation" distance education: Beyond access and convenience. *Journal of Nursing Education, 38,* 246–247.

Billings, D. M. (2000). A framework for assessing outcomes and practices in web-based courses in nursing. *Journal of Nursing Education, 39,* 60–67.

Blakeley, J. A. and Curran-Smith, J. (1998). Teaching community health nursing by distance methods: Development, process, and evaluation. *Journal of Continuing Education in Nursing, 29,* 148–153.

Carlton, K. H., Ryan, M. E., and Siktberg, L. L. (1998). Designing courses for the Internet. A conceptual approach. *Nurse Educator, 23,* 45–50.

Carty, B. and Rosenfeld, P. (1998). From computer technology to information technology. Findings from a national study of nursing education. *Computers in Nursing, 16,* 259–265.

Chandler, G. E. and Hanrahan, P. (2000). Teaching using interactive video: Creating connections. *Journal of Nursing Education, 39,* 73–80.

Colling, K. B. and Rogers, A. E. (1999). Nursing students "surf" the web: Resources for patient teaching. *Journal of Nursing Education, 38,* 286–288.

Coulehan, J. L., Williams, P. C., and Naser, C. (1995). Using electronic mail for a small-group curriculum in ethical and social issues. *Academic Medicine, 70,* 158–160.

Davie, L. and Wells, R. (1991). Empowering the learner through computer-mediated communication. *American Journal of Distance Education, 5,* 15–23.

Edwards, N., Hugo, K., Cragg, B., and Peterson, J. (1999). The integration of problem-based learning strategies in distance education. *Nurse Educator, 24,* 36–41.

Engel, C. E., Browne, E., Nyarango, P., Akor, S., Khwaja, A., Karim, A. A., and Towle, A. (1992). Problem-based learning in distance education: A first exploration in continuing medical education. *Medical Education, 26,* 389–401.

Fetzer, S. J. (2000). A pilot study to investigate the impact of interactional television on student evaluation of faculty effectiveness. *Journal of Nursing Education, 39,* 91–93.

Garrison, D. R. (1985). Three generations of technological innovations in distance education. *Distance Education, 6,* 235–241.

Giani, U. and Martone, P. (1998). Distance learning, problem based learning and dynamic knowledge networks. *International Journal of Medical Informatics, 50,* 273–278.

Gillham, D. (1998). Using hypertext to facilitate nurse education. *Computers in Nursing, 16,* 95–98.

Iwasiw, C., Andrusyszyn, M.-A., Moen, A., Østbye, T., Davie, L., Støvring, T., and Buckland-Foster, I. (2000). Graduate education in nursing leadership through distance technologies: The Canada-Norway nursing connection. *Journal of Nursing Education, 39,* 81–86.

Jadad, A. R. and Gagliardi, A. (1998). Rating health information on the internet. Navigating to knowledge or to Babel? *Journal of the American Medical Association, 279,* 611–614.

Kim, P., Eng, T. R., Deering, M. J., and Maxfield, A. (1999). Published criteria for evaluating health related web sites: Review. *British Medical Journal, 318,* 647–649.

Kirkpatrick, M. K. and Brown, S. (1999). Efficacy of an international exchange via the Internet. *Journal of Nursing Education, 38,* 278–281.

Kirkpatrick, M. K., Brown, S., and Atkins, T. (1998). Electronic education. Using the Internet to integrate cultural diversity and global awareness. *Nurse Educator, 23,* 15–17.

Madorin, S. and Iwasiw, C. (1999). The effects of computer-assisted instruction on the self-efficacy of baccalaureate nursing students. *Journal of Nursing Education, 38,* 282–285.

Mallow, G. E. and Gilje, F. (1999). Technology-based nursing education: Overview and call for further dialogue. *Journal of Nursing Education, 38,* 248–251.

McGonigle, D. and Mastrian, K. (1998). Learning along the way: Cyberspacial quests. *Nursing Outlook, 46,* 81–86.

Milstead, J. A. and Nelson, R. (1998). Preparation for an online asynchronous university doctoral course. Lessons learned. *Computers in Nursing, 16,* 247–258.

Mooney, G. A., Bligh, J. G., Leinster, S. J., and Warenius, H. M. (1995). An electronic study guide for problem-based learning. *Medical Education, 29,* 397–402.

Ribbons, R. M. (1998a). Guidelines for developing interactive multimedia. Applications in nurse education. *Computers in Nursing, 16,* 109–114.

Ribbons, R. M. (1998b). The use of computers as cognitive tools to facilitate higher order thinking skills in nurse education. *Computers in Nursing, 16,* 223–228.

Rogerson, E. C. B. and Harden, R. M. (1999). Seven years on: Distance learning courses for first level registered nurses and midwives. *Nurse Education Today, 19,* 286–294.

Ryan, M., Carlton, K. H., and Ali, N. S. (1999). Evaluation of traditional classroom teaching methods versus course delivery via the World Wide Web. *Journal of Nursing Education, 38,* 272–277.

Sinclair, M. and Gardner, J. (1999). Planning for information technology key skills in nurse education. *Journal of Advanced Nursing, 30,* 1441–1450.

Stanton, F. and Grant, J. (1999). Approaches to experiential learning, course delivery and validation in medicine. A background document. *Medical Education, 33,* 282–297.

Todd, N. A. (1998). Using e-mail in an undergraduate nursing course to increase critical thinking skills. *Computers in Nursing, 16,* 115–118.

Tripp, S. and Roby, W. (1990). Orientation and disorientation in a hypertext lexicon. *Journal of Computer-Based Instruction, 17,* 120–124.

Waddell, D. L., Tronsgard, B. A., Smith, A., and Smith, G. (1999). An evaluation of international nursing education using interactive desktop video conferencing. *Computers in Nursing, 17,* 186–192.

Wambach, K., Boyle, D., Hagemaster, J., Teel, C., Langner, B., Fazzone, P., Connors, H., Smith, C., and Forbes, S. (1999). Beyond correspondence, video conferencing, and voice mail: Internet-based master's degree courses in nursing. *Journal of Nursing Education, 38,* 267–271.

Yucha, C. and Princen, T. (2000). Insights learned from teaching pathophysiology on the World Wide Web. *Journal of Nursing Education, 39,* 68–72.

Introducing Problem-Based Learning: A Process of Adoption or Adaptation?

Barbara Carpio

T he process of educational change presents unique challenges for students, faculty, and institutions as they participate as stakeholders in curriculum transformation. The demands for change in nursing curricula have escalated in the last decade. It is widely acknowledged that a nursing curriculum should overtly and systematically foster the development of the behaviors and skills that graduates will require to fulfill the societal expectations of health care professionals. A content-focused curricula cannot keep pace as the advances in technology and information continue to dramatically change the skill set needed for professional practice. Educators need to alter the curriculum emphasis to process-oriented learning. This will assist learners to develop the values, knowledge, and skills to be critical thinkers, information managers, and problem solvers, as well as lifelong, self-directed learners who continually base their professional practice on critical appraisal of evidence and collaboration with clients and colleagues. Despite the rapid changes in nursing knowledge and technology, care continues to be the core value of nursing practice (Bevis and Watson, 1989), and a student-centered approach to problem-based learning (PBL) should reflect that value. Introducing the PBL Model represents one method of meeting many of the goals of modern nursing education. However, implementing PBL initiates a change much more profound than merely "problematizing" the curriculum content (Venturelli, 1997); it leads to a reconceptualization of the entire teaching/learning process.

Educational change to incorporate PBL calls for a re-examination of the underlying assumptions about the learners and the learning process held by the faculty and the institution, in order to incorporate small group, student-centered, self-directed approaches. Curriculum content must incorporate larger population-based issues, such as the economic, social, cultural, and environmental influences on health, as well as patient care issues of a biomedical and psychosocial nature. Students must be prepared to address the effects of these factors on the health of individuals and populations, and also know how to critique and develop policy for social change. These responsibilities are consistent with the broader scope and definition of practice for nursing in the new millennium (WHO, 1994).

A CONCEPTUAL MODEL FOR STUDENT-CENTERED CURRICULUM DESIGN

Figure 15.1 illustrates a conceptual model intended to assist planners in developing a problem-based nursing curricula. The overarching outcome of nursing education today is to prepare collaborative and reflective practitioners who are lifelong learners and critical thinkers. Nursing graduates must be prepared to meet professional and societal expectations, by demonstrating professional accountability to their clients (individuals, families, groups, and communities) and colleagues for the provision of competency-based and evidence-based practice. Working and learning in small groups provides students with the opportunity, from the beginning of their professional studies, to develop the skills needed for collaborative professional practice with clients and other health care team members.

As the model illustrates, the *learner is at the center* of the educational process of the PBL Model. There is considerable literature about the selection of students who will be successful in PBL curricula. Some authors have addressed the selection methods (Brown, Carpio, and Roberts, 1991; Carpio and Brown, 1993) and the criteria predictive of success (Carpio, O'Mara, and Hezekiah, 1996) in a PBL program. Others have investigated the characteristics of learners that are believed to be important to success such as an awareness and understanding by students of their own learning styles (Carpio et al., 1999) and readiness for self-directed learning (Crook,

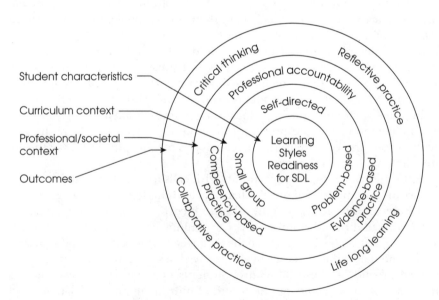

Figure 15.1 A Conceptual Model for Student-Centered Curriculum Design
©1999 B. Carpio and E. Rideout.

1985; Knowles, 1975, 1986; Lunyk-Child et al., 2000). Whether students are to be preselected based on demonstrated readiness for PBL, or will be assisted to develop this ability, the curriculum needs to overtly assist students to develop their skills in this area.

Central to the student-centered, self-directed approach is the gradual and incremental assumption by students of the responsibility for identifying personal learning needs, resources, and strategies. Clinical practice settings must also enact and reinforce shared learning if these skills are to be valued and applied to professional practice upon graduation (Doring, Bramwell-Vial, and Bingham, 1994; Laschinger, 1986, 1992). Inherent in the PBL Model is the need for congruency between classroom learning and professional practice, and clinical role models are key to this process. Although many educational programs purport to encourage collaborative learning in the classroom, there has been some evidence that students in more traditional programs actually become less collaborative over the course of their undergraduate studies, particularly if the observed professional practice model is not consistent with a collaborative team approach to health care (Montecinos, Illesca, & Yañez, 1993). Educators therefore need to be actively involved with learners in clinical practice settings in order to reinforce the link between undergraduate education and professional practice.

DEVELOPING A PBL CURRICULUM AS A PROCESS OF EDUCATIONAL CHANGE

While some nurse educators have the opportunity and challenge of designing new educational programs as wholly integrated PBL curricula, others will undertake a process of curriculum revision and adaptation of the PBL Model into pre-existing programs of study. Whichever the case, change is required and the process of educational change must be initiated.

Fullan (1982) has described educational change as a process that has three phases: initiation, implementation, and continuation. He also describes what might be called the three tasks of change, which represent the product: alteration of beliefs, the use of new teaching approaches, and change or revision of instructional materials. Meaningful and sustainable change requires commitment and innovation to develop the product of change, the new curriculum.

Phase One: The Initiation of Change

The first step in educational change is variously referred to as the initiation, mobilization, or adoption of change, and it refers of the process required to adopt and proceed with change (Fullan, 1982). Several factors have been identified as critical to this step. The first is an awareness of a need for change. The widespread call for reform in nursing education, and the belief that it is not possible to teach and learn all the rapidly expanding content, has made PBL an appealing option for many programs. Concurrently, the prevailing belief has developed that the focus in education should be placed not primarily on content, but on the process of learning and the development of independent learners. Although there is a continuing debate about the method (e.g., Colliver, 2000), the PBL Model has advocates worldwide and, as more and more educators attend conferences, read the literature, and encounter graduates of PBL programs, the stimulus for change continues. Taking stock is a part of this initial step in the change process. This should include acknowledging the strengths and assets of faculty as well as the positive aspects of the present curriculum that should be preserved.

Stakeholders in the Change Process

Advocacy, not merely endorsement, from central administrators is required if the change process is to advance. Although it may be possible to implement PBL within one course within a curriculum, full-scale initiation of a different educational philosophy is not possible without administrative support. Another essential factor is a belief in the change by faculty who will be expected to implement and sustain the innovations. It is faculty members who can provide the pressure and ongoing support required to make change happen. Whether external consultants and change agents, or internal resources are entrusted with the task of managing the process, the commitment of a few key individuals who are viewed positively by other faculty is required for success. As with any change process rewards and incentives are helpful to overcome resistance to change. The degree to which faculty feel involved and supported through the process is influenced by feeling a sense of ownership of the process, which Fullan (1982) calls bureaucratic incentives for innovation impact.

Any change in nursing education will impact on the other systems with which nurses interact, and therefore, the support of professional bodies and the health care community where the program is located will also be needed. Nursing must be accountable to *institutional, provincial,* and *national legislation and policies* governing both education and professional practice, so their support is ultimately needed. For example, keeping in mind the outcomes and competencies dictated by state, provincial, and federal nursing bodies will ensure that accreditation standards are met after the change is in place.

Whichever educational model is adopted, effective communication among the various stakeholders—administrators, faculty, students, community members, and accrediting bodies—is imperative so they all have ongoing access to information about the change process as well as the specific tasks being undertaken. As people work toward change at the individual, group, and faculty level, all the stakeholders should be consulted and informed about curriculum developments.

Helping Change Happen

Taking active steps to initiate change always involves considerable risk. Whether a program chooses a pattern of incremental change in some or all courses, or designs a new and fully integrated PBL curriculum, educational change will require personal energy, resources, clear vision, and commitment, as well as clear understanding of the internal and external forces that are impacting the proposed changes. The key activities of this beginning stage are: linking the educational need for change with the political agenda; developing a clear model and delegating tasks; and identifying advocate(s) who can secure the needed resources and people. It is important to develop a critical mass of faculty who have the actual "lived experience" of being exposed to PBL. Exposure to PBL in an environment that has an established PBL curriculum provides a meaningful introduction to the philosophy as well as the enactment of a new way of learning and teaching. Workshops offered at a number of institutions where PBL is well-established provide the kind of experience required to assess the approach and determine its applicability to individual settings (e.g., McMaster University in Canada; Samford University and the University of Southern Illinois in the USA; the University of Maastricht in Holland; Newcastle University and Griffith University in Australia).

Although the availability of internal and external funds is undeniably an essential consideration when change is contemplated, a lack of resources is often cited as a major barrier to change efforts. Nevertheless, some studies of educational change have found that "cost was inversely related to quality [of innovation]" (Nelson and Sieber, as cited in Fullan, 1982, p. 51), suggesting that change that is otherwise viewed positively should not be deterred because of issues of funding. The potential costs of a PBL curriculum, compared to a more conventional one that uses large group classes and lectures, is a common concern that has been explored in various medical curricula. Mennin and Martinez-Burrola (1986) investigated the faculty costs related to the change to PBL in the medical program at the University of New Mexico, and concluded that total teaching time is not increased in PBL compared to a traditional program, since faculty teach differently but not more. Nieuwenhuijzen Kruseman, Kolle, and Scherpbier (1997) found more teaching staff were required in the PBL program at Maastricht University compared to other Dutch medical programs that used traditional teaching methods. The additional time was needed to participate in nonteaching activities that support the PBL Model, such as student guidance, program evaluation, and faculty development. However, they also concluded that PBL is cost-effective since the PBL students completed their programs more quickly than their peers in traditional programs. In a study conducted at

Newcastle University in Australia, Sefton (1997) found the demands on faculty for scheduled teaching were no greater than in a traditional curriculum, when preparation time for lectures was factored in and when there were ten students in each PBL group. It seems in conclusion that cost may not be the main deterrent to a change to small group PBL.

At the same time it is acknowledged by Mennin and Martinez-Burrola (1986) and Sefton (1997) that there are considerable start-up costs of curricular change, including the re-examination of values and attitudes, design of a new curricular model, creation of curricular materials, and faculty development. Such requirements offer an excellent reason to seek external funding in support of innovation. For example, Samford University in Alabama has developed a center to support the implementation of PBL within all their undergraduate programs which is supported by the Pew Charitable Trusts (Major, 2000).

This phase of initiation has many components, but it is a crucial time in the change process as numerous issues must be addressed to assist faculty and administration in reaching a decision to proceed. As Sefton (1997) states: "From our experience of a large research university, if the dean, faculty leaders and a critical mass of the staff recognize the need for reform, are involved in the process, and support the goals and proposed strategies, difficulties are readily overcome and limited resources do not deter creativity" (p. 173).

Phase Two: The Implementation of Change

Putting plans into action requires renewed and continuing commitment to the desired change. The degree to which true curriculum innovation is possible depends on the degree to which the institution is committed to change, and prepared to support both the outcomes and process of the transition. Regardless of how creative or forwarding thinking change may be, innovation "cannot be assimilated unless its meaning is shared" (Marris, cited in Fullan, 1982). Successful innovation relies on all stakeholders (students, faculty, and community) identifying the need for change and reaching consensus on the nature of that change.

While it is important to have champions of the change, it is imperative that, from the beginning, the process have broad support from the administration and institution. Fullan (1982) warns that "pressure without support" leads to alienation; and that "support without pressure" wastes resources (p. 37). The energy and investment required for implementation is at least as intensive as that expended during the initiation phase.

The institutional as well as personal history of innovative attempts need to be considered. Both faculty and students will be more embracing of educational change if they have had positive experiences in the past. A useful exercise when embarking on curriculum change is to revisit past change to identify strengths as well as pitfalls to avoid. Administrative support and involvement, particularly by the dean/director is also key. To the extent that students and faculty *perceive* that administration is confident positive outcomes will be achieved, they will feel safe in taking the risks involved in making fundamental changes to the way they learn and teach. Staff/faculty development and participation will also directly influence the likelihood of success, and this is related to the perceived costs and benefits.

Implications for Faculty

A curriculum based on small group PBL has a major impact on teacher-teacher relations. The in-depth collaboration that is required of faculty in developing and delivering a small group PBL curricula may challenge relationships among faculty members. Differences in personal values, beliefs, and work habits as well as the variation in orientation of individual teachers may resurface as a challenge to enactment or adoption of proposed changes. For success, these differences among faculty will need to be identified and resolved (Fisher, 1991). Because the learning experience of each tutorial group within a given course or unit will be unique, a concern may be expressed by students and faculty alike about the consistency of learning. Even those who have readily advocated the changes may experience periods of doubt, and will need support to overcome the tendency to revert to past practices. Furthermore, ". . . [I]n the subjective realm of change, false clarity occurs when people *think* that they have changed but have only assimilated the trappings of the new practice. Painful unclarity is experienced when unclear innovations are attempted under conditions which do not support the development of the subjective meaning of change" (Fullan, 1982, p. 28).

In the learning process, the change to PBL may challenge faculty in some unexpected ways. Marris has observed that:

> *Occupational identity represents the accumulated wisdom of how to handle the job, derived from their own experience and the experience of all who have had the job before or have shared it with them. Change threatens to invalidate this experience robbing them of the skills they have learned and confusing their purposes, upsetting the subtle rationalizations and compensations by which they have reconciled the different aspects of the situation (Marris, 1975, p. 16).*

Faculty in health professions programs have traditionally developed their expertise as practitioners/clinicians and/or researchers, but frequently have had limited formal preparation for educational roles that do not call for sharing clinical knowledge and problem-solving expertise (Creedy and Hand, 1994). On the other hand, faculty who have developed expertise in traditional educational roles may be the most reluctant to change! Fullan (1982) underscores the importance of permitting "individual implementers to work out their own meaning [of change]," and further states that "conflict and disagreement are not only inevitable but fundamental to successful change" (p. 91).

Another challenge for some faculty will be the "informality" of the relationships among teachers and students. Functioning as a tutorial leader differs from mentoring individual students in that the tutor must assist students to balance individual learning needs and interests with those of the group, and the priorities of the scenario being studied. In fact, faculty who are truly committed to PBL may find that their active involvement in student learning *increases* rather than decreases because the tutor role calls for continuous modeling of facilitative group behaviors and critical thinking as well as providing formative evaluations to students on their reasoning and problem-solving skills (personal communication, Psychology faculty, University of Colima, Mexico, May, 1999; Nieuwenhuijzen Kriseman et al., 1997). Another aspect of teacher-student relationships is the central role that student evaluations of faculty play in decisions of promotion and tenure. It is crucial to establish a climate of mutual respect and trust to ensure the validity of the process of faculty evaluation.

In order to function as effective tutors in PBL, faculty will need to develop expertise in both group process and encouraging students to discover for themselves "how to learn." The educator needs to be prepared to relinquish control over many aspects of the dissemination of content, yet not abdicate an active involvement in the learning process. Because of these challenges, faculty require support in exploring and testing new teaching behaviors (Holmes and Kaufman, 1994).

Sefton (1997) describes four strategies that are useful in helping faculty make the changes required to implement PBL effectively. First and most important, a faculty development program is needed in which all faculty participate. (Various approaches to faculty development are described in Chapter 8). Second, program planning should be collaborative and participatory, so that large numbers of faculty are involved in the development of problems and other course materials, including evaluation methods and guidelines. Faculty may view the task of developing specific curriculum materials as more concrete and less threatening, and it may be more successful ultimately to focus on tasks perceived to be more manageable (Fullan, 1982). Third, summary spreadsheets of curriculum content that are developed by small working groups need to be distributed and discussed widely. Finally, documents and resources should be made available on the faculty's intranet for information, review, and comment. All these interventions seem to be essential to ensure ongoing involvement and commitment to change.

Implications for Students

Ideally, students should be involved in all steps of curriculum review, evaluation, and revision, and particularly so in a program that purports to be student-centered. In addition to the challenges common to all students entering academically-rigorous health professions education, students entering self-directed learning, PBL programs will need to adjust to a new educational approach, one where faculty are also learning. An additional challenge to students when major curriculum innovations are initiated is a lack of role models, since there are no senior students for the first cohort to consult with, to confirm that the process is "valid." At this point it will be very important for the faculty to demonstrate support for the change, and be responsive to student concerns.

Implications for External Support

There are influences external to the system, beyond the program or institution, that may facilitate or impede implementation of change, such as professional and educational regulatory requirements. Awareness and incorporation of such requirements into planning, and having representatives from such bodies on the planning and development committees are useful ways of ensuring support for change.

While it is important that sufficient resources be allocated to curriculum change, it is also important to recognize that the greater the degree of external support for the innovation, the *less likely* the change will be sustained if the external support is discontinued before the change is well-incorporated into the values and practices of the institution. Therefore, when designing a curriculum, it will be important to consider all three stages of educational change, in order that sufficient internal and external resources are secured to ensure that there are on-going supports for faculty.

Possible Barriers to Change

Innovation may produce change, but it is the consolidation of practices, relationships, and resources that is essential for continuity of systems. An essential step, therefore, is to identify both the openly expressed and the hidden underlying assumptions in order to develop a clear belief system. While it may be necessary, even desirable, to move ahead in small, incremental steps, or to focus on concrete tasks that appear to be less challenging to fundamental beliefs about learning and teaching, the process of educational change must not be viewed as linear. Change of beliefs and attitudes occur over time, and while it is important to move ahead and not lose momentum, people need to know that their beliefs and expertise are respected in the planned change. It is essential to maintain open communication and invite on-going dialogue with stakeholders about the subjective experience of change since, as Glen (1994) suggests, people's "values-in-use" are usually more conservative than "values-as-espoused." Failure to identify the difference between commitment to change and superficial enactment of behaviors can lead to a false sense of success.

Barriers to change may become evident at any step of the process, but it is particularly important to identify them as early as possible since they will certainly limit the sustainability of change in practice. The technological problems in the management of change include lack of expertise, poor timing and lack of institutional support. Deficiencies in developmental soundness of the innovations themselves will also lead to eventual failure. Another potential barrier is negative or unintended outcomes for one or more stakeholder group. Even those who have readily advocated the changes may experience periods of doubt, and will need support to overcome the tendency to revert to past practices (Fullan, 1982).

Phase Three: The Continuation of Change

The change process is not linear, and the decision to continue to "institutionalize" new teaching practices requires renewed commitment based on an evaluation of the outcomes of the change. While it is important that changes that are shown to be ineffective or inefficient be discontinued, in fact many "good" projects do not continue beyond the initiation phase because of lack of interest at the individual and institutional level, failure to secure continued funding and other support for the changes, or recognition of the complexity of change needed to sustain the new practices.

The decision to continue, alter, or discontinue an innovation should be based on clearly evaluated outcomes of change efforts. There are four potential outcomes of the adopted change: a valued and high-quality change is implemented; change is not implemented because it is not valued; change is not implemented because it is of poor quality; or change is implemented but is not valued or is of poor quality.

The primary consideration in a student-centered model of education will be the impact of change on students. It is important to anticipate that students will, at least initially, view change differently from the faculty and will need to be introduced to a new way of looking at learning with patience and support. It is important to not view PBL as the end in itself, rather it is the means to encourage student learning. Student questions and concerns should be openly invited and addressed. Continuous evaluation should be an integral process in curriculum innovation, and both the benefits and costs to students and faculty should be monitored.

Studies have reported that faculty can find the initiation of PBL a more positive experience than they had anticipated, with the opportunity to interact on a more personal level with learners being a chief source of satisfaction (Kaufman and Holmes, 1996; Maxwell and Wilkerson, 1990; Vernon, 1995). Other benefits can include a sense of personal growth and accomplishment derived from the experience. The high visibility and accountability of teachers to learners in a student-centered PBL program presents challenges for educators, but can also provide a dynamic and highly satisfying role for faculty—both professionally and personally.

The benefits to the organization need to also be assessed (Fisher, 1991). Evaluation of faculty, students, and the curriculum itself should be consistent with the philosophy of PBL, i.e., individualized, varied, on-going and formative, as well as summative (DesMarchais and Vu, 1996). Just as the student evaluation measures must be consistent with the philosophy of PBL, the work environment and instruments for faculty evaluation and development must be designed to provide supports and rewards for "good tutoring" (Dolmans, Wolfhagen, Schmidt, and van der Vleuten, 1994).

CONCLUSION

Educational change is social change, and thus is multidimensional and, to some extent, unpredictable. The decision to undertake curriculum innovations in nursing education must be guided by clear understanding and vision of how the change will ultimately have a positive impact on the health of the community. Curriculum revisions must impact on the criteria for selecting and devising learning activities, but educational change will also impact the criteria for clinical practice, teacher-student interactions, and assessment of student learning (Bevis and Watson, 1989). The process of moving from concept to reality is complex and challenging, but problem-based, self-directed, and student-centered learning provides a transformative experience for the students (Callin, 1996), faculty (O'Mara et al., 2000), curriculum (Arthur and Baumann, 1996), and for the institution (King, 1999).

REFERENCES

Arthur, H. and Baumann, A. (1996). Nursing curriculum content: An innovative decision-making process to define priorities. *Nurse Education Today,* *16*(1), 63–68.

Bevis, E. O. and Watson, J. (1989). *Toward a Caring Curriculum: A New Pedagogy for Nursing.* New York: NLN.

Brown, B., Carpio, B., and Roberts, J. (1991). The use of an autobiographical letter in the nursing admission process: Initial reliability and validity. *Canadian Journal of Nursing Research,* *23*(2), 9–20.

Callin, M. (1996). From RN to BScN: Seeing familiar situations in different ways. *Journal of Nursing Education,* *27*, 28–33.

Carpio, B. and Brown, B. (1993). The admissions process of a Bachelor of Science in Nursing programme: Initial reliability and validity of the personal interview. *Canadian Journal of Nursing Research,* *25*(3), 41–52.

Carpio, B., Illesca, M., Ellis, P., Crooks, D., Droghetti, J., Tompkins, C., and Noesgaard, C. (1999). Student and faculty learning styles in a Canadian and a Chilean self-directed, problem-based nursing program. *Canadian Journal of Nursing Research,* *31*(3), 31–50.

Carpio, B., O'Mara, L., and Hezekiah, J. (1996). Predictors of success on the Canadian Nurses Association Testing Service (CNATS) examination. *Canadian Journal of Nursing Research,* *28* (4), 115–123.

Colliver, J. A. (2000). Effectiveness of problem-based learning curricula: Research and theory. *Academic Medicine, 75*(3), 259–266.

Creedy, D. and Hand, B. (1994). The implementation of problem-based learning: Changing pedagogy in nurse education. *Journal of Advanced Nursing, 20*(4), 696–702.

Crook, J. (1985). A validation study of a self-directed learning readiness scale. *Journal of Nursing Education, 24*(7), 274–279.

DesMarchais, J. E. and Vu, N. V. (1996). Developing and evaluating the student assessment system in the pre-clinical problem-based curriculum at Sherbrooke. *Academic Medicine, 26*, 190–199.

Dolmans, D., Wolfhagen, I., Schmidt, H. G., and van der Vleuten, C. L. M. (1994). A rating scale for tutor evaluation in a problem-based curriculum: validity and reliability. *Medical Education, 28*, 550–558.

Doring, A., Bramwell-Vial, A., and Bingham, B. (1994) Staff comfort/discomfort with problem-based learning: A preliminary study. *Nurse Education Today*, 263–266.

Fisher, L. A. (1991). Evaluating the impact of problem-based learning—on the institution and on faculty. In D. Boud and G. Feletti (Eds.), *The Challenge of Problem-Based Learning*. London: Kogan Press.

Fullan, M. (1982). *The Meaning of Educational Change*. Toronto, ON: OISE Press.

Glen, S. (1994). Towards a new model of nursing education. *Nurse Education Today, 15*, 90–95.

Holmes, D. B. and Kaufman, D. M. (1994). Tutoring in problem-based learning: A teacher development process. *Medical Education, 28*, 275–283.

Kaufman, D. M. and Holmes, D. B. (1996). Tutoring in problem-based learning: Perceptions of teachers and students. *Medical Education, 30*, 371–377.

King, S. (1999). Changing to PBL: factoring in the emotion of change. In J. Conway, and A. Williams (Eds.). *Themes and Variations in PBL*, Newcastle, Australia: PROBLARC.

Knowles, M. (1975). *Self-Directed Learning: A Guide for Learners and Teachers*. New York: Association Press.

Knowles, M. (1986). *Using Learning Contracts: Practical Approaches to Individualizing and Structuring Learning*. San Francisco: Jossey-Bass.

Laschinger, H. (1986). Learning styles of nursing students and environmental press in two clinical nursing settings. *Journal of Advanced Nursing, 8*, 289–294.

Laschinger, H. (1992). Impact of nursing environment on the adaptive competencies of baccalaureate nursing students. *Journal of Professional Nursing, 8*, 105–114.

Lunyk-Child, O., Crooks, D., Ellis, P., Ofosu, C., O'Mara, L., and Rideout, L. (2000). Self-directed learning: Faculty and student perceptions. *Journal of Nursing Education*, in press.

Major, C. (2000). *PBL Insight: To Solve, To Learn, Together.* Birmingham, AL: Samford University.

Marris, P. (1975). Loss and Change. New York: Anchor Press/Doubleday.

Maxwell, J. A. and Wilkerson, L. (1990). A study of non-volunteer faculty in a problem-based curriculum. *Academic Medicine, 65*(9), S13–S14.

Mennin, S. P. and Martinez-Burrola, N. (1986). The cost of problem-based learning vs traditional medical education. *Medical Education, 20,* 187–194.

Montecinos, P., Illesca, M., and Yañez, A. (1993). Preferéncias de aprendizaje en estudiantes de una escuela de medicina chilena, estudio longitudinal. *Revista Médica Chilena, 121,* 220–225.

Nieuwenhuijzen Kruseman, A. C., Kolle, L. J. F. Th. M., and Scherpbier, A. J. J. A. (1997). Problem-based learning at Maastricht—An assessment of cost and outcome. *Education for Health, 10*(2), 179–187.

O'Mara, L., Carpio, B., Mallette, C., Down, W., and Brown, B. (2000). Developing a teaching portfolio in nursing education: A reflection. *Nurse Educator, 25*(3), 125–130.

Sefton, A. J. (1997). From a traditional to a problem-based curriculum—Estimating staff time and resources. *Education for Health, 10*(2), 165–178.

Venturelli, J. (1997). *Educacion medica: Nuevos enfoques, metas y métodos.* Washington: PAHO.

Vernon, D. T. A. (1995). Attitudes and opinions of faculty tutors about problem-based learning. *Academic Medicine, 70*(3), 216–223.

WHO (1994). *Nursing beyond the year 2000: Report of a WHO Study Group* (Technical Report Series #860). Geneva: Author.

INDEX

A

Acceptability, 216–217, 283
Access
    to clinical skills laboratory, 273
    to library resources, 276
Accommodators, 61
Accountability, 326
Active learning, 95
Adaptability, 282
Administration, and nursing education, 298–301
Advanced practice nursing, 298
Anatomy laboratory, 266–271
Artifacts, 146
Assessment. *See* Evaluation
Assimilators, 61
Asynchronous computer conferencing, 314
Attestation, 146
Audio teleconferencing, 312
Audiovisual resources, 262, 312
Authenticity, 10
Authentic voices, 124–127
Autobiography, value of, 125
Availability, 128–130, 282

B

Behaviors
    faculty, 195–197, 215
    students, 215
Bruner, Jerome, 25

C

Cajoling, 195
Camaraderie, 82
Carefully structured conversation, 227

Caring, 10
Categories of Reflective Outcomes, 132–135
Chalk and talk approach, 193
Change. *See* Educational change
Clinical competence, 247
Clinical courses, 241–246
Clinical decision making, 38, 41–42
Clinical environment, 250–256
Clinical experiences, 239–241
Clinical information resources, 253, 255
Clinical practice skills, 38, 41–42
Clinical preceptors, 252–253
Clinical reasoning exercise, 217
Clinical settings, 247–249, 255
Clinical skills laboratory (CSL), 271–274
Clinical staff, 248
Clinical teaching, 249–250
Coaching, 195
Cognitive mind maps, 66, 68–69
Cognitive psychology, 25–26
Collections, 274–275
Community health nursing, 297
Community resources, 265
Compact disks, 315
Competencies, for self-directed learning, 55–60
Competency-based practice, 326
Complexity, in problem packages, 168, 181–182
Computer-assisted instruction (CAI) packages, 262–263
Computer laboratories, 276–277
Computer literacy skills, 107–108
Computers. *See* Distance education
Concept mapping, 244

Conflict, managing, 91–92
Consensus, and small group learning,
     88–89
Constructivism, 26–27
Content
     determining, 168, 169–174
     embedding, 175–180
     See also Curriculum
Content expertise, 197–198
Contextual cues, 26
Contextual dependency of learning, 26
Convergers, 61
Courses
     clinical, 241–246
     and small group learning, 80
     See also Content; Curriculum
Course Web pages, 313
Critical incident questionnaire, 63–64, 66
Critical incident reflection, 226. *See also*
     Reflection
Critical reflectors, 133
Critical thinking, 58–59, 240
Culturally diverse learning populations,
     69–70
Curriculum
     and library resources, 275–276
     problem-based learning, 327–335
     and problem packages, 168,
          171–174, 187
Curriculum era, 5

D

Data gaps, 30
Decision making
     clinical, 38, 41–42
     and small group learning, 88–89
Dewey, John, 25
Diaries, 141
Differences, managing, 91–92
Directed paraphrasing, 227–228
Discipline-specific resources, 264
Distance education, 311, 321–322
     advantages of, 320–321
     challenges of, 321
     disadvantages of, 321
     modalities, 311–315
     satisfaction and effectiveness with,
          316–319
     students and faculty, 315–316
Divergers, 61

Diverse learning populations, 69–70
Documentation, of clinical learning
     activities, 242–244
Double jump, 228–232

E

Educational change, 327
     continuation of, 334–335
     implementation of, 330–334
     initiation of, 327–330
Educational environment. *See*
     Environment; Physical
     environment
Elective courses, 24
Electronic mail (e-mail), 313–314
Emancipatory education, 121–123
Empowerment function, 83
Enacted roles, 81
Encoding specificity, 26
Environment
     clinical, 250–256
     in small group learning, 84–88, 97
     See also Physical environment
Epistemic curiosity, 26
Essays, 218
Ethics, 136–137. *See also* Moral/ethical
     knowing era
Evaluation
     information management skills,
          112–113, 115
     small group learning, 92–93
     See also Problem-based learning
     evaluation; Self-evaluation
Evaluation resources, 266
Evaluative feedback
     in problem packages, 186
     in small group learning, 95–96
     from standardized patients, 283
Evidence-based information resources,
     255–256
Evidence-based practice, 6–7, 326
Expectations, tutor, 97
Expected learning outcome, 168, 169
Expected responses, 232
Experiences, clinical, 239–241

F

Facilities, for learning resources, 266–277
Faculty
     in anatomy laboratory, 269

authentic voices, 124–127
and clinical environment, 250–252
and clinical settings, 247–249
and distance education, 315–316,
    318–319
and educational change, 331–332
and information management,
    115–117
as learning resource, 265
and nursing masters programs,
    294–295
and problem-based learning, 37–38,
    193–210, 215
and problem packages, 187–188
and small group learning, 78–79
Faculty development programs, 204–209
    components of, 202–204
    general conclusions, 209–210
Feedback. *See* Evaluative feedback
Format, in problem packages, 174–175
Formative evaluation, 216
Framework for Reflective Action, 131
Frameworks, for reflection, 130–135
Funding, for clinical skills laboratory,
    273–274

G

Goals, in small group learning, 85
Governance function, 83
Graduate education era, 6
Graduate students, 294–295
Group clinical debriefing, 246
Group development, 83–84, 95–96
Group functions, 82–83
Group leadership, 89–91
Group members, roles and
    responsibilities of, 81–82
Group process, 95
    attending to, 201
    issues in, 81–84
    and self-directed learning, 59–60
    See also Small group learning
Groups, in problem-based learning,
    199–201. *See also* Small group
    learning
Group size, 79–80
Guiding, 195

H

Health sciences courses, 24

Holistic knowing era. *See* Relational and
    holistic knowing era
Human resources, 265
Hybrid curricula, 24

I

Incremental learning, 95
Independent study, 31
Individualized learning, 95
Information management, 59
Information management skills, 103, 117
    active engagement strategies,
        111–112
    components of, 103–104
    evaluation of, 112–113, 115
    faculty-library collaboration, 116–117
    faculty role in, 115–116
    need for, 104–106
    outcomes, 107–108
    phased introduction of, 108–111
    in problem-based learning, 106–107
Informational function, 82–83
Information-gathering, 31
Information resources, 265
    clinical, 253, 255
    evidence-based, 255–256
    See also Learning resources
Institutional policies, 328
Integration
    of clinical experiences, 239–240
    of clinical skills resources, 274
    of learning resources, 277
    in problem packages, 168, 180–181
Interdisciplinary masters courses, 301–302
Internet-based tools, 312–315
Interpersonal issues, 96–97
Intragroup issues, 96–97
Intrapersonal issues, 96–97
Invented dialogue, 227

J

Journals, 141–146

K

Knowledge
    accumulation of, 38, 39–41
    and clinical competence, 247
    elaboration of, 25
    See also Nursing knowledge; Prior
        knowledge

L

Leadership
  and problem-based learning, 204
  and small group learning, 89–91
LEARN framework for reflection, 131–132
Learning
  contextual dependency of, 26
  integration of, 168, 180–181
  lifelong, 38, 42–43
  ongoing, 127
  See also Self-directed learning; Small
    group learning
Learning gaps, self-assessment of, 56
Learning issues, identification of, 30
Learning plans, 61–63, 241–242
Learning resource list, 167
Learning resources, 259, 278
  categories of, 259–266
  facilities for, 266–277
  integration of, 277
Learning styles inventory, 60–61
Legislation, 328
Librarians, and information
    management, 116–117
Library, 274–276
Lifelong learning, 38, 42–43
Logs, 141

M

Maintenance roles, 82
Masters programs. *See* Nursing masters
    programs
Materials
  in anatomy laboratory, 266–269
  written, 312
Meta-analyses, 38–39
Methodologies. *See* Teaching
    methodologies
Midwives, nurse, 297–298
Minority populations. *See* Diverse
    learning populations
Model of Structured Reflection
    (MSR), 132
Modified Essay Question (MEQ), 218–222
Moral/ethical knowing era, 7–9
Motivation, in problem packages, 168,
    182–183
Multimedia resources, 263–264
Multiple choice questions, 222

Multiple methods guideline, 216
Multiple truths era, 12

N

National legislation and policies, 328
Nonreflectors, 133
Normative function, 83
No surprises rule, 216
Nurse midwives, 297–298
Nurse practitioners, 297–298
Nursing, in twenty-first century, 1–5
Nursing courses, 24
Nursing education. *See also* Distance
    education; Information
    management skills; Learning
    resources; Nursing knowledge;
    Nursing masters programs;
    Problem-based learning;
    Problem-based learning
    evaluation; Problem packages;
    Reflection; Self-directed
    learning; Small group
    learning; Standardized patients
Nursing knowledge, 16–17
  curriculum era, 5
  evidence-based practice, 6–7
  graduate education era, 6
  moral/ethical knowing era, 7–9
  multiple truths era, 12
  relational and holistic knowing era,
    9–12
  research era, 5
  technological knowing era, 12–16
  theory era, 6
  See also Knowledge
Nursing masters programs, 293–294, 306
  future of, 305–306
  graduate students and faculty, 294–295
  interdisciplinary courses, 301–302
  outcomes, 302, 304–305
  problem-based learning in, 295–301

O

Objective Structured Clinical
    Examination (OSCE), 223–225
Ongoing learning, 127
Openness, of problems, 175
Organization, of anatomy laboratory
    resources, 269–270

Outcomes
  information management skills,
    107–108
  nursing masters programs, 302,
    304–305
  problem-based learning, 38–43, 326
  problem packages, 168, 169
  reflection, 132–135, 137–141,
    153–154

P

Patient data, 166
Patients. *See* Standardized patients
Peers, and reflection, 127
Peer-to-peer learning, 95
People resources, 265
Performance evaluation. *See* Evaluation
Personal characteristics, for clinical
    settings, 248–249
Person-to-person electronic mail,
    313–314
Perspective transformation, 123
Physical environment
  anatomy laboratory, 270
  clinical skills laboratory, 271–272
  library, 275
  for small group learning, 80
Pilot, of problem package, 187
Policies, 328
Portfolios
  problem-based learning, 225–226
  professional, 146–150
Practitioners, nurse, 297–298
Prescribed roles, 81
Print resources, 261–262
Prior knowledge, activation of, 25
Problem development. *See* Problem
    packages
Problem packages, 29, 165, 188–189
  complexity, 181–182
  components of, 166–167
  content, 169–174, 175–180
  evaluative feedback, 186
  expected learning outcomes, 169
  format, 174–175
  integration, 180–181
  as learning resource, 260–261
  openness, 175
  pilot, 187

  problem writing skills, 187–188
  relevance and motivation, 182–183
  revision and refinement, 187
  student activity, 183–185
  supplementary resource material,
    186
Problem writing skills, 187–188
Problem-based learning (PBL), 21–22,
    43–44, 325
  clinical courses, 241–246
  clinical environment, 250–256
  clinical experiences, 239–241
  clinical setting, 247–249
  clinical teaching, 249–250
  conceptual model, 326–327
  definition, 22–24
  and educational change, 327–335
  faculty perceptions of, 37–38, 195
  faculty role, 193–210
  information management in, 106–107
  outcomes of, 38–43
  small group learning in, 75, 76–79
  student perceptions of, 33–37, 38, 194
  theoretical foundation, 24–27
  use of, 27–33
  See also Distance education; Nursing
    masters programs; Problem
    packages
Problem-based learning evaluation,
    215, 234
  clinical reasoning exercise, 217
  essays, 218
  guidelines, 215–217
  Modified Essay Question, 218–222
  multiple choice questions, 222
  Objective Structured Clinical
    Examination, 223–225
  portfolios, 225–226
  progress testing, 226
  self-selected strategies, 226–228
  triple jump, 228–233
  tutorial performance, 233–234
Problem-solving, enhancement of, 240
Process
  problem-based learning, 197–198
  reflection, 137–141
  support, 253
  See also Group process
Production, 146

Professional accountability, 326
Professional development, 96
Professional portfolios, 146–150
Professional socialization, 241
Progress testing, 226
Provincial policies, 328
Purpose, in small group learning, 85

Q

Qualitative studies, 35–37
Quantitative studies, 33–35

R

Recruitment, of standardized patients, 284–286
Reference resources, 261–265
Refinement, of problem package, 187
Reflection, 57–58
    authentic voices, 124–127
    critical incident, 227
    critical processes, 121–123
    critiquing, 154–156
    ethics of, 136–137
    exploring, 120–121
    facilitating, 128–135
    future challenges, 119–120
    process and outcomes, 137–141
    research, 153–154
    samplings of, 156–157
    skills for, 123–124
    strategies, 141–152
Reflective practice. *See* Reflection
Reflective writing, 244, 246
Reflectors, 133
Relational and holistic knowing era, 9–12
Relevance
    of clinical experiences, 239–241
    of problems, 168, 182–183
    of small group learning, 76
Reliability, 216–217, 282
Reproductions, 146
Research, on reflection, 153–154
Research era, 5
Resource material, supplementary, 186
Resources. *See* Standardized patients; *specific resources*
Revision, of problem package, 187

S

Scenarios, 166
Self-assessment. *See* Self-evaluation
Self-directed learning, 38, 42–43, 51, 71
    challenges, 53–54
    and clinical courses, 241–246
    and clinical experiences, 240–241
    competencies for, 55–60
    definition of, 52–53
    in diverse learning populations, 69–70
    foundations of, 51–52
    resources for, 60–69, 70
Self-evaluation
    clinical courses, 246
    reflection, 151–152
    self-directed learning 56–57
Self-oriented roles, 82
Self-study, motivation for, 182–183
Settings, clinical, 247–249, 255
Skills. *See specific skills*
Small group learning, 75, 98
    benefits, 93, 95–96
    decision making/achieving consensus, 88–89
    drawbacks, 96–97
    group process issues, 81–84
    leadership issues, 89–91
    management of differences, tensions, and conflict, 91–92
    new group environments, 84–88
    performance evaluation in, 92–93
    in problem-based learning, 75, 76–79
    and reflection, 151
    relevance of, 76
    structural issues and group function, 79–80
Socialization, 82, 241
Staff, 248, 265, 273
Standardized patients
    advantages of, 282–283
    disadvantages of, 283–284
    example, 288–289
    history of, 281–282
    recruitment and training of, 284–286
    student interaction with, 286–288
Students
    and clinical assignments, 242
    and clinical setting, 248

and distance education, 315–316
and educational change, 332–333
graduate, 294–295
and problem-based learning, 33–37, 38, 194, 215, 216
and problem packages, 168, 183–185
and reflection, 123–124, 156–157
and small group learning, 77–78, 97
and standardized patients, 286–288
Subjective roles, 81
Summative evaluation, 216
Supplementary resource material, 186
Support, 82, 253, 271, 333
Synchronous online tutorials, 314–315

T

Task completion, 82–83
Task roles, 82
Teaching, clinical, 249–250
Teaching methodologies, for technological knowing era, 13–16
Teaching skills, and clinical setting, 247–248
Team-building skills, 95
Technological knowing era, 12–16
Technology, and nursing masters programs, 305–306. *See also* Distance education

Telecommunications, 312
Tensions, managing, 91–92
Theory era, 6
Time-out, 91–92
Time restrictions, 283
Training, of standardized patients, 284–286
Transcendent, 10
Transpersonal, 10
Triple jump, 228–233
Tutor guide, 166
Tutorial performance, 233–234
Tutor skills and expectations, 97

U

Unleash Your Creativity, 228

V

Validity, 216–217
Video teleconferencing, 312
Vygotsky, Lev, 26

W

Web pages, 313
Writing, reflective, 244, 246
Writing skills. *See* Problem writing skills
Written materials, 312